MEDICAL ABBREVIATIONS:

14,000 Conveniences at the Expense of Communications and Safety

Ninth Edition

Neil M Davis, MS, PharmD, FASHP

Professor Emeritus, Temple University
    School of Pharmacy, Philadelphia, PA,
Editor-in-Chief, Hospital Pharmacy
President, Safe Medication Practices
    Consulting, Inc.

published by

Neil M Davis Associates
1143 Wright Drive
Huntingdon Valley, PA 19006-2721

Phone (215) 947-1752 (9 AM-6 PM EST, Mon-Fri)
FAX (215) 938-1937
Web site http://www.neilmdavis.com
E-mail med@neilmdavis.com

Contents

Chapter 1
Introduction

L isted are 14,000 current acronyms, symbols, and other abbreviations and 20,000 of their possible meanings. This list has been compiled to assist individuals in reading and transcribing medical records, medically-related communications, and prescriptions. The list, although current and comprehensive, represents a portion of abbreviations in use and their many possible meanings as new ones are being coined every day.

WARNING

Abbreviations are a convenience, a time saver, a space saver, and a way of avoiding the possibility of misspelling words. However, a price can be paid for their use. Abbreviations are sometimes not understood, misread, or are interpreted incorrectly. Their use lengthens the time needed to train individuals in the health fields, wastes the time of healthcare workers in tracking down their meaning, at times delays the patient's care, and occasionally results in patient harm.

The publication of this list of abbreviations is not an endorsement of their legitimacy. It is not a guarantee that the intended meaning has been correctly captured, or an indication that they are in common use. Where uncertainty exists, the one who wrote the abbreviation must be contacted for clarification.

There are many variations in how an abbreviation can be expressed. Anterior-posterior has been written as AP, A.P., ap, and A/P. Since there are few standards and those who use abbreviations do not necessarily follow these standards, this book only shows anterior-posterior as AP. This is done to make it easier to find the meaning of an abbreviation as all the meanings of AP are listed together. This elimination of unnecessary duplication also keeps the book at a convenient size, thus enabling it to be sold at a reasonable price. Lower-case letters are used when firm custom dictates as in Ag, Na, mCi, etc. The first letter of trademarks are capitalized, whereas nonproprietary names appear in lowercase.

The abbreviation AP is listed as meaning doxorubicin and cisplatin. The reason for this apparent disparity is that the official generic names (United States Adopted Names) are shown rather than the trade names Adriamycin® and Platinol AQ®. In the case of LSD, the official name, lysergide, is given, rather than the chemical name, lysergic acid diethylamide. The Latin derivations for older medical and pharmaceutical abbreviations (TID, *ter in die,* three times daily) may be found in *Remington.*[1]

Healthcare organizations are wisely advised by the Joint Commission on Accreditation of Healthcare Organizations to formulate an approved list of abbreviations. Every attempt should be made to restrict this list to common abbreviations that are understood by all health professionals who must work with medical records. There are certain dangerous abbreviations that should not be approved, and a warning should be issued about their use (see Table 1 as well as notes in the text). A second list should be published by the healthcare organizations containing dangerous abbreviations that were purposely omitted from the approved list. The reasons for their omission should be stated.

Many inherent problems associated with abbreviations contribute to or cause errors. Reports of such errors have been published routinely.[2-5]

Abbreviations and symbols can easily be misread or interpreted in a unintended manner. For example:

(1) "HCT250 mg" was intended to mean hydrocortisone 250 mg but was interpreted as hydrochlorothiazide 50 mg (HCTZ50 mg).

(2) Flucytosine was improperly abbreviated as 5 FU, causing it to be read as fluorouracil. Flucytosine is abbreviated 5 FC and fluorouracil is 5 FU.

(3) Floxuridine was improperly abbreviated as 5 FU, causing it to be read as fluorouracil. Floxuridine is abbreviated FUDR and fluorouracil is 5 FU.

Table 1. Examples of dangerous abbreviations

Problem term	Reason	Suggested term
O.D. for once daily	Interpreted as right eye	Write "once daily"
q.o.d. for every other day	Interpreted as meaning "every once a day" or read as q.i.d.	Write "every other day"
q.d. for once daily	Read or interpreted as q.i.d.	Write "once daily"
q.n. for every night	Read as every hour	Write "every night," "HS" or nightly
q hs for every night	Read as every hour	Use "HS" or "at bedtime"
TIW for three times a week	Interpreted as T/W (Tuesday & Wednesday); as twice a week; as TID (three times daily)	Write "three times a week"
U for Unit	Read as 0, 4, 6, or cc	Write "unit"
O.J. for orange juice	Read as OD or OS	Write "orange juice"
µg (microgram)	When handwritten, misread as mg	Write "mcg"
sq or sub q for subcutaneous	The q is read as every	Use "subcut"
Chemical symbols	Not understood or misunderstood	Write full name
Lettered abbreviations for drug names or drug protocols	Not understood or misunderstood	Use generic or trade name(s)
Apothecary symbols or terms	Not understood or misunderstood	Use metric system
per os for by mouth	OS read as left eye	Use "by mouth," "orally," or "PO"
D/C for discharge	Interpreted as discontinue (orders for discharge medications result in premature discontinuance of current medication)	Write "discharge"
Ṫ/d for one per day	Read as T.I.D.	Use "once daily"
/ (a slash mark) for with, and, or per	Read as a one	Use, "and," "with," or "per"

3

(4) MTX was thought to be mechlorethamine. MTX is methotrexate and mechlorethamine is abbreviated HN2.

(5) The abbreviation "U" for unit is the most dangerous one in the book, having caused numerous tenfold insulin overdoses. The word unit should never be abbreviated. The handwritten U for unit has been mistaken for a zero, causing tenfold errors. The handwritten U has also been read as the number four, six, and as "cc."

(6) OD, meant to signify once daily, has caused Lugol's solution to be given in the right eye.

(7) OJ meant to signify orange juice, looked like OS and caused saturated solution of potassium iodide to be given in the left eye.

(8) IVP, meant to signify intravenous push (Lasix 20 mg IVP), caused a patient to be given an intravenous pyelogram which is the usual meaning of this abbreviation.

(9) Na Warfarin (sodium warfarin) was read as "No Warfarin."

(10) The abbreviation "s̄" for "without" has been thought to mean "with" (c̄).

(11) The order for PT, intended to signify a laboratory test order for prothrombin time, resulted in the ordering of a physical therapy consultation.

(12) The abbreviation "TAB," meant to signify Triple Antibiotic (a coined name for a hospital sterile topical antibiotic mixture), caused patients to have their wounds irrigated with a diet soda.

(13) A slash mark (/) has been mistaken for a one, causing a patient to receive a 100 unit overdose of NPH insulin when the slash was used to separate an order for two insulin doses:

6 units regular insulin/20 units NPH insulin

(14) Vidarabine, an antiviral agent, was ordered as ara-A; however, ara-C, which is cytarabine, an antineoplastic agent, was given.

(15) On several occasions, pediatric strength diphtheria-

tetanus toxoids (DT) have been confused with adult strength tetanus-diphtheria toxoids (Td).

(16) DTP is commonly understood to refer to diphtheria-tetanus-pertussis vaccine, but in some hospitals it is also used as shorthand for a sedative cocktail of Demerol, Thorazine, and Phenergan. Several cases have occurred where a child was vaccinated rather than given the sedative mixture.

(17) What does the abbreviation MR mean? Some will guess measles-rubella vaccine (M-R-Vax II, Merck), while others will assume mumps-rubella vaccine (Biavax II, Merck).

(18) The abbreviation TIW (three times a week) was thought to mean Tuesday and Wednesday when the I was read as a slash mark. Due to confirmation bias (you see what you know), this uncommon abbreviation is seen as the more commonly used TID (three times a day).

(19) PCA, meant to be procainamide, was interpreted as patient-controlled analgesia.

(20) PGE$_1$ (alprostadil, Caverject) was read as P6 E1 (Alcon's ophthalmic pilocarpine and epinephrine solution).

(21) A nurse transcribed an oral order for the antibiotic aztreonam as AZT, which was subsequently thought to be the antiviral drug zidovudine.

(22) An order for TAC 0.1%, intended to mean triamcinolone cream, was interpreted as tetracaine, Adrenalin, and cocaine solution.

(23) An order for SPA (salt poor albumin) was overlooked because it was not recognized as a drug order.

(24) Therapy was delayed and considerable professional time was wasted when an order for "Bactrim SS q 12 h on S/S" had to be clarified (Bactrim Single Strength every 12 hours on Saturday and Sunday).

A prescription could be written with directions as follows: "OD OD OD," to mean one drop in the right eye once daily!

Abbreviations should not be used for drug names as they are particularly dangerous. As previously illustrated, there is the possibility that the writer may, through mental error, confuse two abbreviations and use the wrong one. Similarly, the reader may attribute the wrong meaning to an abbreviation. To further confound the problem, some drug name abbreviations have multiple meanings (see ATR, CPM, CPZ, GEM, NITRO, and PBZ in Table 2). The abbreviation AC has been used for three different cancer chemotherapy combinations to mean Adriamycin and either cyclophosphamide, carmustine, or cisplatin.

Beside causing medication errors and incorrect interpretation of medical records, abbreviations can create problems because treatment is delayed while a health professional seeks clarification for the meaning of the abbreviation used. Abbreviations should not be used to designate drugs or combinations of drugs.

Certain abbreviations in the book are followed by a warning, "this is a dangerous abbreviation." This warning could be placed after many abbreviations, but was reserved for situations where errors have been published because these abbreviations were used or where the meaning is critical and not likely to be known. Such warning statements should also appear after every abbreviation for a drug or drug combination.

Abbreviations for medical facility names create problems as they are usually not recognized by the readers in other geographic areas. A clue to the fact that one is dealing with such an abbreviation is when it ends with MC, for Medical Center; MH, for Memorial Hospital; CH, for Community Hospital; UH, for University Hospital; and H, for Hospital.

When an abbreviation cannot be found in this book or when the listed meaning(s) do not make sense, there is a possibility that the abbreviation has been misread. As an example, a reader could not find the meaning of HHTS. On closer examination it really was +HTS, not HHTS. Also EWT could not be identified because it was really ENT.

Chapter 5 contains a cross-referenced list of 2,900 generic and trademark names. The list contains names of commonly prescribed and new drugs. Trademarks have their first letter capitalized whereas generic names are in lower case. This list will enable readers to obtain the generic name for trademark products or trademarks for generic names. It will also serve as a spelling check.

Table 2. Examples of abbreviations that have contradictory or ambiguous meanings

AMI	= amifostine; amitriptyline
APC	= advanced pancreatic cancer; advanced prostate cancer
ATR	= atropine; atracurium;
AZT	= zidovudine; azathioprine
BO	= bowel open; bowel obstruction
CF	= cystic fibrosis; Caucasian female; calcium leucovorin (citrovorum factor); complement fixation; cancer-free; cardiac failure; coronary flow; contractile force; Christmas factor; count fingers; cisplatin and fluorouracil
CPM	= cyclophosphamide; chlorpheniramine maleate
CPZ	= chlorpromazine; Compazine
DW	= dextrose in water; distilled water; deionized water
ESLD	= end-stage liver disease; end-stage lung disease
GEM	= gemfibrozil; gemcitabine
HD	= Hansen's disease; Hodgkin's disease; Huntington's disease
ICA	= internal carotid artery; intracranial abscess; intracranial aneurysm
LFD	= lactose-free diet; low fat diet; low fiber diet
MS	= morphine sulfate; multiple sclerosis; mitral stenosis; musculoskeletal; medical student; minimal support; muscle strength; mental status; milk shake; mitral sound; morning stiffness
MTD	= maximum tolerated dose; minimum toxic dose
NBM	= no bowel movement; normal bowel movement; nothing by mouth
NITRO	= nitroglycerin; sodium nitroprusside
OLB	= open-liver biopsy; open-lung biopsy
PBZ	= phenylbutazone; pyribenzamine; phenoxybenzamine
PORT	= postoperative radiotherapy; postoperative respiratory therapy
PVO	= peripheral vascular occlusion; portal vein occlusion; pulmonary venous occlusion
RS	= Reiter's syndrome; Reye's syndrome; Raynaud's disease (syndrome)
S & S	= swish and spit; swish and swallow
SDBP	= seated, standing, or supine diastolic blood pressure
STF	= special tube feeding; standard tube feeding
VAP	= vincristine, Adriamycin, and prednisone; vincristine, Adriamycin, and procarbazine; vincristine, actinomycin D, and Platinol AQ; vincristine, asparaginase, and prednisone

Coded drug names and abbreviations for drug names are found in the chapter on abbreviations (Chapter 3).

Chapter 6 is a table of normal laboratory values. Both the conventional and international values are listed. Each laboratory publishes a list of its normal values. These local lists should be reviewed to see if there are significant differences.

The Council of Biology Editors (CBE), in their 1983 edition of the *CBE Style Manual* listed about 600 abbreviations gathered from 15 internationally recognized authorities and organizations.[6] The majority of these symbols and abbreviations tend to be more scientifically oriented than those which would appear in medical records. In the few situations where the CBE abbreviations differ from what is presented in this book, the CBE abbreviation has been placed in parentheses after the meaning. As is the practice in the United States, mL has been used rather than ml and the spelling of liter, meter, etc. is used rather than litre and metre, even though ml, litre, and metre are listed in the *CBE Style Manual*. A new edition of the *CBE Style Manual* was published in 1995.[7] Again, in this edition, emphasis is placed on scientific abbreviations.

An examination of the 14,000 abbreviations and their 20,000 meanings is a testimonial to the problems and dangers associated with most undefined abbreviations.

The assistance of Ann Sandt Kishbaugh, Matthew Davis, Danial Baker, Suzette Knight, and Evelyn Canizares and all the others that helped is gratefully acknowledged.

References

1. Gennaro AR, ed. Remington's Pharmaceutical Sciences, 19th ed. Easton, PA: Mack Publishing Co, 1995.

2. Davis NM, Cohen MR. Medication errors: causes and prevention. Huntingdon Valley, PA: Neil M. Davis Associates; 1983.

3. Cohen MR. Medication error reports. Hosp Pharm (appears monthly from 1975 to the present).

4. Cohen MR. Medication errors. Nursing 99 (appears monthly, starting in Nursing 77, to the present).

5. Davis NM. Med Errors. Am J Nursing (appears monthly from 1994 to 1995).

6. CBE Style Manual, 5th ed. Bethesda, MD: Council of Biology Editors; 1983.

7. Scientific Style and Format: The CBE Manual for Authors, Editors, and Publishers, 6th Ed. Council of Biological Editors-Cambridge University Press. Cambridge UK, New York, Victoria Australia: 1995.

Chapter 2

A Healthcare Controlled Vocabulary

Presently there are no standards for physician's orders, consultations, written prescriptions, standing orders, computer order sets, nurse's medication administration records, pharmacy profiles, hospital formularies, etc. Because in the healthcare field everyone does their own thing, there are many variations. These variations in the way abbreviations are expressed are not always understood and at times are misinterpreted. They cause delays in initiating therapy, cause accidents, waste time for everyone in clarifying these documents, lengthen the time it takes to train those working in the healthcare field, lengthen hospital stays, and waste money.

A controlled vocabulary similar to what is used in the aviation industry is needed. Everyone in the aviation industry "follows the book," and uses a controlled vocabulary. All pilots and air traffic controllers say, "alpha", "bravo", "charley." They do not go off on their own and say "adam", "beef", "candy!" They say "one three," not thirteen, because thirteen sounds like thirty. Radio transmission in the aviation industry is not easy to decipher, yet because precision is critical everything possible is done to eliminate error. To prevent errors all radio transmissions are given only in English, every transmission is given in the same order and must be immediately repeated by the receiver to make sure it was heard correctly. Written and oral communication in the medical professions are just as critical and are also not easy to decipher, so establishing a controlled vocabulary is also necessary in this industry.

Listed below are three organizations that have ongoing projects related to standardizing medical terminology:

Computer-Based Patient Record Institute, Inc.
1000 East Woodfield Rd. Suite 102
Schuamburg, IL 60173

The United States Pharmacopeial Convention, Inc.
12601 Twinbrook Parkway
Rockville, MD, 20852

National Library of Medicine
Unified Medical Language System
8600 Rockville Pike
Bethesda, MD, 20894

Listed below is the start of a Healthcare Controlled Vocabulary. The basis for this controlled vocabulary is established standard terminology and the result of 35 years of studying medication errors by this author.

It is anticipated that a Healthcare Controlled Vocabulary, with professional organizations' input and backing, will grow and someday evolve into an "official standard." Your suggestions and comments are vital to this growth and eventual recognition. It is always safest to avoid the use of abbreviations unless a standard has been established and is well-publicized in your work environment.

Standard	What not to use or do	Comments
100 mg (100 space mg)	100mg (100 no space mg)	The USP* standard way of expressing a strength is to leave a space between the number and its units. Leaving this space makes it easier to read the number as can be seen below. 1mg 1 mg 10mg 10 mg 100mg 100 mg
1 mg	1.0 mg	This is a USP standard. When a trailing zero is used, the decimal point is sometimes not seen thus causing a tenfold overdose. These overdoses have caused injury and death.
0.1 mL	.1 mL	When the decimal point is not seen, this is read as 1 mL, causing a ten fold overdose.
once daily (Do not abbreviate.)	The abbreviation OD	The classic meaning for OD is right eye. Liquids intended to be given once daily are mistakenly given in the right eye.
	The abbreviation QD	When the Q is dotted too aggressively it looks like Q.I.D. and the medication is given four times daily. When a lower case q is used, the tail of the q has come up between the q and the d to make it look like qid. In the United Kingdom, Q.D. means four times daily
unit (Do not abbreviate. Write "unit" using a lower-case u)	The abbreviation U	The handwritten U is mistaken for a zero when poorly written causing a 10 fold overdose (i.e. 6 U regular insulin is read as 60). The poorly written U has also been read as 4, 6, and cc. Write "unit," leaving a space between the number and the word unit.

(continued)

13

Standard	What not to use or do	Comments
mg (Lower case mg with no period)	mg., Mg., Mg, MG, mgm, mgs	The USP standard expression is the mg
mL (lower case m with a capital L, no period)	mL., ml, ml, mls, mLs, cc	The USP standard expression is the mL
Use generic names or trademarks	Do not abbreviate drug names or combinations of drugs, such as CPZ, PBZ, NTG, MS, 5FC, MTX, 6MP, MOPP, ASA, HCTZ, etc.	Abbreviated drug names and acronyms are not always known to the reader; at times they have more than one possible meaning, or are thought to be another drug.
	Do not use shortened names or chemical names	When the chemical name "6 mercaptopurine" has been used, six doses of mercaptopurine have been mistakenly administered. The generic name, mercaptopurine, should be used. When an unofficial shortened version of the name norfloxacin, norflox was used, Norflex was mistakenly given. An order for Aredia was read as Adriamycin, as some professionals abbreviated the name Adriamycin as "Adria" which looks like Aredia.
The metric system	The apothecary system (grains, drams, minims, ounces, etc.)	The Apothecary system is so rarely used it is not recognized or understood. The symbol for minim (♏) is read as mL; the symbol for one dram (ℨi) is read as 3 tablespoons, and gr (grain) is read as gram.
Use properly placed commas for numbers above 999, as in 10,000, or 5,000,000	5000000	Many people have difficulty in reading large numbers such as 5000000. The use of commas helps the reader to read these numbers correctly.

Standard	What not to use or do	Comments
600 mg When possible, do not use decimal expressions. 25 mcg	0.6 g 0.025 mg	A USP standard. The elimination of decimals lessens the chance for error. Mistakes are made when reading numbers less than 1 with decimals.
Do not use the term "bolus" in conjunction with the administration of potassium chloride injection. Use specific concentrations and the time in which the drug should be administered.		Some physicians will erroneously indicate that potassium chloride injection should be "bolused" or be given "IV push," vaguely meaning that it should not be dripped in slowly. Many deaths have been reported when prescribers have been taken literally and the potassium chloride was given by bolus or IV push. Orders should be specific such as, "20 mEq of potassium chloride in 50 mL of 5% dextrose to run over 30 minutes."
use "and"	Do not use a slash mark or the symbol "&"	A slash mark looks like a one. An order written "6 units regular insulin/20 units NPH insulin," was read as 120 units of NPH insulin. The symbol "&" has been read as a 4.
Orally transmitted medical orders should be read back as heard for verification.	Do not assume that one has spoken or heard correctly.	During oral communications, speakers misspeak and/or transcribers mishear. To minimize these errors, the transmitter must speak clearly and slowly, the transcriber must repeat what was transcribed, and the transmitter must listen attentively when this is being done. Errors are less likely to occur when the prescription is complete.

(continued)

Standard	What not to use or do	Comments
When prescriptions are written or orally transmitted they must be complete. • dosage form must be specified • strength must be specified • directions must be specified • included in the directions must be the purpose or indication.	Incomplete orders	Prescribers on occasion think of one drug and mistakenly order another. Nurses and pharmacists on occasion misread prescriptions because of error, poor handwriting or poor oral communications, or look-alike or sound-alike drugs.[1] When the prescription is complete and the purpose or indication is included, these errors are less likely to occur. Listing the purpose or indication on the prescription label will assist in increasing patient adherence.
Written communications must be legible.	Illegible handwriting	Prescribers who cannot or will not write legibly must either print (if this would be legible), type, use a computer, or have an employee write for them and then immediately verify and sign the document.
Prescribe specific doses.	Do not prescribe 2 ampuls or 2 vials	There is often more than one size or concentration of drug available. Failing to be specific will lead to unintended doses being administered.
Establish a list of approved abbreviations with no abbreviation having more than one possible meaning within a context.	Everyone using their own abbreviations.	To understand the scope of this problem examine the contents of this book for abbreviations that have many meanings and for obscure abbreviations which would not generally be recognized.
Use h or hr for hour	°	An order written as q 4° has been read as q 40 or the symbol ° has not been understood.
Specify amount of drug to be given in a single dose.[2]	Specify total amount of drug to be administered over a period of time.	Orders such as . . . . 1,600 mg over 4 days have caused death when mistakenly given as a single dose. Order should state . . . 400 mg once daily for four days (2-1-99 to 2-4-99)

*USP = United States Pharmacopeia
1. Davis NM. Look-alike and sound alike drug names. Hosp Pharm 1997;32:1558–70
2. Kohler DR, Montello MJ, Green I, et al. Standardizing the expression and nomenclature of cancer treatment regimens. Am J Health-

Chapter 3

Lettered Abbreviations and Acronyms

Where an abbreviation contains numbers, symbols, punctuation, spaces, etc., they are *not* considered during alphabetizing. Entries beginning with a *Greek letter* are alphabetized where the name of the letter would be found alphabetically.

The letter-by-letter (dictionary) system of alphabetizing is used.

Trademarks (proprietary names) have their first letter capitalized, whereas nonproprietary (generic) names are in lower-case letters.

The listing of symbols and numbers can be found in Chapter 4.

See WARNING in chapter 1.

A

A	accommodation
	Acinetobacter
	adenine
	age
	alive
	ambulatory
	angioplasty
	anterior
	anxiety
	apical
	arterial
	artery
	Asian
	assessment

A+	blood type A positive
A−	blood type A negative
A′	ankle
@	at
(a)	axillary temperature
$\bar{a}$	before
A_1	aortic first heart sound
A_2	aortic second sound
A250	5% albumin 250 mL
A1000	5% albumin 1000 mL
A II	angiotensin II
AA	acetic acid
	achievement age
	active assistive
	acute asthma
	African-American
	Alcoholics Anonymous
	alcohol abuse
	alopecia areata
	alveolar-arterial gradient

amino acid
anaplastic astrocytomas
anti-aerobic
antiarrhythmic agent
aortic aneurysm
aplastic anemia
arm ankle (pulse ratio)
ascending aorta
audiologic assessment
Australia antigen
authorized absence
automobile accident
cytarabine (ara-C) and doxorubicin (Adriamycin)

aa of each

A&A aid and attendance
arthroscopy and arthrotomy
awake and aware

A-a alveolar arterial (gradient)

a/A arterial-alveolar (gradient)

AAA abdominal aortic aneurysmectomy (aneurysm)
acute anxiety attack
aromatic amino acids

A&AA active and active assistive

AAAE amino acid activating enzyme

AAAHC Accreditation Association of Ambulatory Health Care

AAC Adrenalin, atropine, and cocaine
advanced adrenocortical cancer
antimicrobial agent-associated colitis

AACG acute angle closure glaucoma

AAD acid-ash diet
antibiotic-associated diarrhea

A$_1$AD alpha$_1$-antitrypsin deficiency

AADA Abbreviated Antibiotic Drug Application

[A-a]Do$_2$ alveolar-arterial oxygen tension gradient

AAE active assistance exercise
acute allergic encephalitis

AAECS amino acid enriched cardioplegic solution

A/AEX active assistive exercise

AAF African American female

AAFB alcohol acid-fast bacilli

AAG alpha-1-acid glycoprotein

AAH acute alcoholic hepatitis

AAI acute alcohol intoxication arm-ankle indices

AAL anterior axillary line

AAM African American male amino acid mixture

AAMI age associated memory impairment

AAMS acute aseptic meningitis syndrome

AAN AIDS-associated neutropenia
analgesic abuse nephropathy
analgesic-associated nephropathy
attending's admission notes

AAO alert, awake, & oriented

AAO × 3 awake and oriented to time, place, and person

AAOC antacid of choice

AAP acute anterior poliomyelitis
assessment adjustment pass

AAPC antibiotic-associated pseudomembranous colitis

AAPMC antibiotic-associated pseudomembranous colitis

a/ApO$_2$ arterial-alveolar oxygen tension ratio

AAPSA age-adjusted prostate-specific antigen

AAR antigen-antiglobulin reaction

	automated anesthesia record		absolute band counts
AAROM	active-assistive range of motion		absolute basophil count
			advanced breast cancer
AAS	acute abdominal series		airway, breathing, and circulation
	androgenic-anabolic steroid		all but code (resuscitation order)
	Ann Arbor stage (Hodgkin's disease staging system)		aneurysmal bone cyst
			antigen binding capacity
	aortic arch syndrome		apnea, bradycardia, and cyanosis
	atlantoaxis subluxation		applesauce, bananas, and cereal (diet)
	atypical absence seizure		
AASCRN	amino acid screen		argon beam coagulator
AAT	activity as tolerated		aspiration, biopsy and cytology
	alpha-antitrypsin		
	androgen ablation therapy		artificial beta cells
	at all times		avidin-biotin complex
	atypical antibody titer	ABCD	amphotericin B cholesteryl sulfate complex (Amphotec; amphotericin B colloid dispersion)
A_1AT	alpha$_1$-antitrypsin		
A_1AT-P_i	alpha$_1$-antitrypsin (phenotyping)		
AAU	acute anterior uveitis		
AAV	adeno-associated vector	ABCDE	botulism toxoid pentavalent
	adeno-associated virus		
AAVV	accumulated alveolar ventilatory volume	ABD	after bronchodilator
			type of plain gauze dressing
AAWD	antiandrogen withdrawal		
AB	abortion	Abd	abdomen
	Ace® bandage		abdominal
	antibiotic		abductor
	antibody	ABDCT	atrial bolus dynamic computer tomography
	Aphasia Battery		
	apical beat	ABD GR	abdominal girth
	armboard	ABD PB	abductor pollicis brevis
	products meeting bioequivalence requirements for generic pharmaceuticals	ABD PL	abductor pollicis longus
		ABE	acute bacterial endocarditis
			adult basic education
A/B	acid-base ratio		botulism equine trivalent antitoxin
	apnea/bradycardia		
$A > B$	air greater than bone (conduction)	ABECB	acute bacterial exacerbations of chronic bronchitis
A & B	apnea and bradycardia		
	assault and battery	ABEP	auditory brain stem-evoked potentials
AB+	AB positive blood type		
AB−	AB negative blood type	ABF	aortobifemoral (bypass)
ABC	abbreviated blood count	ABG	air/bone gap

	aortoiliac bypass graft
	arterial blood gases
	axiobuccogingival
ABH	Ativan, Benadryl, and Haldol
ABI	ankle brachial index (ankle-to-arm systolic blood pressure ratio)
	atherothrombotic brain infarction
ABID	antibody identification
A Big	atrial bigeminy
ABK	aphakic bullous keratopathy
ABL	abetalipoproteinemia
	allograft bound lymphocytes
	axiobuccolingual
ABLB	alternate binaural loudness balance
ABLC	amphotericin B lipid complex (Abelcet)
A/B Mods	apnea/bradycardia moderate stimulation
ABMS	autologous bone marrow support
A/B MS	apnea/bradycardia mild stimulation
ABMT	autologous bone marrow transplantation
ABN	abnormality(ies)
abnl bld	abnormal bleeding
ABNM	American Board of Nuclear Medicine
abnor.	abnormal
ABO	absent bed occupant
	blood group system (A, AB, B, and O)
ABP	ambulatory blood pressure
	androgen binding protein
	arterial blood pressure
ABPA	allergic bronchopulmonary aspergillosis
ABPM	allergic bronchopulmonary mycosis
	ambulatory blood pressure monitoring
ABR	absolute bed rest

	auditory brain (evoked) responses
ABS	absent
	absorbed
	absorption
	Accuchek® blood sugar
	acute brain syndrome
	admitting blood sugar
	antibody screen
	at bedside
A/B SS	apnea/bradycardia self-stimulation
ABT	aminopyrine breath test
	antibiotic therapy
ABVD	Adriamycin®, bleomycin, vinblastine, and dacarbazine (DTIC)
ABW	actual body weight
ABx	antibiotics
AC	abdominal circumference
	acetate
	acromioclavicular
	activated charcoal
	acute
	air conditioned
	air conduction
	anchored catheter
	antecubital
	anticoagulant
	arm circumference
	assist control
	before meals
	doxorubicin (Adriamycin) and cyclophosphamide
A/C	anterior chamber of the eye
	assist/control
A & C	alert and cooperative
A_{1C}	glycosylated hemoglobin A
5-AC	azacitidine
9AC	9-aminocamptothecin
ACA	acrodermatitis chronica atrophicans
	acyclovir
	adenocarcinoma
	against clinical advice
	aminocaproic acid
	anterior cerebral artery

anterior communicating artery

anticanalicular antibodies

AC/A accommodation convergence–accommodation (ratio)

ACABS acute community-acquired bacterial sinusitis

ACAS acute community-acquired sinusitis

ACAT acyl coenzyme A: cholesterol acyltransferase

ACB alveolar-capillary block
antibody-coated bacteria
aortocoronary bypass
before breakfast

AcB assist with bath

AC & BC air and bone conduction

ACBE air contrast barium enema

ACC acalculous cholecystitis
accident
accommodation
adenoid cystic carcinomas
administrative control center
advanced colorectal cancer
ambulatory care center
amylase creatinine clearance
automated cell count

AcCoA acetyl-coenzyme A

ACCR amylase creatinine clearance ratio

ACCU acute coronary care unit

ACCU✔ Accucheck® (blood glucose monitoring)

ACD absolute cardiac dullness
absorbent cover dressing
acid-citrate-dextrose
allergic contact dermatitis
anemia of chronic disease
anterior cervical diskectomy
anterior chamber diameter
anterior chest diameter

before dinner

dactinomycin (actinomycin D)

AC-DC bisexual (homo- and heterosexual

ACDDS Alcoholism/Chemical Dependency Detoxification Service

ACDF anterior cervical diskectomy fusion

ACDK acquired cystic disease of the kidney

ACDs anticonvulsant drugs

ACE adrenocortical extract
adverse clinical event
aerosol cloud enhancer
angiotensin-converting enzyme
doxorubicin (Adriamycin), cyclophosphamide, and etoposide

ACEI angiotensin-converting enzyme inhibitor

ACF aberrant crypt focus
accessory clinical findings
acute care facility
anterior cervical fusion

ACG accelerography
angiocardiography

ACGME Accreditation Council for Graduate Medical Education

ACH adrenal cortical hormone
aftercoming head
arm girth, chest depth, and hip width

ACh acetylcholine

ACHA air-conduction hearing aid

AChE acetylcholinesterase

ACHES abdominal pain, chest pain, headache, eye problems, and severe leg pains (early danger signs of oral contraceptive adverse effects)

AC & HS before meals and at bedtime

ACI adrenal cortical insufficiency

	aftercare instructions	ACQ	acquired
	autologous chondrocyte implantation	ACR	adenomatosis of the colon and rectum
ACIOL	anterior chamber intraocular lens		anterior chamber reformation
ACIP	Advisory Committee on Immunization Practices (of the Centers for Disease Control and Prevention)	ACRC	anticonstipation regimen
			advanced colorectal cancer
ACJ	acromioclavicular joint	ACS	acute chest syndrome
A/CK	Accuchek®		acute confusional state
ACL	anterior cruciate ligament		acute coronary syndromes
aCL	anticardiolipin (antibody)		American Cancer Society
ACLF	adult congregate living facility		anodal-closing sound
			before supper
ACLR	anterior cruciate ligament repair	ACSL	automatic computerized solvent litholysis
ACLS	advanced cardiac (cardio-pulmonary) life support	ACSVBG	aortocoronary saphenous vein bypass graft
ACM	alternative/ complementary medicine	ACSW	Academy of Certified Social Workers
		ACT	activated clotting time
	Arnold-Chiari malformation		aggressive comfort treatment
ACME	aphakic cystoid macular edema		allergen challenge test
			anticoagulant therapy
ACMT	advanced combined modality therapy		assertive community treatment (program)
		ACT-D	dactinomycin
ACMV	assist-controlled mechanical ventilation	Act Ex	active exercise
ACN	acute conditioned neurosis	ACTG	AIDS Clinical Trial Group
ACNU	nidran	ACTH	corticotropin (adrenocorticotrophic hormone)
ACOA	Adult Children of Alcoholics	ACT-Post	activated clotting time post-filter
A COMM A	anterior communicating artery	ACT-Pre	activated clotting time pre-filter
ACP	acid phosphatase ambulatory care program	ACTSEB	anterior chamber tube shunt encircling band
ACPA	anticytoplasmic antibodies	ACU	ambulatory care unit
AC-PH	acid phosphatase	ACV	acyclovir
ACPO	acute colonic pseudo-obstruction		amifostine, cisplatin, and vinblastine
ACPP	adrenocorticopolypeptide		assist control ventilation
ACPPD	average cost per patient day		atrial/carotid/ventricular
ACPP PF	acid phosphatase prostatic fluid	A-C-V	A wave, C wave, and V wave

ACVD	acute cardiovascular disease		apparent diffusion coefficient
ACVP	doxorubicin (Adriamycin), cyclophosphamide, vincristine, and prednisone	ADCC	average daily consumption antibody-dependent cellular cytotoxicity
ACW	apply to chest wall	A.D.C.	mnemonic for formatting
acyl-CoA	acyl coenzyme A	VAAN	physician orders:
AD	accident dispensary	DIML	**A**dmit, **D**iagnosis,
	admitting diagnosis		**C**ondition, **V**itals,
	advance directive (living will)		**A**ctivity, **A**llergies, **N**ursing procedures,
	air dyne		**D**iet, **I**ns and outs,
	alternating days (this is a		**M**edication, **L**abs
	dangerous abbreviation)	ADD	adduction
	Alzheimer's disease		attention deficit disorder
	androgen deprivation		average daily dose
	antidepressant	ADDH	attention deficit disorder
	atopic dermatitis		with hyperactivity
	axis deviation	ADDL	additional
	right ear	ADDM	adjustment disorder with
A&D	admission and discharge		depressed mood
	alcohol and drug	ADDP	adductor pollicis
	ascending and descending	ADDs	AIDS (acquired immune
	vitamins A and D		deficiency syndrome)-
ADA	adenosine deaminase		defining diseases
	American Diabetes Association	ADDU	alcohol and drug dependence unit
	Americans with Disabilities Act	ADE	acute disseminated encephalitis
	anterior descending artery		adverse drug event
ADAM	adjustment disorder with anxious mood	ADEM	acute disseminating encephalomyelitis
ADAS	Alzheimer's Disease Assessment Scale	ADE-NOCA	adenocarcinoma
ADAS COG	Alzheimer's Disease Assessment Scale-Cognitive Subscale	ADEPT	antibody-directed enzyme prodrug therapy
ADAT	advance diet as tolerated	AEDP	assisted end diastolic pressure
ADAU	adolescent drug abuse unit	ADFU	agar diffusion for fungus
ADB	amorous disinhibited behavior	ADG	atrial diastolic gallop axiodistogingival
ADC	Aid to Dependent Children	ADH	antidiuretic hormone atypical ductal
	AIDS (acquired immune deficiency syndrome) dementia complex	ADHD	hyperplasia attention-deficit
	anxiety disorder clinic		hyperactivity disorder

ADI	allowable (acceptable) daily intake	ADT	alternate-day therapy
	axiodistoincisal		androgen deprivation treatment (therapy)
A-DIC	doxorubicin and dacarbazine		anticipate discharge tomorrow
Adj Dis	adjustment disorder		any damn thing (a placebo)
Adj D/O	adjustment disorder		Auditory Discrimination Test
ADL	activities of daily living	ADTP	Adolescent Day Treatment Program
ad lib	as desired		Alcohol Dependence Treatment Program
	at liberty		
ADM	administered (dose)	A5D5W	alcohol 5%, dextrose 5% in water for injection
	admission		
	adrenomedullin	ADX	audiological diagnostic
	doxorubicin	AE	above elbow (amputation)
ADME	absorption, distribution, metabolism, and excretion		accident and emergency (department)
			acute exacerbation
ADO	axiodisto-occlusal		adaptive equipment
Ad-OAP	doxorubicin, vincristine, cytarabine, and prednisone		adverse event
			air entry
			antiembolitic
ADOL	adolescent		arm ergometer
ADP	arterial demand pacing		aryepiglottic (fold)
	adenosine diphosphate	A&E	accident and emergency (department)
ADPKD	autosomal dominant polycystic kidney disease		
		AEA	above elbow amputation
			anti-endomysium antibody
ADPV	anomaly of drainage of pulmonary vein	AEB	as evidenced by
			atrial ectopic beat
ADQ	abductor digiti quinti	AEC	at earliest convenience
	adequate	AECB	acute exacerbations of chronic bronchitis
ADR	acute dystonic reaction		
	adverse drug reaction	AECG	ambulatory electrocardiogram
	alternative dispute resolution		
		AED	antiepileptic drug
	doxorubicin (Adriamycin)		automated external defibrillator
ADRIA	doxorubicin (Adriamycin)	AEDD	anterior extradural defects
		AEDP	automated external defibrillator pacemaker
ADS	admission day surgery		
	anatomical dead space	AEEU	admission entrance and evaluation unit
	anonymous donor's sperm		
	antibody deficiency syndrome	AEG	air encephalogram
			Alcohol Education Group
ADs	advance directives (living wills)	AEIOU TIPS	mnemonic for the diagnosis of coma:
ADSU	ambulatory diagnostic surgery unit		

	Alcohol, Encephalopathy, Insulin, Opiates, Uremia, Trauma, Infection, Psychiatric, and Syncope	AF/FL	atrial fibrillation/atrial flutter
AELBM	after each loose bowel movement	aFGF	acidic fibroblast growth factor
AEM	active electrode monitor	AFI	acute febrile illness
	ambulatory electrogram monitor		amniotic fluid index
	antiepileptic medication	A fib	atrial fibrillation
AEP	auditory evoked potential	AFIP	Armed Forces Institute of Pathology
AEq	age equivalent	AFKO	ankle-foot-knee orthosis
AER	acoustic evoked response	AFL	atrial flutter
	albumin excretion rate	AFLP	acute fatty liver of pregnancy
	auditory evoked response	A Flu	atrial flutter
Aer. M.	aerosol mask	AFM	acute *Plasmodium falciparum* malaria
AERS	adverse event reporting system		atomic force microscopy
			doxorubicin (Adriamycin), fluorouracil, and methotrexate
Aer. T.	aerosol tent	AFM×2	double aerosol face mask
AES	adult emergency service	AFO	ankle fixation orthotic
	anti-embolic stockings		ankle-foot orthosis
AEs	adverse events	AFOF	anterior fontanel–open and flat
AET	alternating esotropia	AFP	acute flaccid paralysis
	atrial ectopic tachycardia		alpha-fetoprotein
AF	acid-fast		anterior faucial pillar
	afebrile		ascending frontal parietal
	amniotic fluid	AFQT	Armed Forces Qualification Test
	anterior fontanel	AFRD	acute febrile respiratory disease
	antifibrinogen		
	aortofemoral	Aft/Dis	aftercare/discharge
	ascitic fluid	AFV	amniotic fluid volume
	atrial fibrillation	AFVSS	afebrile, vital signs stable
AFB	acid-fast bacilli	AFX	air-fluid exchange
	aorto-femoral bypass	AG	abdominal girth
	aspirated foreign body		adrenogenital
AFBG	aortofemoral bypass graft		aminoglycoside
AFBY	aortofemoral bypass (graft)		anion gap
			antigen
AFC	adult foster care		anti-gravity
	air filled cushions		atrial gallop
AFDC	Aid to Family and Dependent Children	Ag	silver
		A/G	albumin to globulin ratio
AFE	amniotic fluid embolization	AGA	accelerated growth area
AFEB	afebrile		acute gonococcal arthritis
AFEU	ante partum fetal evaluation unit		

	antigliadin antibody		amenorrhea-hyperprolac-tinemia
	appropriate for gestational age		antihyaluronidase
	average gestational age		auditory hallucinations
AGAS	accelerated graft atherosclerosis	A&H	accident and health (insurance)
AG/BL	aminoglycoside/beta-lactam	AHA	acetohydroxamic acid (Lithostat®)
AGCUS	atypical glandular cells of undetermined significance		acquired hemolytic anemia
			autoimmune hemolytic anemia
AGD	agar gel diffusion		
AGE	acute gastroenteritis	AHAs	alpha hydroxy acids
	advanced glycation end product	AHase	antihyaluronidase
		AHB$_c$	hepatitis B core antibody
	angle of greatest extension	AHC	acute hemorrhagic conjunctivitis
	anterior gastroenterostomy		acute hemorrhagic cystitis
	irreversible advanced glycosylation end products		Adolescent Health Center
		AHCA	American Healthcare Association
AGF	angle of greatest flexion	AHCPR	Agency for Health Care Policy and Research
AGG	agammaglobulinemia	AHD	antecedent hematological disorder
aggl.	agglutination		
AGI	alpha-glucosidase inhibitor		arteriosclerotic heart disease
AGL	acute granulocytic leukemia		autoimmune hemolytic disease
A GLAC-TO-LK	alpha galactoside leukocytes	AHE	acute hemorrhagic encephalomyelitis
AGN	acute glomerulonephritis	AHEC	Area Health Education Center
AgNO$_3$	silver nitrate		
AgNORs	argyrophilic nucleolar organizer regions (staining)	AHF	antihemophilic factor
		AHF-M	antihemophilic factor (human), method M, (monoclonal purified)
α$_1$-AGP	alpha$_1$-acid glycoprotein		
AGPT	agar-gel precipitation test	AHFS	American Hospital Formulary Service
AGS	adrenogenital syndrome		
AG SYND	adrenogenital syndrome	AHG	antihemophilic globulin
AGTT	abnormal glucose tolerance test	AHGS	acute herpetic gingival stomatitis
AGU	aspartylglycosaminuria	AHHD	arteriosclerotic hyper-tensive heart disease
AGVHD	acute graft-versus-host disease		
		AHI	apnea/hypopnea index
AGVI	Ahmed glaucoma valve implantation	AHJ	artificial hip joint
		AHL	apparent half-life
AH	abdominal hysterectomy	AHM	ambulatory Holter monitoring
	amenorrhea and hirsutism		

AHMO	anterior horizontal mandibular osteotomy		disease
			aortoiliac disease
AHN	adenomatous hyperplastic nodule		artificial insemination donor
	Assistant Head Nurse		automatic implantable defibrillator
AHP	acute hemorrhagic pancreatitis	AIDH	artificial insemination donor husband
AHS	adaptive hand skills	AIDKS	acquired immune
	allopurinol hypersensitivity syndrome		deficiency syndrome with Kaposi's sarcoma
AHST	autologous hematopoietic stem cell transplantation	AIDS	acquired immune deficiency syndrome
		AIE	acute inclusion body encephalitis
AHT	alternating hypertropia		
	autoantibodies to human thyroglobulin	AIF	aortic-iliac-femoral
		AIH	artificial insemination with husband's sperm
AHTG	antihuman thymocyte globulin	AIHA	autoimmune hemolytic anemia
AI	accidentally incurred		
	apical impulse	AIHD	acquired immune hemolytic disease
	allergy index		
	aortic insufficiency	AIIS	anterior inferior iliac spine
	artificial insemination		
	artificial intelligence	AILD	angioimmunoblastic lymphadenopathy with dysproteinemia
A & I	Allergy and Immunology (department)		
AIA	Accommodation Independence Assessment	AIMS	Abnormal Involuntary Movement Scale
			Arthritis Impact Measurement Scales
	allergen-induced asthma		
	allyl isopropyl acetamide	AIN	acute interstitial nephritis
	anti-insulin antibody		anal intraepithelial neoplasia
	aspirin-induced asthma		
AI-Ab	anti-insulin antibody	AINS	anti-inflammatory non-steroidal
AIBF	anterior interbody fusion		
AICA	anterior inferior cerebellar artery	AIOD	aortoiliac occlusive disease
	anterior inferior communicating artery	AION	anterior ischemic optic neuropathy
AICD	activation-induced cell death	AIP	acute infectious polyneuritis
	automatic implantable cardioverter/ defibrillator		acute intermittent porphyria
		AIPC	androgen-independent prostate cancer
AICS	acute ischemic coronary syndromes	AIR	accelerated idioventricular rhythm
AID	absolute iron deficiency		
	acute infectious	AIS	Abbreviated Injury Score

	adolescent idiopathic scoliosis	ALAD	abnormal left axis deviation
	anti-insulin serum	ALARA	as low as reasonably achievable
AISA	acquired idiopathic sideroblastic anemia	ALAT	alanine transaminase (alanine aminotransferase; SGPT)
AIS/ISS	Abbreviated Injury Scale/ Injury Severity Score		
AIT	auditory integration therapy	ALAX	apical long axis
		ALB	albumin
AITN	acute interstitial tubular nephritis		albuterol
			anterior lenticular bevel
AITP	autoimmune thrombocytopenia purpura	ALC	acute lethal catatonia
			alcohol
			alcoholic liver cirrhosis
AIU	absolute iodine uptake		allogeneic lymphocyte cytotoxicity
	adolescent inpatient unit		
AIVR	accelerated idioventricular rhythm		alternate level of care
			Alternate Lifestyle Checklist
AJ	ankle jerk		
AJCC	American Joint Committee on Cancer		axiolinguocervical
		ALCA	anomalous left coronary artery
AJO	apple juice only		
AJR	abnormal jugular reflex	ALCL	anaplastic large-cell lymphoma
AK	above knee (amputation)		
	actinic keratosis	ALC R	alcohol rub
	artificial kidney	ALD	adrenoleukodystrophy
AKA	above-knee amputation		alcoholic liver disease
	alcoholic ketoacidosis		aldolase
	all known allergies	ALDH	aldehyde dehydrogenase
	also known as	ALDOST	aldosterone
AKS	alcoholic Korsakoff syndrome	ALF	acute liver failure
			assisted living facility
	arthroscopic knee surgery	ALFT	abnormal liver function tests
AKU	artificial kidney unit	ALG	antilymphoblast globulin
AL	acute leukemia		antilymphocyte globulin
	argon laser	ALH	atypical lobular hyperplasia
	arterial line		
	assisted living	ALI	argon laser iridotomy
	axial length	A-line	arterial catheter
	left ear	ALK	alkaline
Al	aluminum		automated lamellar keratoplasty
ALA	alpha-linolenic acid (α-linolenic acid)		
		ALK ∅	alkaline phosphatase
	alpha-lipoic acid	ALK ISO	alkaline phosphatase isoenzymes
	aminolevulinic acid		
	anti-lymphocyte antibody	ALK-P	alkaline phosphatase
ALAC	antibiotic-loaded acrylic cement	ALK PHOS ISO	alkaline phosphatase isoenzyme

ALL	acute lymphoblastic leukemia		autolymphocyte therapy
	acute lymphocytic leukemia	2 alt	every other day (this is a dangerous abbreviation)
	allergy	ALTB	acute laryngotracheobron-chitis
ALLD	arthroscopic lumbar laser diskectomy	ALTE	acute (aberrant, apparent) life threatening event
ALLO	allogeneic	*alt hor*	every other hour (this is a dangerous abbreviation)
Allo-BMT	allogenic bone marrow transplantation	ALUP	Alupent
ALM	acral lentiginous melanoma	ALVAD	abdominal left ventricular assist device
	alveolar lining material autoclave-killed *Leishmania major*	ALWMI	anterolateral wall myocardial infarct
		ALZ	Alzheimer's disease
ALMI	anterolateral myocardial infarction	AM	adult male amalgam
ALN	anterior lower neck		anovulatory menstruation
	anterior lymph node		morning (a.m.)
	axillary lymph nodes		myopic astigmatism
ALND	axillary lymph node dissection	AMA	against medical advice
ALNM	axillary lymph node metastasis		American Medical Association
ALO	axiolinguo-occlusal		antimitochondrial antibody
Al(OH)₃	aluminum hydroxide	AMAC	adults molested as children
ALOS	average length of stay		
ALP	alkaline phosphatase	AMAD	morning admission
	argon laser photocoagulation	AM/ADM	morning admission
	Alupent	AMAG	adrenal medullary autograft
ALSG	Australian Leukemia Study Group	AMAL	amalgam
ALTP	argon laser trabeculo-plasty	AMAP	American Medical Accreditation Program
ALPZ	alprazolam (Xanax)		as much as possible
ALR	adductor leg raise	Amask	aerosol mask
ALRI	acute lower-respiratory-tract infection	AMAT	anti-malignant antibody test
	anterolateral rotary instability		Arm Motor Ability Test
		A-MAT	amorphous material
ALS	acute lateral sclerosis	AMB	ambulate
	advanced life support		ambulatory
	amyotrophic lateral sclerosis		amphotericin B
			as manifested by
ALT	alanine transaminase (SGPT)	AMBER	advanced multiple beam equalization radiography
	argon laser trabeculo-plasty	AMC	arm muscle circumference

	arthrogryposis multiplex congenita	AMM	agnogenic myeloid metaplasia
AM/CR	amylase to creatinine ratio	AMML	acute myelomonocytic leukemia
AMD	age-related macular degeneration	AMMOL	acute myelomonoblastic leukemia
	arthroscopic microdiskectomy	AMN	adrenomyeloneuropathy
	axiomesiodistal	amnio	amniocentesis
	dactinomycin (actinomycin D)	AMN SC	amniotic fluid scan
	methyldopa (alpha methyldopa)	AMOL	acute monoblastic leukemia
AME	agreed medical examination	AMP	adenosine monophosphate
	anthrax meningoencephalitis		ampere
	apparent mineralocorticoid excess (syndrome)		ampicillin
			ampul
			amputation
		A-M pr	Austin-Moore prosthesis
		AMPT	metyrosine (alphameth-ylpara tyrosine)
	Aviation Medical Examiner	AMR	acoustic muscle reflex
			alternating motion rates
AMegL	acute megakaryoblastic leukemia	AMRI	anterior medial rotary instability
AMES-LAN	American sign language	AMS	acute mountain sickness
			aggravated in military service
AMF	aerobic metabolism facilitator		altered mental status
			amylase
	autocrine motility factor		aseptic meningitis syndrome
AMG	acoustic myography		atypical mole syndrome
	aminoglycoside		auditory memory span
	axiomesiogingival	m-AMSA	amsacrine (acridinyl anisidide)
	Federal Republic of German's equivalent to United States Food, Drug, and Cosmetic Act	AMSIT	portion of the mental status examination: A—appearance, M—mood, S—sensorium, I—intelligence, T—thought process
AMGA	American Medical Group Association		
AMI	acute myocardial infarction	AMT	Adolph's Meat Tenderizer
	amifostine (Ethyol)		allogeneic (bone) marrow transplant
	amitriptyline		aminopterin
	axiomesioincisal		amount
AMKL	acute megakaryocytic leukemia	AMTS	Abbreviated Mental Test Score
AML	acute myelogenous leukemia	AMU	accessory-muscle use
	angiomyolipoma		
	anterior mitral leaflet		

AMV	alveolar minute ventilation	ANOVA	analysis of variance
	assisted mechanical ventilation	ANP	Adult Nurse Practitioner atrial natriuretic peptide (anaritide acetate)
AMY	amylase		axillary node–positive
AMY/CR	amylase/creatinine ratio	ANPR	advanced notice of proposed rule making
AN	acoustic neuromas	ANS	answer
	amyl nitrate		autonomic nervous system
	anorexia nervosa		
	Associate Nurse	ANSER	Aggregate Neurobehavioral Student Health and Education Review
	avascular necrosis		
ANA	antinuclear antibody		
ANAD	anorexia nervosa and associated disorders	ANT	anterior
			enpheptin (2-amino-5-nitrothiazol)
ANADA	Abbreviated New Animal Drug Application		
		ante	before
ANAG	acute narrow angle glaucoma	ANTI A:AGT	anti blood group A antiglobulin test
ANA SWAB	anaerobic swab	Anti bx	antibiotic
		anti-GAD	antibodies to glutamic acid decarboxylase
ANC	absolute neutrophil count		
ANCA	antineutrophil cytoplasmic antibody	anti-HBc	antibody to hepatitis B core antigen (HBcAg)
anch	anchored		
ANCN	absolute neutrophil count nadir	anti-HBe	antibody to hepatitis B e antigen (HBeAg)
ANCOVA	analysis of covariance	anti-HBs	antibody to hepatitis B surface antigen (HBsAg)
AND	anterior nasal discharge axillary node dissection		
		ant sag D	anterior sagittal diameter
ANDA	Abbreviated New Drug Application	ANTU	alpha naphthylthiourea
		ANUG	acute necrotizing ulcerative gingivitis
anes	anesthesia		
ANF	antinuclear factor	ANV	acute nausea and vomiting
	atrial natriuretic factor		
ANG	angiogram	ANX	anxiety
ANG II	angiotensin II		anxious
ANGIO	angiogram	AO	Agent Orange
ANH	acute normovolemic hemodilution		anterior oblique
			aorta
	artificial nutrition and hydration		aortic opening
			aortography
ANISO	anisocytosis		axio-occlusal
ANK	ankle		plate, screw (orthopedics)
	appointment not kept		right ear
ANLL	acute nonlymphoblastic leukemia	A-O	atlanto-occipital (joint)
		A/O	alert and oriented
ANM	Assistant Nurse Manager	A & O	alert and oriented
ANN	axillary node–negative		

A&O × 3	awake and oriented to person, place, and time	AOR	Alvarado Orthopedic Research
A&O × 4	awake and oriented to person, place, time, and object		at own risk
			auditory oculogyric reflex
AOAA	aminooxoacetic acid	AORT REGURG	aortic regurgitation
AOAP	as often as possible		
AOB	alcohol on breath	AORT STEN	aortic stenosis
AOBS	acute organic brain syndrome		
		AOS	ambulatory outpatient surgery
AOC	abridged ocular chart		
	advanced ovarian cancer		anode opening sound
	amoxicillin, omeprazole, and clarithromycin		antibiotic order sheet
			aortic ostial stenoses
	anode opening contraction	AOSC	acute obstructive suppurative cholangiotomy
	antacid of choice		
	area of concern		
AOCD	anemia of chronic disease	AOSD	adult-onset Still's disease
AOCL	anodal opening clonus		
AOD	adult onset diabetes	AOTe	anodal opening tetanus
	alleged onset date	AP	abdominoperineal
	arterial occlusive disease		acute pancreatitis
	Assistant-Officer-of-the-Day		aerosol pentamidine
			alkaline phosphatase
AODA	alcohol and other drug abuse		angina pectoris
			antepartum
AODM	adult onset diabetes mellitus		anterior-posterior (x-ray)
			apical pulse
A of 1	assistance of one		appendectomy
A of 2	assistance of two		appendicitis
AOI	area of induration		arterial pressure
ao-il	aorta-iliac		atrial pacing
AOL	augmentation of labor		attending physician
AOLC	acridine-orange leukocyte cytospin		doxorubicin (Adriamycin); cisplatin (Platinol AQ)
AOLD	automated open lumbar diskectomy	A&P	active and present
			anterior and posterior
AOM	acute otitis media		assessment and plans
	alternatives of management		auscultation and percussion
AONAD	alert, oriented, and no acute distress	A/P	ascites/plasma ratio
		$A_2 > P_2$	second aortic sound greater than second pulmonic sound
AOO	anodal opening odor		
	continuous arterial asynchronous pacing	APA	antiphospholipid antibody
AOP	anemia of prematurity	APAA	anterior parietal artery aneurysm
	anodal opening picture		
	aortic pressure		
	apnea of prematurity		

APACHE	Acute Physiology and Chronic Health Evaluation	
APAD	anterior-posterior abdominal diameter	
APAG	antipseudomonal aminoglycosidic penicillin	
APAP	acetaminophen (N acetyl-para-aminophenol)	
APB	abductor pollicis brevis atrial premature beat	
APBSCT	autologous peripheral blood stem cell transplantation	
APC	absolute phagocyte count activated protein C acute pharyngoconjunctiivitis (fever) adenoidal-pharyngeal-conjunctival adenomatous polyposis of the colon and rectum advanced pancreatic cancer advanced prostate cancer antigen-presenting cell aspirin, phenacetin, and caffeine atrial premature contraction autologous packed cells	
APCD	adult polycystic disease	
APCIs	atrial peptide clearance inhibitors	
APCKD	adult polycystic kidney disease	
APD	acid peptic disease action potential duration afferent pupillary defect anterior-posterior diameter atrial premature depolarization automated peritoneal dialysis pamidronate disodium (aminohydroxypropylidene diphosphate)	
APDC	Anxiety and Panic Disorder Clinic	
APDT	acellular pertussis vaccine with diphtheria and tetanus toxoids	
APE	absolute prediction error acute psychotic episode acute pulmonary edema Adriamycin, cisplatin (Platinol), and etoposide anterior pituitary extract	
APER	abdominoperineal excision of the rectum	
APG	ambulatory patient group Apgar (score)	
APGAR	appearance (color), pulse (heart rate), grimace (reflex irritability), activity (muscle tone), and respiration (score reflecting condition of newborn)	
APH	adult psychiatric hospital alcohol-positive history antepartum hemorrhage	
APHIS	Animal and Plant Health Inspection Service	
API	Asian-Pacific Islander	
APIS	Acute Pain Intensity Scale	
APIVR	artificial pacemaker-induced ventricular rhythm	
APKD	adult polycystic kidney disease adult-onset polycystic kidney disease	
APL	abductor pollicis longus accelerated painless labor acute promyelocytic leukemia anterior pituitary-like (hormone) chorionic gonadotropin	
AP & L	anteroposterior and lateral	
APLA	anti-phospholipid antibody	

APLD	automated percutaneous lumbar diskectomy		streptokinase activator complex)
APMPPE	acute posterior multifocal placoid pigment epitheliopathy	APSD	Alzheimer's presenile dementia
		APSP	assisted peak systolic pressure
APMS	acute pain management service	aPTT	activated partial thromboplastin time
APN	acute panautonomic neuropathy	APU	ambulatory procedure unit
	acute pyelonephritis		antepartum unit
APO	adverse patient occurrence	APUD	amine precursor uptake and decarboxylation
	apolipoprotein A-1		
	doxorubicin (Adriamycin), prednisone, and vincristine (Oncovin)	APVC	partial anomalous pulmonary venous connection
APO(a)	apolipoprotein (A)		
APOE	apolipoprotein E	APVR	aortic pulmonary valve replacement
APOE-4	apolipoprotein-E (gene)	APW	aortopulmonary window
APOLT	auxiliary partial orthotopic liver transplantation	aq	water
		AQ	accomplishment quotient
		aq dest	distilled water
APOPPS	adjustable postoperative protective prosthetic socket	A quad	atrial quadrageminy
		AR	Achilles reflex
APP	amyloid precursor protein		acoustic reflex
APPG	aqueous procaine penicillin G (dangerous terminology; since it is for intramuscular use only, write as penicillin G procaine)		active resistance
			airway resistance
			alcohol related
			ankle reflex
			aortic regurgitation
			Argyll Robertson (pupil)
appr.	approximate		assisted respiration
appt.	appointment		at risk
APPY	appendectomy		aural rehabilitation
APR	abdominoperineal resection		autorefractor
		Ar	argon
APRT	abdominopelvic radiotherapy	A&R	adenoidectomy with radium
			advised and released
APRV	airway pressure release ventilation	A-R	apical-radial (pulses)
		ARA	adenosine regulating agent
APS	Acute Physiology Scoring (system)	ara-A	vidarabine
	adult protective services	ara-AC	fazarabine
	Adult Psychiatric Service	ara-C	cytarabine
	antiphospholipid syndrome	ARAD	abnormal right axis deviation
APSAC	anistreplase (anisoylated plasminogen	ARAS	ascending reticular activating system

	atherosclerotic renal-artery stenosis	ARMD	age-related macular degeneration
ARB	angiotensin II receptor blocker	ARMS	amplification refractory mutation system
	any reliable brand	ARN	acute retinal necrosis
ARBOR	arthropod-borne virus	AROM	active range of motion
ARBOW	artificial rupture of bag of water		artifical rupture of membranes
ARC	abnormal retinal correspondence	ARP	absolute refractory period
	AIDS-related complex		alcohol rehabilitation program
	Alcohol Rehabilitation Center	ARPF	anterior release posterior fusion
	anomalous retinal correspondence	ARPKS	autosomal recessive polycystic kidney disease
	American Red Cross		
ARCBS	American Red Cross Blood Services	ARR	absolue risk reduction
ARD	acute respiratory disease		arrive
	adult respiratory distress	ARROM	active resistive range of motion
	antibiotic removal device		
	antibiotic retrieval device	ARRT	American Registry of Radiologic Technologists
	aphakic retinal detachment		
ARDMS	American Registry of Diagnostic Medical Sonographers	ARS	antirabies serum
		ART	Accredited Record Technician
ARDS	adult respiratory distress syndrome		Achilles (tendon) reflex test
ARE	active-resistive exercises		acoustic reflex threshold(s)
ARF	acute renal failure		arterial
	acute respiratory failure		assessment, review, and treatment
	acute rheumatic fever		assisted reproductive technology
ARG	alkaline reflux gastritis		
	arginine		automated reagin test (for syphilis)
ARHL	age-related hearing loss		
ARHNC	advanced resected head and neck cancer	ARTIC	articulation
		Art T	art therapy
ARI	acute renal insufficiency	ARU	alcohol rehabilitation unit
	acute respiratory infection	ARV	AIDS related virus
	aldose reductase inhibitor	ARW	Accredited Rehabilitation Worker
ARL	average remaining lifetime		
		ARWY	airway
ARLD	alcohol-related liver disease	AS	activated sleep
			anabolic steroid
ARM	anxiety reaction, mild		anal sphincter
	artificial rupture of membranes		androgen suppression

35

ankylosing spondylitis
anterior synechia
aortic stenosis
atherosclerosis
atropine sulfate
AutoSuture®
doctor called through answering service
left ear

ASA — American Society of Anesthesiologists
argininosuccinate
aspirin (acetylsalicylic acid)
atrial septal aneurysm

ASA I — American Society of anesthesiologists' classification
Healthy patient with localized pathological process

ASA II — A patient with mild to moderate systemic disease

ASA III — A patient with severe systemic disease limiting activity but not incapacitating

ASA IV — A patient with incapacitating systemic disease

ASA V — Moribund patient not expected to live. (These are American Society of Anesthesiologists' patient classifications. Emergency operations are designated by "E" after the classification.)

5-ASA — mesalamine (5-aminosalicylic acid) (this is a dangerous abbreviation as it is mistaken for five aspirin tablets)

ASAA — acquired severe aplastic anemia

ASACL — American Society of Anesthesiologists Classification

AS/AI — aortic stenosis/aortic insufficiency

A's and B's — apnea and bradycardia

ASAP — as soon as possible

ASAT — aspartate transaminase (aspartate aminotransferase) (SGOT)

ASB — anesthesia standby
asymptomatic bacteriuria

ASBO — adhesive small-bowel obstruction

ASC — altered state of consciousness
ambulatory surgery center
anterior subcapsular cataract
antimony sulfur colloid
apocrine skin carcinoma
ascorbic acid

ASCAD — atherosclerotic coronary artery disease

ASCCC — advanced squamous cell cervical carcinoma

ASCCHN — advanced squamous cell carcinoma of the head and neck

ASCI — acute spinal cord injury

ASCO — American Society of Clinical Oncology

ASCR — autologous stem cell rescue

ASCS — autologous stem cell support

ASCT — autologous stem cell transplantation

ASCUS — atypical squamous cell of undetermined significance

ASCVD — arteriosclerotic cardiovascular disease

ASCVR — arteriosclerotic cardiovascular renal disease

ASD — aldosterone secretion defect
atrial septal defect

ASD I	atrial septal defect, primum	ASO	aldicarb sulfoxide
ASD II	atrial septal defect, secundum		allele-specific oligodeoxynucleotide (probes)
ASDH	acute subdural hematoma		antistreptolysin-O titer
ASE	abstinence symptom evaluation		arteriosclerosis obliterans
	acute stress erosion		automatic stop order
ASF	anterior spinal fusion	As₂O₃	arsenic trioxide
ASFR	age-specific fertility rate	ASOT	antistreptolysin-O titer
ASH	asymmetric septal hypertrophy	ASP	acute suppurative parotitis
AsH	hypermetropic astigmatism		acute symmetric polyarthritis
			asparaginase
ASHD	arteriosclerotic heart disease		aspartic acid
ASI	Anxiety Status Inventory	ASPVD	arteriosclerotic peripheral vascular disease
ASIA	American Spinal Injury Association (Score)	ASR	aldosterone secretion rate
	A-Complete—No preservation of any motor and/or sensory function below the zone of injury		automatic speech recognition
		ASS	anterior superior supine
			assessment
		asst	assistant
	B-Incomplete—Preserved sensation	AST	allergy skin test
			Aphasia Screening Test
	C-Incomplete—Preserved motor (non-functional)		aspartate transaminase (SGOT)
			astemizole
	D-Incomplete—Preserved motor (functional)		astigmatism
		AstdVe	assisted ventilation
	E-Complete Recovery	ASTH	asthenopia
ASIH	absent, sick in hospital	ASTI	acute soft tissue injury
ASIMC	absent, sick in medical center	AS TOL	as tolerated
		ASTIG	astigmatism
ASIS	anterior superior iliac spine	ASTRO	astrocytoma
		ASTZ	antistreptozyme test
ASK	antistreptokinase	ASU	acute stroke unit
ASKase	antistreptokinase		ambulatory surgical unit
ASL	American Sign Language	ASV	antisnake venom
	antistreptolysin (titer)	ASVD	arteriosclerotic vessel disease
ASLO	antistreptolysin-O		
ASLV	avian sarcoma and leukosis virus (Rous virus)	ASYM	asymmetric (al)
		ASX	asymptomatic
		AT	activity therapy (therapist)
AsM	myopic astigmatism		Addiction Therapist
ASMA	anti-smooth muscle antibody		antithrombin
			applanation tonometry
ASMI	anteroseptal myocardial infarction		ataxia-telangiectasia
			atraumatic

37

	atrial tachycardia	ATM	acute transverse myelitis
AT 10	dihydrotachysterol		atmosphere
ATA	atmosphere absolute	At ma	atrial milliamp
ATB	antibiotic	ATN	acute tubular necrosis
	atypical tuberculosis	ATNC	atraumatic normocephalic
ATC	acute toxic class	aTNM	autopsy staging of
	aerosol treatment chamber		cancer
	alcoholism therapy classes	ATNR	asymmetrical tonic neck
	all-terrain cycle		reflex
	antituberculous	ATO	arsenic trioxide
	chemoprophylaxis	ATP	addiction treatment
	around the clock		program
	Arthritis Treatment Center		adenosine triphosphate
ATCC	American Type Culture		anterior tonsillar pillar
	Collection		autoimmune thrombo-
ATD	antithyroid drug(s)		cytopenia purpura
	anticipated time of	ATPase	adenosine triphosphatase
	discharge	ATPS	ambient temperature &
	asphyxiating thoracic		pressure, saturated with
	dystrophy		water vapor
	autoimmune thyroid	ATR	Achilles tendon reflex
	disease		atracurium (Tracrium)
ATE	adipose tissue extraction		atrial
ATEM	analytical transmission		atropine
	electron microscopy	ATRA	all-*trans* retinoic acid
At Fib	atrial fibrillation		(tretinoin-Vesanoid®)
ATFL	anterior talofibular	atr fib	atrial fibrillation
	ligament	ATRO	atropine
AT III FUN	antithrombin III	ATRX	acute transfusion reaction
	functional	ATU	alcohol treatment unit
ATG	antithymocyte globulin	ATV	all-terrain vehicle
ATHR	angina threshold heart	ATS	antimony trisulfide
	rate		antitetanic serum (tetanus
ATI	Abdominal Trauma Index		antitoxin)
	acute traumatic ischemia		anxiety tension state
ATL	Achilles tendon	ATSO	admit to (the) service of
	lengthening	ATSO4	atropine sulfate
	adult T-cell leukemia	ATT	antitetanus toxoid
	anterior temporal		arginine tolerance test
	lobectomy	ATTN	attention
	anterior tricuspid leaflet	ATTR	amyloid transtyretin
	antitension line	at. wt	atomic weight
	atypical lymphocytes	AU	allergenic (allergy) units
ATLL	adult T-cell leukemia		arbitrary units
	lymphoma		both ears
ATLS	acute tumor lysis	Au	gold
	syndrome	A/U	at umbilicus
	advanced trauma life	198Au	radioactive gold
	support	AUB	abnormal uterine bleeding

AuBMT	autologous bone marrow transplant	AVE	aortic valve echocardiogram
AUC	area under the curve	AVF	arteriovenous fistula
AUC$_t$	area under the curve to last time point		augmented unipolar foot (left leg)
AUD	amplifiable units of DNA (deoxyribonucleic acid)	avg	average
		AVGS	autologous vein graft stent
	arthritis of unknown diagnosis	AVGs	ambulatory visit groups
	auditory	AVH	acute viral hepatitis
AUD COMP	auditory comprehension	AVHB	atrioventricular heart block
AUG	acute ulcerative gingivitis	AVJR	atrioventricular junctional rhythm
AUGIB	acute upper gastrointestinal bleeding	AVL	augmented unipolar left (left arm)
AUIC	area under the inhibitory curve	AVLT	auditory verbal learning test
AUL	acute undifferentiated leukemia	AVM	arteriovenous malformation
AUR	acute urinary retention	AVN	arteriovenous nicking
AUS	acute urethral syndrome		atrioventricular node
	artificial urinary sphincter		avascular necrosis
	auscultation	AVNR	atrioventricular nodal re-entry
AUTO SP	automatic speech	AVNRT	atrioventricular node recovery time
AV	anteverted		
	anticipatory vomiting		atrioventricular nodal re-entry tachycardia
	arteriovenous	A-VO$_2$	arteriovenous oxygen difference
	atrioventricular		
	auditory visual	AVOC	avocation
	auriculoventricular	AVP	arginine vasopressin
A:V	arterial-venous (ratio in fundi)	AVR	aortic valve replacement
			augmented unipolar right (right arm)
AVA	aortic valve atresia		
	arteriovenous anastomosis	AVRP	atrioventricular refractory period
AVB	atrioventricular block		
AVC	acrylic veneer crown	AVRT	atrioventricular reciprocating tachycardia
AVD	aortic valve disease		
	apparent volume of distribution	AVS	atriovenous shunt
		AVSD	atrioventricular septal defect
	arteriosclerotic vascular disease	AVSS	afebrile, vital signs stable
AVDP	asparaginase, vincristine, daunorubicin, and prednisone	AVT	atrioventricular tachycardia
	avoirdupois		atypical ventricular tachycardia
AVDO$_2$	arteriovenous oxygen difference		

AvWS	acquired von Willebrand's syndrome		
AW	abdominal wall		
	abnormal wave		
	airway		
A/W	able to work		
A&W	alive and well	B	bacillus
AWA	alcohol withdrawal assessment		bands
			bilateral
	as well as		black
A waves	atrial contraction wave		bloody
AWB	autologous whole blood		bolus
AWDW	assault with a deadly weapon		both
			botulism (Vaccine B is botulism toxoid)
AWI	anterior wall infarct		brother
AWMI	anterior wall myocardial infarction		buccal
AWO	airway obstruction	Ⓑ	both
AWOL	absent without leave	B+	blood type B positive
AWP	airway pressure	B−	blood type B negative
	average wholesale price	B_1	thiamine HCl
AWRU	active wrist rotation unit	B I	Billroth I (gastric surgery)
AWS	alcohol withdrawal seizures	B II	Billroth II (gastric surgery)
		B_2	riboflavin
	alcohol withdrawal syndrome	B_3	nicotinic acid
		b/4	before
AWU	alcohol withdrawal unit	B_5	pantothenic acid
ax	axillary	B_6	pyridoxine HCl
AXB	axillary block	B_7	biotin
AXC	aortic cross clamp	B_8	adenosine phosphate
ax-fem.fem.	axilla-femoral-femoral (graft)	B_9	benign
		B_{12}	cyanocobalamin
AXND	axillary node dissection	Ba	barium
AXR	abdomen x-ray	BA	backache
AXT	alternating exotropia		Baptist
AY	acrocyanotic (infant color)		benzyl alcohol
AZA	azathioprine (Imuran®)		bile acid
AZA-CR	azacitidine		biliary atresia
5-AZC	azacitidine		blood agar
AzdU	azidouridine		blood alcohol
AZE	azelastine hydrochloride		bone age
AZM	acquisition zoom magnification		Bourns assist
			branchial artery
AZQ	diaziquone		broken appointment
AZT	zidovudine (azidothymidine)		bronchial asthma
			buccoaxial
A-Z test	Aschheim-Zondek test	B > A	bone greater than air
	(diagnostic test for	B < A	bone less than air
	pregnancy)	B & A	brisk and active

BAA	beta-adrenergic agonist	BALF	bronchoalveolar lavage fluid
BAAM	Beck airway airflow monitor	B-ALL	B cell acute lymphoblastic leukemia
Bab	Babinski		
BAC	benzalkonium chloride	BaM	barium meal
	blood alcohol concentration	BAN	British Approved Name
		BAND	band neutrophil (stab)
	bronchioloalveolar carcinoma	BANS	back, arm, neck and scalp
		BAO	basal acid output
	buccoaxiocervical	BAP	blood agar plate
BACI	bovine anti-cryptosporidium immunoglobulin	BAPT	Baptist
		Barb	barbiturate
		BARN	bilateral acute retinal necrosis
BACM	blocking agent corticosteroid myopathy	BAR Troche	Benadryl, Ativan, and Reglan troche
BACON	bleomycin, doxorubicin, lomustine, vincristine, and mechlorethamine	BAS	bile acid sequestrants boric acid solution
		BaS	barium swallow
BACOP	bleomycin, Adriamycin®, cyclophosphamide, vincristine, and prednisone	BASA	baby aspirin (81 mg chewable tablets of aspirin)
		BASIS	Basic Achievement Skills Individual Screener
BACs	bacterial artificial chromosomes	BASK	basket cells
		baso.	basophil
BACT	bacteria	BASO STIP	basophilic stippling
	base activated clotting time		
BAD	dipolar affective disorder	BAT	Behavioral Avoidance Test
BADL	basic activities of daily living		borreliacidal-antibody test
			brightness acuity tester
BaE	barium enema	BATO	boronic acid adduct of technetium oxime
BAE	bronchial artery embolization		
		batt	battery
BAEDP	balloon aortic end diastolic pressure	BAVP	balloon aortic valvuloplasty
BAEP	brain stem auditory evoked potential	BAU	bioequivalent allergy units
		BAV	bicuspid aortic valve
BAERs	brain stem auditory evoked responses	BAW	bronchoalveolar washing
BAG	buccoaxiogingival	BB	baby boy
BAHA	bone-anchored hearing aid		backboard
BAI	breath-actuated inhalers		back to back
BAL	balance		bad breath
	blood alcohol level		bed bath
	British antilewisite (dimercaprol)		bed board
			beta-blocker
	bronchoalveolar lavage		blanket bath
BALB	binaural alternate loudness balance		blood bank

	blow bottle		bladder cancer
	blue bloaters		blood culture
	body belts		Blue Cross
	both bones		bone conduction
	breakthrough bleeding		Bourn control
	breast biopsy		breast cancer
	brush biopsy		buccocervical
	buffer base		buffalo cap (cap for
B&B	bismuth and bourbon		intravenous line)
	bowel and bladder	B/C	because
B/B	backward bending		blood urea nitrogen/
BBA	born before arrival		creatinine ratio
BBB	baseball bat beating	B&C	bed and chair
	blood-brain barrier		biopsy and curettage
	bundle branch block		board and care
BBBB	bilateral bundle branch		breathed and cried
	block	BCA	balloon catheter
BBC	Brown-Buerger		angioplasty
	cystoscope		basal cell atypia
BBD	baby born dead		bicinchoninic acid
	before bronchodilator		brachiocephalic artery
	benign breast disease	BCAA	branched-chain amino acids
BBFA	both bones forearm	BC < AC	bone conduction less than
BBFP	blood and body fluid		air conduction
	precautions	BC > AC	bone conduction greater
BBI	Bowman Birk inhibitor		than air conduction
BBIC	Bowman Birk inhibitor	B. cat	*Branhamella catarrhalis*
	concentrate	B-CAVe	bleomycin, lomustine
BBL	bottle blood loss		(CCNU), doxorubicin
BBM	banked breast milk		(Adriamycin), and
BBOW	bulging bag of water		vinblastine (Velban)
BBP	butyl benzyl phthalate	BCB	Brilliant cresyl blue
BBR	bibasilar rales		(stain)
BBS	Berg Balance Scale	BCBR	bilateral carotid body
	bilateral breath sounds		resection
BBSE	bilateral breath sounds	BC/BS	Blue Cross/Blue Shield
	equal	BCC	basal cell carcinoma
BBSI	Brigance Basic Skills		birth control clinic
	Inventory	BCCa	basal cell carcinoma
BBT	basal body temperature	BCD	basal cell dysplasia
BB to	belly button to medial		bleomycin,
MM	malleolus		cyclophosphamide, and
B Bx	breast biopsy		dactinomycin
BC	back care		borderline of cardial
	battered child		dullness
	bed and chair	BCDH	bilateral congenital
	beta carotene		dislocated hip
	bicycle	BCE	basal cell epithelioma
	birth control		beneficial clinical event

B cell	large lymphocyte	BCSS	bone cell stimulating substance
BCF	basic conditioning factor		
	Baylor core formula	BCT	Bag Carrying Test
BCG	bacille Calmette-Guérin vaccine		breast-conserving therapy
		BCU	burn care unit
	bicolor guaiac	BCUG	bilateral cystourethrogram
BCH	benign coital headache	BD	band neutrophil
BCHA	bone-conduction hearing aid		base deficit
			base down
BCI	blunt carotid injury		behavior disorder
BCL	basic cycle length		Behçet's disease
	bio-chemoluminescence		bile duct
B/C/L	BUN,(blood urea nitrogen),creatinine, lytes (electrolytes)		birth date
			birth defect
			blood donor
BCLP	bilateral cleft lip and palate		brain dead
			bronchial drainage
BCM	below costal margin		bronchodilator
	birth control medication		buccodistal
	birth control method		United Kingdom abbreviation for twice a day
	body cell mass		
BCME	bis (chloromethyl) ether		
BCNP	Board Certified Nuclear Pharmacist	B-D	Becton Dickinson and Company
BCNU	carmustine	BDAE	Boston Diagnostic Aphasia Examination
BCOC	bowel care of choice		
	bowel cathartic of choice	BDBS	Bonnet-Dechaume-Blanc syndrome
BCP	biochemical profile		
	birth control pills	BDC	burn-dressing change
	blood cell profile	BDD	body dysmorphic disorder
	carmustine, cyclophos-phamide, and prednisone		bronchodilator drugs
		BDE	bile duct exploration
		BDF	bilateral distal femoral
BCPAP	Broun's continuous positive airway pressure		black divorced female
		BDI	Beck Depression Inventory
BCQ	breast central quadrantectomy	BDI SF	Beck's Depression Inventory-Short Form
BCR	bulbocavernosus reflex		
BCRS	Brief Cognitive Rate Scale	BDL	below detectable limits
			bile duct ligation
BCRT	breast conservation followed by radiation therapy	BDM	black divorced male
		BDNF	brain-derived neurotrophic factor
BCS	battered child syndrome	B-DOPA	bleomycin, dacarbazine, vincristine (Oncovin), prednisone, and doxorubicin (Adriamycin)
	breast conserving surgery		
	Budd-Chiari syndrome		
BCSF	bone cell stimulating factor		

BDP	beclomethasone dipropionate	BF	black female
			bone fragment
	best demonstrated practice		boyfriend
BDR	background diabetic retinopathy		breakfast fed
			breast-feed
BDV	Borna disease virus	B/F	bound-to-free ratio
BE	bacterial endocarditis	%BF	percentage of body fat
	barium enema	BFA	baby for adoption
	Barrett's esophagus		basilic forearm
	base excess		bifemoral arteriogram
	below elbow	BFC	benign febrile convulsion
	bread equivalent	bFGF	basic fibroblast growth factor
	breast examination		
B↑E	both upper extremities	BFL	breast firm and lactating
B↓E	both lower extremities	B-FLY	butterfly
B & E	brisk and equal	BFM	black married female
BEA	below elbow amputation	BFNC	benign familial neonatal convulsions
BEAC	carmustine (BiCNU), etoposide, cytarabine (ara-C), and cyclophosphamide	BFP	biologic false positive
			blue fluorescent protein
		BFR	blood filtration rate
BEAM	brain electrical activity mapping		blood flow rate
		B. frag	*Bacillus fragilis*
	carmustine BCNU), etoposide, cytarabine (ara-C), and methotrexate	BFT	bentonite flocculation test
			biofeedback training
		BFU$_e$	erythroid burst-forming unit
BEAR	Bourn's electronic adult respirator	BG	baby girl
			basal ganglia
			blood glucose
BEC	bacterial endocarditis		bone graft
BED	biochemical evidence of disease	B-G	Bender Gestalt (test)
		BGA	Bundesgesundheitsamt (German drug regulatory agency)
	biological equivalent dose		
BEE	basal energy expenditure	B-GA-LACTO	beta galactosidase
BEF	bronchoesophageal fistula		
BEH	benign essential hypertension	BGC	basal-ganglion calcification
Beh Sp	behavior specialist	BGCT	benign glandular cell tumor
BEI	butanol-extractable iodine		
BEL	blood ethanol level	BGDC	Bartholin gland duct cyst
BEP	bleomycin, etoposide, and cisplatin (Platinol)	BGDR	background diabetic retinopathy
		BGL	blood glucose level
	brain stem evoked potentials	BGM	blood glucose monitoring
BE-PEG	balanced electrolyte with polyethylene glycol	BGT	Bender-Gestalt test
		BGTT	borderline glucose tolerance test
BEV	billion electron volts		
	bleeding esophageal varices	BH	bowel habits

	breath holding	BIG 6	analysis of 6 serum
BHA	butylated hydroxyanisole		components (see
BHC	benzene hexachloride		SMA 6)
bHCG	beta human chorionic	BIGEM	bigeminal
	gonadotropin	BIH	benign intracranial
BHD	carmustine, hydroxyurea,		hypertension
	and dacarbazine		bilateral inguinal hernia
B-HEXOS-	beta hexosaminidase A	BIL	bilateral
A-LK	leukocytes		brother-in-law
BHI	biosynthetic human	BILAT	bilateral short leg case
	insulin	SLC	
	brain-heart infusion	BILAT	bilateral salpingo-
BHN	bridging hepatic necrosis	SXO	oophorectomy
BHR	bronchial hyperrespon-	Bili	bilirubin
	siveness (hyperactivity)	BILI-C	conjugated bilirubin
BHP	boarding home placement	BIL MRY	bilateral myringotomy
BHS	beta-hemolytic	BIMA	bilateral internal
	streptococci		mammary arteries
	breath-holding spell	BIN	twice a night (this is a
BHT	breath hydrogen test		dangerous abbreviation)
	butylated hydroxytoluene	BIND	Biological Investigational
BI	Barthel Index		New Drug
	base in	BIO	binocular indirect
	Boehringer Ingelheim		ophthalmoscopy
	Pharmaceuticals, Inc.	BIOF	biofeedback
	bowel impaction	BIP	bipolar affective disorder
	brain injury		bleomycin, ifosfamide,
Bi	bismuth		and cisplatin (Platinol)
BIA	bioelectrical impedance		brain injury program
	analysis	BiPAP	bilevel positive airway
	biospecific interaction		pressure
	analysis	BiPD	biparietal diameter
BIB	brought in by	BIPP	bismuth iodoform paraffin
BIBA	brought in by ambulance		paste
BIC	brain injury center	BIR	back internal rotation
BICAP	bipolar electrocoagulation	BIRB	Biomedical Institutional
	therapy		Review Board
Bicarb	bicarbonate	BIS	Bispectral Index
BiCNU®	carmustine	Bi-SLT	bilateral, sequential single
BICROS	bilateral contralateral		lung transplantation
	routing of signals	bisp	bispinous diameter
BICU	burn intensive care unit	BIT	behavioral inattention test
BID	brought in dead	BIVAD	bilateral ventricular assist
BID	twice daily		device
BIDA	amonafide	BIW	twice a week (this is a
BIDS	bedtime insulin, daytime		dangerous abbreviation)
	sulfonylurea	BIZ-PLT	bizarre platelets
BIF	bifocal	BJ	Bence Jones (protein)
BIG	botulism immune globulin		biceps jerk

	body jacket	BLEED	ongoing *b*leeding, *l*ow
	bone and joint		blood pressure, *e*levated
	Bristoljet® syringe		prothrombin time,
BJE	bone and joint		*e*rratic mental status,
	examination		and unstable comorbid
	bones, joints, and		*d*isease (risk factors for
	extremities		continued
BJI	bone and joint infection		gastrointestinal
BJM	bones, joints, and muscles		bleeding)
BJP	Bence Jones protein	BLEO	bleomycin sulfate
BK	below knee (amputation)	BLESS	bath, laxative, enema,
	bradykinin		shampoo, and shower
	bullous keratopathy	BLG	bovine beta-lactoglobulin
BKA	below knee amputation	BLIC	beta-lactamase inhibitor
BKC	blepharokerato-		combination
	conjunctivitis	BLIP	beta-lactamase inhibiting
bkft	breakfast		protein
Bkg	background	BLL	bilateral lower lobe
BKTT	below knee to toe (cast)		blood lead level
BKWC	below knee walking cast		brows, lids, and lashes
BKWP	below-knee walking	BLLS	bilateral leg strength
	plaster (cast)	BLM	bleomycin sulfate
BL	baseline (fetal heart rate)	BLN	bronchial lymph nodes
	bioluminescence	BLOBS	bladder obstruction
	bland	BLOC	brief loss of
	blast cells		consciousness
	blood level	BLPB	beta-lactamase-producing
	blood loss		bacteria
	blue	BLPO	beta-lactamase-producing
	bronchial lavage		organism
	Burkitt's lymphoma	BLQ	both lower quadrants
B/L	brother-in-law	BLR	blood flow rate
BLA	Biological License	BLS	basic life support
	Application	BLT	blood-clot lysis time
BLB	Boothby-Lovelace-		brow left transverse
	Bulbulian (oxygen	B.L. unit	Bessey-Lowry units
	mask)	BM	bacterial meningitis
	bronchoscopic lung		black male
	biopsy		bone marrow
BLBK	blood bank		bone metastases
BLBS	bilateral breath sounds		bowel movement
BL = BS	bilateral equal breath		breast milk
	sounds	BMA	biomedical application
bl cult	blood culture		bismuth subsalicylate,
B-L-D	breakfast, lunch, and		metronidazole, and
	dinner		amoxicillin
bldg	bleeding		bone marrow aspirate
bld tm	bleeding time	BMB	bone marrow biopsy
BLE	both lower extremities	BMC	bone marrow cells

	bone marrow culture	BN	bladder neck
	bone mineral content	BNC	binasal cannula
BMD	Becker muscular dystrophy		bladder neck contracture
	bone marrow depression	BNCT	boron neutron capture therapy
	bone mineral density	BNE	but not exceeding
BME	basal medium Eagle (diploid cell culture)	BNF	British National Formulary
	biomedical engineering	BNI	blind nasal intubation
	brief maximal effort	BNL	below normal limits
BMET	basic metabolic panel (laboratory tests, see SMA-7)		breast needle localization
		Bn M	bone marrow
BMF	between meal feedings	BNO	bladder neck obstruction
	black married female		bowels not open
BMG	benign monoclonal gammopathy	BNP	brain natriuretic peptide
		BNPA	binasal pharyngeal airway
BMI	body mass index	BNR	bladder neck retraction
BMJ	bones, muscles, joints	BNS	benign nephrosclerosis
BMK	birthmark	BNT	Boston Naming Test
BMM	black married male	BO	base out
	bone marrow micrometastases		because of
			behavior objective
BMMM	bone marrow micrometastases		body odor
B-MODE	brightness modulation		bowel obstruction
			bowel open
BMP	behavior management plan		bucco-occlusal
		B & O	belladonna & opium (suppositories)
BMPs	bone-morphogenic proteins	BOA	behavioral observation audiometry
BMR	basal metabolic rate		born on arrival
	best motor response		born out of asepsis
BMRM	bilateral modified radical mastectomy	BOB	ball on back
		BOC	beats of clonus
BMS	Bristol-Myers Squibb Company	BOD	bilateral orbital decompression
BMT	bilateral myringotomy and tubes	Bod Units	Bodansky units
		BOE	bilateral otitis externa
	bismuth subsalicylate, metronidazole, and tetracycline	BOH	bundle of His
		BOLD	bleomycin, vincristine (Oncovin®), lomustine, and dacarbazine
	bone marrow transplant		
BMTN	bone marrow transplant neutropenia	BOM	benign ovarian mass
			bilateral otitis media
BMTT	bilateral myringotomy with tympanic tubes	BOMA	bilateral otitis media, acute
BMTU	bone marrow transplant unit	BOME	bilateral otitis media with effusion
BMU	basic multicellular unit	BOMP	bleomycin, vincristine

	(Oncovin), mitomycin, and cisplatin (Platinol AQ)	BPF	bronchopleural fistula
BoNT/A	Botulinum neurotoxin type A	BPH	benign prostatic hypertrophy
BOO	bladder outlet obstruction	BPG	bypass graft
BOOP	bronchitis obliterans with organized pneumonia	BPI	bactericidal/permeability increasing (protein)
BOP	bleeding on probing		Brief Pain Inventory
BOR	bowels open regularly	BPIG	bacterial polysaccharide immune globulin
	bronchia-oto-renal (syndrome)	BPL	benzylpenicilloylpolylysine
BOS	base of support	BPLA	blood pressure, left arm
BOSS	Becker orthopedic spinal system	BPM	beats per minute
			breaths per minute
BOT	base of tongue	BPN	bacitracin, polymyxin B, and neomycin sulfate
BOU	burning on urination	BPO	benzoyl peroxide
BOUGIE	bougienage		bilateral partial oophorectomy
BOVR	Bureau of Vocational Rehabilitation	BPP	biophysical profile
BOW	bag of water	BPPP	bilateral pedal pulses present
BOW-I	bag of water-intact		
BOW-R	bag of water-ruptured	BP,P,R,T,	blood pressure, pulse, respiration, and temperature
BP	bathroom privileges		
	bed pan		
	bench press	BPPV	benign paroxysmal postural vertigo
	benzoyl peroxide	BPR	blood per rectum
	bipolar		blood pressure recorder
	birthplace	BPRS	Brief Psychiatric Rating Scale
	blood pressure		
	British Pharmacopeia	BPS	bilateral partial salpingectomy
	bullous pemphigoid		
	bypass		blood pump speed
BP-200	Bourn's Infant Pressure Ventilator	BPs	systolic blood pressure
		BPSD	bronchopulmonary segmental drainage
BPA	birch pollen allergy		
BPAD	bipolar affective disorder	BPV	benign paroxysmal vertigo
BPb	whole blood lead concentration		benign positional vertigo
			bovine papilloma virus
BPI	bipolar disorder, Type I	Bq	becquerel
BPII	bipolar type II disorder	BQL	below quantifiable levels
BPD	benzoporphyrin derivative	BQR	brequinar sodium
	biparietal diameter	BR	bathroom
	borderline personality disorder		bedrest
			Benzing retrograde
	bronchopulmonary dysplasia		birthing room
			blink reflex
BPd	diastolic blood pressure		bowel rest

	breech	BRU	basic remodeling unit (osteon)
	bridge		
	bright red	BRVO	branch retinal vein occlusion
	brown		
Br	bromide	BS	barium swallow
	bromine		bedside
BRA	bananas, rice (rice cereal), and applesauce (diet)		before sleep
			Bennett seal
	brain		blind spot
BRADY	bradycardia		blood sugar
BRANCH	branch chain amino acids		Blue Shield
BRAO	branch retinal artery occlusion		bone scan
			bowel sounds
BRAT	bananas, rice (rice cereal), applesauce, and toast		breath sounds
		B & S	Bartholin and Skene (glands)
	Baylor rapid autologous transfuser		bending and stooping
	blunt thoracic abdominal trauma	BS×4	bowel sounds in all four quadrants
BRATT	bananas, rice (rice cereal), applesauce, tea, and toast	BSA	body surface area
			bowel sounds active
BRB	blood-retinal barrier	BSAB	Balthazar Scales of Adaptive Behavior
	bright red blood		
BRBR	bright red blood per rectum	BSAb	broad-spectrum antibiotics
		BSB	bedside bag
BRBPR	bright red blood per rectum		body surface burned
		BSC	bedside care
BRC	bladder reconstruction		bedside commode
BRCM	below right costal margin		burn scar contracture
		BSCC	bedside commode chair
BRex	breathing exercise		Bjork-Shiley convexoconcave (valves)
Br Fdg	breast-feeding		
BRJ	brachial radialis jerk		
BRM	biological response modifiers	BSD	baby soft diet
			bedside drainage
BRN	brown	BSE	bovine spongiform encephalopathy
BRO	brother		
BROM	back range of motion		breast self-examination
BRONK	bronchoscopy	BSEC	bedside easy chair
BRP	bathroom privileges	BSepF	black separated female
BR RAO	branch retinal artery occlusion	BSepM	black separated male
		BSER	brain stem evoked responses
BR RVO	branch retinal vein occlusion		
		BSF	black single female
BRS	baroreceptor reflex sensitivity		busulfan
		BSG	Bagolini striated glasses
BrS	breath sounds		brain stem gliomas
BRSV	bovine respiratory syncytial virus	BSGA	beta streptococcus group A

BSI	body substance isolation		brief stimulus therapy
	brain stem injury	BSU	Bartholin, Skene's,
BSL	blood sugar level		urethra (glands)
BS L	breath sounds diminished,		behavioral science unit
base	left base	BSu	blood sugar
BSM	black single male	BSUTD	baby shots up to date
	blood safety module		Base Service Unit
BSN	Bachelor of Science in	BSW	Bachelor of Social Work
	Nursing		bedscale weight
	bowel sounds normal	BT	bedtime
BSNA	bowel sounds normal and		behavioral therapy
	active		bituberous
BSNMT	Bachelor of Science in		bladder tumor
	Nuclear Medicine		Blalock-Taussig (shunt)
	Technology		bleeding time
BSNT	breast soft and nontender		blood type
BSNUTD	baby shots not up to date		blood transfusion
BSO	bilateral salpingo-		brain tumor
	oophorectomy		breast tumor
	l-buthionine sulfoximine		bowel tones
bSOD	bovine superoxide	Bt	*Bacillus thuringiensis*
	dismutase	B/T	between
BSOM	bilateral serous otitis	Bt#	bottle number
	media	BTA	below the ankle
BSP	body substance		bladder tumor antigen
	precautions		bladder tumor-associated
	Bromsulphalein®		analytes
BSPA	bowel sounds present and	BTB	back to bed
	active		beat-to-beat (variability)
BSPM	body surface potential		break-through bleeding
	mapping	BTBV	beat to beat variability
BSR	bowels sounds regular	BTC	bilateral tubal cautery
BSRI	Bem Sex Role Inventory		bladder tumor check
BSRT (R)	Bachelor of Science in		by the clock
	Radiologic Technology	BTE	Baltimore Therapeutic
	(Registered)		Equipment
BSS	Baltimore Sepsis Scale		behind-the-ear (hearing
	bedside scale		aid)
	bismuth subsalicylate		bisected, totally embedded
	black silk sutures	BTF	blenderized tube feeding
BSS®	balanced salt solution	BTFS	breast tumor frozen
BSSG	sitogluside		section
BSSO	bilateral sagittal split	BTG	beta thromboglobulin
	osteotomy	B-Thal	beta thalassemia
BSSS	benign sporadic sleep	BTHOOM	beats the hell out of me
	spikes		(better stated as
BSST	breast self-stimulation test		"differed diagnosis")
BST	bedside testing	BTI	biliary tract infection
	bovine somatotropin		bitubal interruption

BTKA	bilateral total knee arthroplasty		blood volume
		BVAD	biventricular assist device
BTL	bilateral tubal ligation	BVD	bovine viral diarrhea
BTM	bilateral tympanic membranes	BVE	blood volume expander
		BVF	bulboventricular foramen
	bismuth subcitrate, tetracycline, and metronidazole	BVH	biventricular hypertrophy
		BVL	bilateral vas ligation
		BVM	bag valve mask
BTMEAL	between meals	BVMG	Bender Visual-Motor Gestalt (test)
BTO	bilateral tubal occlusion	
BTP	bismuth tribromophenate	BVO	branch vein occlusion
	breakthrough pain	BVR	Bureau of Vocational Rehabilitation
BTPABA	bentiromide	
BTPS	body temperature pressure saturated	BVRO	bilateral vertical ramus osteotomy
BTR	bladder tumor recheck	BVRT	Benton Visual Retention Test
BTS	Blalock-Taussig shunt	
BTSH	bovine thyrotropin	BVT	bilateral ventilation tubes
BTU	behavior therapy unit	BW	birth weight
BTW	back to work		bite-wing (radiograph)
BTW M	between meals		body water
BTX	Botulinum toxin		body weight
BU	base up (prism)	B & W	Black and White (milk of magnesia & aromatic cascara fluidextract)
	below umbilicus	
	Bodansky units	
	burn unit	BWA	bed wetter admission
	busulfan	BWCS	bagged white cell study
BUA	broadband ultrasound attenuation	BWF	Blackwater fever
		BWFI	bacteriostatic water for injection
BuCy	busulfan and cyclophosphamide	
		BWidF	black widowed female
BUD	budesonide (Rhinocort)	BWidM	black widowed male
BUdR	bromodeoxyuridine	BWS	battered woman syndrome
BUE	both upper extremities	BWs	bite-wing (x-rays)
BUFA	baby up for adoption	BWX	bite-wing x-ray
BUN	blood urea nitrogen	Bx	biopsy
	bunion	B x B	back to back
BUO	bleeding of undetermined origin	BX BS	Blue Cross and Blue Shield
BUR	back-up rate (ventilator)	BXM	B cell crossmatch
Burd	Burdick suction	ΦBZ	phenylbutazone
BUS	Bartholin, urethral, and Skene's glands	BZD	benzodiazepine
		BZDZ	benzodiazepine
BUSV	Bartholin urethral Skeins vagina	
BUT	biopsy urease test	
	break up time	
BV	bacterial vaginitis	
	biological value	

C

C	ascorbic acid
	carbohydrate
	Catholic
	Caucasian
	Celsius
	centigrade
	clubbing
	conjunctiva
	constricted
	cyanosis
	cytosine
	hundred
$\bar{c}$	with
C′	cervical spine
C+	with contrast
C−	without contrast
C_1–C_7	cervical vertebra 1 through 7
C_1–C_8	cervical nerves 1 through 8
C_1 to C_9	precursor molecules of the complement system
C_1 to C_{12}	cranial nerves 1 to 12
C3	complement C3
C4	complement C4
CI-CV	Drug Enforcement Agency scheduled substances class one through five
C_{II}	second cranial nerve
CA	cancelled appointment
	Candida albicans
	carcinoma
	cardiac arrest
	carotid artery
	celiac artery
	cellulose acetate (filter)
	Certified Acupuncturist
	chronologic age
	Cocaine Anonymous
	community-acquired
	compressed air
	continuous aerosol
	coronary angioplasty
	coronary artery
Ca	calcium
C/A	conscious, alert
CA 125	cancer antigen 125
C&A	Clinitest® and Acetest®
CAA	colo-anal anastamosis
	crystalline amino acids
CAB	catheter-associated bacteriuria
	cellulose acetate butyrate
	combined androgen blockade
	coronary artery bypass
CAB-BAGE	coronary artery bypass graft
CABG	coronary artery bypass graft
CaBI	calcium bone index
CaBP	calcium-binding protein
CABS	coronary artery bypass surgery
CAC	cardioacceleratory center
	Certified Alcohol Counselor
	Community Action Center
CACI	computer-assisted continuous infusion
$CaCl_2$	calcium chloride
$CaCO_3$	calcium carbonate
CACP	cisplatin
CAD	cadaver (kidney donor)
	computer-aided diagnosis
	coronary artery disease
CADAC	Certified Alcohol and Drug Abuse Counselor
CADASIL	cerebral autosomal dominant arteriopathy with subcortical infarcts and leukoencephalopathy
CADD®	Computerized Ambulatory Drug Delivery (pump)
CADP	computer-assisted design of prosthesis
CADXPL	cadaver transplant
CAE	cellulose acetate electrophoresis

coronary artery endarterectomy

cyclophosphamide, doxorubicin (Adriamycin), and etoposide

CAEC cardiac arrhythmia evaluation center

CaEDTA calcium disodium edetate

CAF chronic atrial fibrillation
controlled atrial flutter/fibrillation
cyclophosphamide, doxorubicin (Adriamycin), and fluorouracil

CAFF controlled atrial fibrillation/flutter

CAFT Clinitron® air fluidized therapy

CAG chronic atrophic gastritis
closed angle glaucoma
continuous ambulatory gamma globin (infusion)
coronary arteriography

CaG calcium gluconate

CAGE a questionnaire for alcoholism evaluation (JAMA 1984; 252: 1905-7) C Have you ever felt the need to cut down on your drinking? A Have you ever felt annoyed by criticism of your drinking? G Have you ever felt guilty about your drinking? E Have you ever taken a drink (eye opener) first thing in the morning?

CAH chronic active hepatitis
chronic aggressive hepatitis
congenital adrenal hyperplasia

CAHB chronic active hepatitis B

CAI carbonic anhydrase inhibitors
carboxyamide aminoimidazoles
computer-assisted instructions

'caid Medicaid

CAIV cold-adapted influenza virus vaccine

CAL callus
calories (cal)
chronic airflow limitation

C_alb albumin clearance

cal ct calorie count

CALD chronic active liver disease

CALGB Cancer and Leukemia Group B

CALLA common acute lympho-blastic leukemia antigen

CAM Caucasian adult male
cell adhesion molecules
child abuse management
complementary and alternative medicine
confusion assessment method
cystic adenomatoid malformation

CAMCOG Cambridge Cognitive Examination

CAMD computer-aided molecular design

CAMF cyclophosphamide, Adriamycin, methotrexate, and fluorouracil

CAMP cyclophosphamide, doxorubicin (Adriamycin), methotrexate, and procarbazine

cAMP cyclic adenosine monophosphate

CAMs cell adhesion molecules

CAN contrast-associated nephropathy
cord around neck

CA/N child abuse and neglect

CANC	cancelled
c-ANCA	antineutrophil cytoplasmic antibody
CANDA	computer-assisted new drug application
CANP	Certified Adult Nurse Practitioner
CAO	chronic airway (airflow) obstruction
CaO₂	arterial oxygen concentration

CANC — cancelled
c-ANCA — antineutrophil cytoplasmic antibody
CANDA — computer-assisted new drug application
CANP — Certified Adult Nurse Practitioner
CAO — chronic airway (airflow) obstruction
CaO_2 — arterial oxygen concentration
CaOx — calcium oxalate
CAP — cancer of the prostate
capsule
chaotic atrial tachycardia
chemistry admission profile
chloramphenicol
community-acquired pneumonia
compound action potentials
cyclophosphamide, doxorubicin (Adriamycin), and cisplatin
CaP — cancer of the prostate
Ca/P — calcium to phosphorus ratio
CAPB — central auditory processing battery
CAPD — chronic ambulatory peritoneal dialysis
CAPLA — computer-assisted product license application
CAPS — caffeine, alcohol, pepper, and spicy food (dietary restrictions)
CAPWA — computerized arterial pulse waveform analysis
CAR — cardiac ambulation routine
CARB — carbohydrate
CARBO — Carbocaine®
carboplatin
CARD — Cardiac Automatic Resuscitative Device
C-arm — fluoroscopy image intensifier

CARN — Certified Addiction Registered Nurse
CART — classification and regression tree
CAS — carotid artery stenosis
cerebral arteriosclerosis
Chemical Abstracts Service
Clinical Asthma Score
combined androgen suppression
computer-assisted surgery
CASA — cancer-associated serum antigen
Center on Addiction and Substance Abuse
computer-assisted semen analysis
CaSC — carcinoma of the sigmoid colon
CASHD — coronary arteriosclerotic heart disease
CASP — Child Analytic Study Program
CASS — computer-aided sleep system
CAST® — color allergy screening test
CAT — Cardiac Arrest Team
carnitine acetyl transferase
cataract
Children's Apperception Test
coital alignment technique
computed axial tomography
methcatinone
CATH — catheter
catheterization
Catholic
CATS — catecholamines
CAU — Caucasian
CAV — computer-aided ventilation
congenital absence of vagina
cyclophosphamide, doxorubicin (Adriamycin), and vincristine

CAV-1	canine adenovirus type 1		common bile duct
CAVB	complete atrioventricular block	CBDE	common bile duct exploration
CAVC	common artrioventricular canal	CBE	child birth education
CAVE	cyclophosphamide, doxorubicin, (Adriamycin)	CBER	Center for Biologics Evaluation and Research
	vincristine, and etoposide	CBF	cerebral blood flow
		CBFS	cerebral blood flow studies
CAVH	continuous arteriovenous hemofiltration	CBFV	cerebral blood flow velocity
CAVHD	continuous arteriovenous hemodialysis	CBG	capillary blood glucose
CAV-P-VP	cyclophosphamide, doxorubicin (Adriamycin),	CBGM	capillary blood glucose monitor
	vincristine, cisplatin, and etoposide	CBI	continuous bladder irrigation
CAVR	continuous arteriovenous rewarming	CBM	cryopreserved bone marrow
CAVS	calcific valve stenosis	CBN	chronic benign neutropenia
CAVU	continuous arteriovenous ultrafiltration		collected by nurse
CAX	central axis	CBP	chronic benign pain
CB	cesarean birth		copper-binding protein
	chronic bronchitis	CBPS	coronary bypass surgery
	code blue	CBR	carotid bodies resected
	conjugated bilirubin (direct)		chronic bedrest
c/b	complicated by		clinical benefit responders
C & B	chair and bed		complete bedrest
	crown and bridge	CBRAM	controlled partial rebreathing-anesthesia method
CBA	chronic bronchitis and asthma	CB RRR s̄	cardiac beat, regular rhythm and rate
	cost-benefit analysis	M/R/G	without murmurs, rubs, or gallops
	County Board of Assistance	CBrS	clear breath sounds
CBAVD	congenital bilateral absence of the vas deferens	CBS	Charles Bonnet's syndrome
			chronic brain syndrome
CBC	carbenicillin		coarse breath sounds
	complete blood count		Cruveilhier-Baumgarten syndrome
	contralateral breast cancer	CBT	cognitive behavioral therapy
CBCDA	carboplatin		
CBCL	Child Behavior Checklist	CBU	cumulative breath units
CBCT	community based clinical trials	CBV	central blood volume
		CBZ	carbamazepine
CBD	closed bladder drainage	CBZE	carbamazepine epoxide

C

CC	cardiac catheterization			child care clinic
	Catholic			Comprehensive Cancer
	cerebral concussion			Center
	chief complaint	C/cc		colonies per cubic
	choriocarcinoma			centimeter
	chronic complainer	CC & C		colony count and culture
	circulatory collapse	CCC-A		Certificate of Clinical
	clean catch (urine)			Competence in
	comfort care			Audiology
	coracoclavicular	CCC-SP		Certificate of Clinical
	cord compression			Competence in Speech-
	corpus collosum			Language Pathology
	creatinine clearance	CCD		charged-coupled device
	critical condition			childhood celiac disease
	cubic centimeter (cc),	CCDC		Certified Chemical
	(mL)			Dependency Counselor
	with correction (with	CCDS		color-coded duplex
	glasses)			sonography
C_c	concentration of drug in	CCE		clubbing, cyanosis, and
	the central compartment			edema
C/C	cholecystectomy and			countercurrent
	operative			electrophoresis
	cholangiogram	CCF		cephalin cholesterol
	complete upper and lower			flocculation
	dentures			compound comminuted
CCII	Clinical Clerk–2nd year			fracture
C & C	cold and clammy			congestive cardiac failure
CCA	calcium-channel			crystal-induced
	antagonist			chemotactic factor
	circumflex coronary	CCFE		cyclophosphamide,
	artery			cisplatin, fluorouracil,
	common carotid artery			and estramustine
	concentrated care area	CCFs		chronic-care facilities
	countercurrent	CCG		Children's Cancer
	chromatography			Group
	critical care area	CCH		community care home
CCAP	capsule cartilage articular			Cook County Hospital
	preservation	CCHD		complex congenital heart
CCAT	common carotid artery			disease
	thrombosis			cyanotic congenital heart
CCB	calcium channel			disease
	blocker(s)	CCHF		Congo-Crimean
	Community Care Board			hemorrhagic fever
	corn, callus, and bunion	CCI		chronic coronary
CCC	Cancer Care Center			insufficiency
	central corneal clouding			corrected count increment
	(Grade 0+ to 4+)	CCK		cholecystokinin
	Certificate of Clinical	CCK-OP		cholecystokinin
	Competency			octapeptide

CCK-PZ	cholecystokinin pancreozymin		carotid compression tomography
CCL	cardiac catheterization laboratory		Certified Cardiographic Technician
	critical condition list		closed cerebral trauma
CCl₄	carbon tetrachloride		closed cranial trauma
CCM	calcium citrate malate		congenitally corrected transposition (of the great vessels)
	children's case management		
	cyclophosphamide, lomustine (CCNU; CeeNU), and methotrexate		crude coal tar
		CCTGA	congenitally corrected transposition of the great arteries
CCMSU	clean catch midstream urine	CCT in PET	crude coal tar in petroleum
CCMU	critical care medicine unit	CCTV	closed circuit television
CCN	continuing care nursery	CCU	coronary care unit
CCNS	cell cycle-nonspecific		critical care unit
CCNU	lomustine	CCUA	clean catch urinalysis
CCO	continuous cardiac output	CCUP	colpocystourethropexy
C-collar	cervical collar	CCV	Critical Care Ventilator (Ohio)
CCP	crystalloid cardioplegia		
CCPD	continuous cycling (cyclical) peritoneal dialysis		critical closing volume
		CCW	childcare worker
			counterclockwise
CCR	cardiac catheterization recovery	CCWR	counterclockwise rotation
		CCX	complications
	continuous complete remission	CCY	cholecystectomy
		CD	cadaver donor
	counterclockwise rotation		candela
C_cr	creatinine clearance		Castleman's disease
CCRC	Certified Clinical Research Coordinator		celiac disease
			cervical dystonia
	continuing care residential community		cesarean delivery
			character disorder
CCRN	Certified Critical Care Registered Nurse		chemical dependency
			childhood disease
CCRT	combined chemo-radiotherapy		chronic dialysis
			closed drainage
CCRU	critical care recovery unit		clusters of differentiation
CCS	cell cycle-specific		common duct
	certified coding specialist		communication disorders
CC & S	cornea, conjunctiva, and sclera		complicated delivery
			conjugate diameter
CCSK	clear cell sarcoma of the kidney		continuous drainage
			convulsive disorder
CCSP	Certified Chiropractic Sports Physician		Crohn's disease
			cumulative doses
CCT	calcitriol		cyclodextran

	cytarabine and daunorubicin		*Clostridium difficile* disease
Cd	cadmium		cytidine deaminase
	concentration of drug	CDDP	cisplatin
C/D	cigarettes per day	CDE	canine distemper encephalitis
	cup to disk ratio		Certified Diabetes Educator
CD4	antigenic marker on helper/inducer T cells (also called OKT 4, T4, and Leu3)		common duct exploration
		CDER	Center for Drug Evaluation and Research (FDA)
CD8	antigenic marker on suppressor/cytotoxic T cells (also called OKT 8, T8, and Leu 8)	CDG	carbohydrate-deficient glycoprotein
C&D	curettage and desiccation	CDGE	constant denaturant gel electrophoresis
	cystectomy and diversion	CDGP	constitutional delay of growth and puberty
	cytoscopy and dilatation	CDH	chronic daily headache
CDA	Certified Dental Assistant		congenital diaphragmatic hernia
	chenodeoxycholic acid (chenodiol)		congenital dislocation of hip
	congenital dyserythro-poietic anemia		congenital dysplasia of the hip
2-CDA	cladribine (Leustatin; chlorodeoxyadenosine)	CDI	Children's Depression Inventory
CDAD	*Clostridium difficile*-associated diarrhea		clean, dry, and intact
CDAI	Crohn's Disease Activity Index		color Doppler imaging
			Cotrel Duobosset Instrumentation
CDAK	Cordis Dow Artificial Kidney	CDIC	*Clostridium difficile*-induced colitis
CDAP	continuous distended airway pressure	C Dif	*Clostridium difficile*
CDB	cough and deep breath	CDK	climatic droplet keratopathy
CDC	calculated day of confinement		cyclin-dependent kinase
	cancer detection center	CDKI	cyclin-dependent kinase inhibitor
	carboplatin, doxorubicin, and cyclophosphamide	CDLE	chronic discoid lupus erythematosus
	Centers for Disease Control and Prevention	CdLS	Cornelia de Lange's syndrome
	Certified Drug Counselor	CDP	chemical dependence profile
	chenodeoxycholic acid (chenodiol)		Child Development Program
	Clostridium difficile colitis		crystalline degradation product
CDCA	chenodeoxycholic acid (chenodiol)		
CDD	Certificate of Disability for Discharge		

58

	cytidine diphosphate		contrast echocardiology
CDQ	corrected development quotient	C&E	consultation and examination
CDR	clinical data repository		cough and exercise
	Clinical Dementia Rating		curettage and electrodesiccation
	continuing disability review	CEA	carcinoembryonic antigen
CDRH	Center for Devices and Radiological Health		carotid endarterectomy
			cost-effectiveness analysis
CDR(H)	cup-to-disk ratio horizontal	CEB	calcium entry blocker
CDRs	complementary determining regions		carboplatin, etoposide, and bleomycin
		CEBV	chronic Epstein-Barr virus
CDR(V)	cup-to-disk ratio vertical	CEC	capillary electrochromatography
CDS	closed door seclusion		
	color Doppler sonography		Council for Exceptional Children
CDSC	Communicable Disease Surveillance Centre (United Kingdom)	CECD	congenital endothelial corneal dystrophy
CDSPIES	congestive heart failure, drugs, spasm, pneumothorax, infection, embolism, and secretions (differential diagnosis mnemonic)	CECT	contrast-enhanced computed tomography
		CED	cystoscopy-endoscopy dilation
		CEE	conjugated equine estrogen (Premarin; conjugated estrogen)
CDT	carbohydrate-deficient transferrin	CEF	chick embryo fibroblast
		CEFOT	cefotaxime
	Chemical Dependency Technician	CEFOX	cefoxitin
		CEFTAZ	ceftazidime
CDTM	collaborative drug therapy management	CEFUR	cefuroxime
		CEI	continuous extravascular infusion
CDU	chemical dependency unit		
CDV	canine distemper virus		converting enzyme inhibitor
	cardiovascular		
CDX	chlordiazepoxide	CEL	cardiac exercise laboratory
cdyn	dynamic compliance		
CE	California encephalitis	CELP	chronic erosive lichen planus
	capillary electrophoresis		
	cardiac enlargement	CEMD	consultative examination by physician
	cardiac enzymes		
	cardioesophageal	CEN	Certified (Nurse)– Emergency Room
	cataract extraction		
	central episiotomy	CENOG	computerized electroneuro- ophthalmogram
	chemoembolization		
	cholesterol ester		
	community education	CEO	chief executive officer
	consultative examination	CEP	cardiac enzyme panel
	continuing education		cognitive evoked potential

	congenital erythropoietic porphyria		cisplatin and fluorouracil
	countercurrent electrophoresis		complement fixation
			contractile force
	cyclophosphamide, etoposide, and cisplatin (Platinol)		count fingers
			cystic fibrosis
		C&F	cell and flare
CEPH	cephalic		chills and fever
	cephalosporin	CFA	common femoral artery
CEPH FLOC	cephalin flocculation		complete Freund's adjuvant
CEPP (B)	cyclophosphamide, etopside, procarbazine, prednisone, and bleomycin		cryptogenic fibrosing alveolitis
			cystic fibrosis anthropathy
		CFAC	complement-fixing antibody consumption
CER	conditioned emotional response	C-factor	cleverness factor
		CFCs	chlorofluorocarbons
CE&R	central episiotomy and repair	CFD	color-flow Doppler
			computational fluid dynamics
CERA	cortical evoked response audiometry	CFF	critical fusion (flicker) frequency
CERD	chronic end-stage renal disease	CFFT	critical flicker fusion threshold
CERULO	ceruloplasmin	CFI	confrontation fields intact
CERV	cervical	CFIDS	chronic fatigue immune dysfunction syndrome
CES	Cauda equina syndrome		
	central excitatory state	CFL	cisplatin, fluorouracil, and leucovorin calcium
	cognitive environmental stimulation		
		CFLX	ciprofloxacin
	estrogen, conjugated (conjugated estrogen substance)		circumflex
		CFM	cerebral function monitor
CESB	chronic electrical stimulation of the brain		close fitting mask
			craniofacial microsomia
CESD	Center for Epidemiologic Studies – Depression		cyclophosphamide, fluorouracil, and mitoxantrone
CESI	cervical epidural steroid injection	CFNS	chills, fever, and night sweats
CETP	cholesterol ester transfer protein	CFP	cystic fibrosis protein
		CFPT	cyclophosphamide, fluorouracil, prednisone, and tamoxifen
CEV	cyclophosphamide, etoposide, and vincristine		
		CFR	case-fatality rates
CF	calcium leucovorin (citrovorum factor)		*Code of Federal Regulations*
	cancer-free		coronary flow reserve
	cardiac failure	CFS	cancer family syndrome
	Caucasian female		
	Christmas factor		

	Child and Family Service	CGM	central gray matter
	childhood febrile seizures	CGMP	Current Good Manufacturing Practices
	chronic fatigue syndrome		
CFT	chronic follicular tonsillitis	cGMP	cyclic guanine monophosphate
	complement fixation test	CGN	chronic glomerulonephritis
CFTR	cystic fibrosis transmembrane (conductance) regulator	C-GRD	coffee-ground
		CGRP	calcitonin gene-related peptide
	cystic fibrosis transmembrane receptor	CGS	cardiogenic shock
CFU	colony-forming units		catgut suture
CFU-E	colony-forming unit– erythroid		centimeter-gram-second system
CFU-G	colony-forming unit– granulocyte	CGTT	cortisol glucose tolerance test
CFU-G/M	colony-forming unit– granulocyte/macro- phage	cGy	centigray
		CH	chest
			chief
CFU-M	colony-forming unit– macrophage		child (children)
			chronic
CFU-S	colony-forming unit–spleen		cluster headache
			congenital hypothyroidism
CG	cardiogreen (dye)		convalescent hospital
	caregiver		crown-heal
	cholecystogram	C_h	hepatic clearance
	contact guarding	ch^1	Christ Church chromosone
	contralateral groin	CH_{50}	total hemolytic complement
CGA	comprehensive geriatric assessment	C&H	cocaine and heroin
	contact guard assist	CHA	compound hypermetropic astigmatism
CGB	chronic gastrointestinal (tract) bleeding		congenital hypoplastic anemia
CGD	chronic granulomatous disease	CHAD	cyclophosphamide, altretamine, (hexamethylmelamine), doxorubicin (Adriamycin), and cisplatin (DDP)
CGF	continuous gavage feeding (infant feeding)		
CGI	Clinical Global Impressions (scale)		
CGIC	Clinical Global Impression of Change	CHAI	continuous hepatic artery infusion
CGI-S	Clinical Global Impressions, Severity of Illness	CHAM-OCA	cyclophosphamide, hydroxyurea, dactinomycin, methotrexate, vincristine, leucovorin, and doxorubicin
CGL	chronic granulocytic leukemia		
	with correction/with glasses		

CHAM-PUS Civilian Health and Medical Program of the Uniformed Services

CHAP child health associate practitioner

cyclophosphamide, altretamine, (hexamethylmelamine), doxorubicin (Adriamycin), and cisplatin (Platinol AQ)

CHARGE coloboma (of eyes), hearing deficit, choanal atresia, retardation of growth, genital defects (males only), and endocardial cushion defect

CHART continuous hyperfractionated accelerated radiotherapy

CHB complete heart block

CHBHA congenital Heinz body hemolytic anemia

CHC concentric hypertrophic cardiomyopathy

CH₃-CCNU semustine

cHct central hematocrit

CHD center hemodialysis
changed diaper
childhood diseases
chronic hemodialysis
common hepatic duct
congenital heart disease
coordinate home care

CHE chronic hepatic encephalopathy

CHEF clamped homogeneous electric field

CHEM 7 laboratory tests for glucose, blood urea nitrogen, creatinine, potassium, sodium, chloride, and carbon dioxide

CHEMO chemotherapy

ChemoRx chemotherapy

CHESS chemical shift suppression

CHF congestive heart failure
Crimean hemorrhagic fever

CHFV combined high frequency of ventilation

CHG change

CHI closed head injury
creatinine-height index

CHIN community health information network

CHIP comprehensive health insurance plan
iproplatin

Chix chickenpox

CHL conductive hearing loss

ChloMP chlorambucil, mitoxantrone, and prednisolone

ChlVPP chlorambucil, vinblastine, procarbazine, and prednisone

CHN central hemorrhagic necrosis
Chinese herb nephropathy
community nursing home

CHO carbohydrate
Chinese hamster ovary

C_{H_2O} free-water clearance

C_2H_5OH alcohol (ethyl alcohol)

chol cholesterol

c̄ hold withhold

CHOP cyclophosphamide, doxorubicin, vincristine (Oncovin), prednisone

CHOP-Bleo cyclophosphamide, doxorubicin (hydroxydaunorubicin), vincristine (Oncovin), prednisone, and bleomycin

CHPB Canadian Health Protection Branch (the equivalent of the U.S. Food and Drug Administration)

CHPX chickenpox

CHR Cercaria-Hullen reaction
chronic

CHRPE congenital hypertrophy of

	the retinal pigment epithelium		Change with Caregiver Input
CHRS	congenital hereditary retinoschisis	CIBP	chronic intractable benign pain
CHS	Chediak-Higashi syndrome contact hypersensitivity	CIC	cardioinhibitory center circulating immune complexes
CHT	closed head trauma		clean intermittent catheterization
CHU	closed head unit		
CHUC	Certified Health Unit Coordinator		completely in the canal (hearing aid)
CHVP	cyclophosphamide, doxorubicin (hydroxydaunorubicin), teniposide (VM26), and prednisone		coronary intensive care
		CICE	combined intracapsular cataract extraction
		CICU	cardiac intensive care unit
CHW	community health workers	CICVC	centrally inserted central venous catheter
CHWG	chewing gum		
CI	cardiac index	CID	cervical immobilization device
	cesium implant		
	Clinical Instructor		combined immunodeficiency
	cochlear implant		
	commercial insurance		cytomegalic inclusion disease
	complete iridectomy		
	confidence interval	CIDP	chronic inflammatory demyelinating polyradiculoneuropathy
	continuous infusion		
	coronary insufficiency		
Ci	curie(s)	CIDS	cellular immunodeficiency syndrome
CIA	calcaneal insufficiency avulsion		
			continuous insulin delivery system
	chronic idiopathic anhidrosis	CIE	chemotherapy induced emesis
CIAA	competitive insulin autoantibodies		
			congenital ichthyosiform erythroderma
CIAED	collagen induced autoimmune ear disease		
			counterimmunoelectrophoresis
CIB	Carnation Instant Breakfast®		crossed immunoelectrophoresis
		CIEA	continuous infusion epidural analgesia
	crying-induced bronchospasm		
	cytomegalic inclusion bodies	CIEP	counterimmunoelectrophoresis crossed immunoelectrophoresis
CIBD	chronic inflammatory bowel disease		
		CIG	cigarettes
CIBI	Clinician Interview Based Impression (of change)	CIH	continuous infusion haloperidol
CIBIC	Clinician Interview-Based Impression of Change	CIHD	chronic ischemic heart disease
CIBIC-plus	Clinician's Interview-Based Impression of	CII	continuous insulin infusion

63

CIIA	common internal iliac artery		mide, and doxorubicin (Adriamycin)
CIL	carbamazepine-induced lupus	Cis-DDP	cisplatin
CIM	change in menses	CIS-R	Clinical Interview Schedule, Revised
	chemotherapy-induced mucositis	CI-Stim	cochlear implant stimulation
	corticosteroid-induced myopathy	CIT	conventional immunosuppressive therapy
CIMCU	cardiac intermediate care unit		conventional insulin therapy
CIN	cervical intraepithelial neoplasia	CITP	capillary isotachophoresis
	chemotherapy induced neutropenia	CIU	chronic idiopathic urticaria
	chronic interstitial nephritis	CIV	common iliac vein
C_{IN}	insulin clearance		continuous intravenous (infusion)
CIND	cognitive impairment, no dementia	CIVI	continuous intravenous infusion
CINE	chemotherapy-induced nausea and emesis	CIXU	constant infusion excretory urogram
	cineangiogram	CIWA-Ar	Clinical Institute Withdrawal Assessment for Alcohol–revised
CINV	chemotherapy-induced nausea and vomiting		
CIO	corticosteroid-induced osteoporosis	CJD	Creutzfeldt-Jakob disease
CIOMS	The Council for International Organization of Medical Sciences	cJET	congenital junctional ectopic tachycardia
		CJR	centric jaw relation
		CK	check
CIP	Cardiac Injury Panel		creatine kinase
	critical illness polyneuropathy	CK-BB	creatine kinase BB band (primarily in brain)
CIPD	chronic intermittent peritoneal dialysis	CKC	cold knife conization
		CK-ISO	creatine kinase isoenzyme
Circ	circulation	CK-MB	creatine kinase MB fraction (primarily in cardiac muscle)
	circumcision		
	circumference		
circ. & sen.	circulation and sensation	CK MM	creatine kinase MM fraction (primarily in skeletal muscle)
CIS	carcinoma in situ	CKW	clockwise
	continuous interleaved sampling	Cl	chloride
CI&S	conjunctival irritation and swelling	CL	central line
			chemoluminescence
CISC	clean intermittent self-catheterization		clear liquid
			cleft lip
			cloudy
CISCA	cisplatin, cyclophospha-		critical list

	cycle length	CLEIA	chemiluminescent enzyme immunoassay
	lung compliance		
C_L	compliance of the lungs	CLEP	college level examination program
CLA	community living arrangements	CLF	cholesterol-lecithin flocculation
	conjugated linoleic acid	CLG	clorgyline
		CLH	chronic lobular hepatitis
CLAMSS	cleavage- and ligation-associated mutation-specific sequencing	Cl_h	hepatic clearance
		CLI	clomipramine
			critical leg ischemia
CLAS	congenital localized absence of skin	CLIA	Clinical Laboratory Improvement Act
CLASS	computer laser assisted surgical system	Cl_{int}	intrinsic clearance
		CLL	chronic lymphocytic leukemia
CLASS I	congestive heart failure with no limitation with ordinary activity, (New York Heart Association Classification)	CLLE	columnar-lined lower esophagus
		cl liq	clear liquid
		Cl_{nr}	nonrenal clearance
CLASS II	congestive heart failure with slight limitation of physical activity	CLO	Campylobacter-like organism
			close
			cod liver oil
CLASS III	congestive heart failure with marked limitation of physical activity	CL & P	cleft lip and palate
		CL PSY	closed psychiatry
		Cl_r	renal clearance
CLASS IV	congestive heart failure with inability to engage in any physical activity without symptoms	Cl Red	closed reduction
		CLRO	community leave for reorientation
Clav	clavicle	CLS	capillary leak syndrome
CLB	chlorambucil		community living skills
	coccidian-like body	CLSE	calf lung surfactant extract (Infasurf®)
CLBBB	complete left bundle branch block	CLT	chronic lymphocytic thyroiditis
CLBD	cortical Lewy body disease		complex lymphedema therapy
CLBP	chronic low back pain		cool lace tent
CLC	cork leather and celastic (orthotic)	Cl_T	total body clearance
CL/CP	cleft lip and cleft palate	CLV	cutaneous leukocytoclastic vasculitis
CLD	chronic liver disease		
	chronic lung disease	CL VOID	clean voided specimen
Cl_d	dialysis clearance	clysis	hypodermoclysis
CLE	centrilobular emphysema	cm	centimeter
	congenital lobar emphysema	CM	capreomycin
			cardiac monitor
	continuous lumbar epidural (anesthetic)		case management
			case manager

Caucasian male
centimeter (cm)
chondromalacia
cochlear microphonics
common migraine
continuous microwave
continuous murmur
contrast media
costal margin
cow's milk
culture media
cutaneous melanoma
cystic mesothelioma
tomorrow morning (this is a dangerous abbreviation)

cm1	circumflex marginal 1
cm2	circumflex marginal 2
cm^2	square centimeters
cm^3	cubic centimeter
CMA	Certified Medical Assistant
	compound myopic astigmatism
	cost-minimization analysis
	cow's milk allergy
CMAF	centrifuged microaggregate filter
CMAPs	compound muscle action potentials
C_{max}	maximum concentration of drug
CMB	carbolic methylene blue
CMBBT	cervical mucous basal body temperature
CMC	carboxymethylcellulose
	carpal metacarpal (joint)
	chloramphenicol
	chronic mucocutaneous candidosis
	closed mitral commissurotomy
CMD	congenital muscular dystrophy
	cytomegalic disease
CMDRH	Center for Medical Devices and Radiological Health (of

the Food and Drug Administration)

CME	cervicomediastinal exploration (examination)
	continuing medical education
	cystoid macular edema
CMER	current medical evidence of record
CMF	cyclophosphamide, methotrexate and fluorouracil
CMFP	cyclophosphamide, methotrexate, fluorouracil, and prednisone
CMFT	same as CMF with tamoxifen
CMFVP	cyclophosphamide, methotrexate, fluorouracil, vincristine, and prednisone
CMG	cystometrogram
CMGM	chronic megakaryocytic granulocytic myelosis
CMGN	chronic membranous glomerulonephritis
CMH	current medical history
CMHC	community mental health center
CMHN	Community Mental Health Nurse
CMI	cell-mediated immunity
	clomipramine
	Cornell Medical Index
CMID	cytomegalic inclusion disease
C_{min}	minimum concentration of drug
CMIR	cell-mediated immune response
CMJ	carpometacarpal joint
CMK	congenital multicystic kidney
CML	cell-mediated lympholysis
	chronic myelogenous leukemia
	chronic myeloid leukemia

CMM	Comprehensive Major Medical (insurance)		Charot-Marie-Tooth (phenotype)
	cutaneous malignant melanoma		choline magnesium trisalicylate (Trilisate)
CMME	chloromethyl methyl ether		combined modality therapy
CMML	chronic myelomacrocytic leukemia		continuing medication and treatment
CMMS	Columbia Mental Maturity Scale		cutis marmorata telangiectasia
CMO	cardiac minute output		
	Chief Medical Officer	CMTX	chemotherapy treatment
	comfort measures only (resuscitation order)	CMUA	continuous motor unit activity
	consult made out	CMV	cisplatin, methotrexate, and vinblastine
C-MOPP	cyclophosphamide, mechlorethamine, vincristine (Oncovin), procarbazine, and prednisone		controlled mechanical ventilation
			conventional mechanical ventilation
CMP	cardiomyopathy		cool mist vaporizer
	chondromalacia patellae		cytomegalovirus
	cushion mouthpiece	CMVIG	cytomegalovirus immune globulin
CMPF	cow's milk, protein-free		
CMPT	cervical mucous penetration test	CMVS	culture midvoid specimen
		CN	congenital nystagmus
CMR	cerebral metabolic rate		cranial nerve
CMRNG	chromosomally mediated resistant *Neisseria gonorrhoeae*		tomorrow night (this is a dangerous abbreviation)
		Cn	cyanide
CMRO	chronic multifocal recurrent osteomyelitis	C/N	contrast-to-noise ratio
		CN II–XII	cranial nerves 2 through 12
CMRO$_2$	cerebral metabolic rate for oxygen	CNA	Certified Nurse Aide
			chart not available
CMS	children's medical services	C$_{Na}$	sodium clearance
	circulation motion sensation	CNAG	chronic narrow angle glaucoma
	chocolate milkshake	CNAP	continuous negative airway pressure
	constant moderate suction	CNB	core-needle biopsy
CMSUA	clean midstream urinalysis	CNC	clinical nurse coordinator
			Community Nursing Center
CMT	carpometatarsal (joint)	CNCbl	cyanocobalamin
	Certified Massage Therapist	CND	canned
	Certified Medical Transcriptionist		cannot determine
	Certified Music Therapist		chronic nausea and dyspepsia
	cervical motion tenderness	CNDC	chronic nonspecific diarrhea of childhood

CNE	chronic nervous exhaustion	CNSHA	congenital nonspherocytic hemolytic anemia
	could not establish	CNT	could not tell
C-NES	conversion nonepileptic seizures		could not test
		CNTA	combined neurosurgical and transfacial approach
CNF	cyclophosphamide, mitoxantrone (Novatantrone), and fluorouracil		
		CNTF	ciliary neurotrophic factor
		CNV	choroidal neovascularization
CNH	central neurogenic hypernea		
		CNVM	choroidal neovascular membrane
	contract nursing home		
CNHC	chronodermatitis nodularis helicis chronicus	CO	carbon monoxide
			cardiac output
	community nursing home care		castor oil
			centric occlusion
CNL	chemonucleolysis		Certified Orthoptist
CNLD	chronic neonatal lung disease		cervical orthosis
			court order
CNM	certified nurse midwife	Co	cobalt
CNMT	Certified Nuclear Medicine Technologist	C/O	check out
			complained of
CNN	congenital nevocytic nevus		complaints
			under care of
CNO	Chief Nursing Officer	CO₂	carbon dioxide
	community nursing organization	CO₃	carbonate
		COA	children of alcoholic
CNOP	cyclophosphamide, mitoxantrone (Novantrone), vincristine (Oncovin), and prednisone		coenzyme A
		CoA	coarctation of the aorta
		COAD	chronic obstructive airway disease
			chronic obstructive arterial disease
CNOR	Certified Nurse, Operating Room		
		COAG	chronic open angle glaucoma
CNP	capillary nonprofusion		
CNPS	cardiac nuclear probe scan	COAGSC	coagulation screen
		COAP	cyclophosphamide, vincristine (Oncovin), cytarabine (ara-C), and prednisone
CNRN	Certified Neurosurgical Registered Nurse		
CNS	central nervous system		
	Certified Nutrition Specialist	COAR	coarctation
		COARCT	coarctation
	Clinical Nurse Specialist	COB	cisplatin, vincristine (Oncovin), and bleomycin
	coagulase-negative staphylococci		
	Crigler-Najjar syndrome	COBE	chronic obstructive bullous emphysema
CNSD	Certified Nutrition Support Dietitian	COBS	chronic organic brain syndrome

COBT	chronic obstruction of biliary tract	COMLA	cyclophosphamide, vincristine (Oncovin), methotrexate, calcium leucovorin, and cytarabine (ara-C)
COC	chain of custody		
	combination oral contraceptive		
	continuity of care	COMP	complications
COCCIO	coccidioidomycosis		composite
COCM	congestive cardiomyopathy		compound
			compress
COD	cataract, right eye		cyclophosphamide, vincristine (Oncovin), methotrexate, and prednisone
	cause of death		
	codeine		
	coefficient of oxygen delivery		
		COMT	catechol-o-methyl transferase
	condition on discharge		
CODE 99	patient in cardiac or respiratory arrest	CON	catheter over a needle
			certificate of need
COD-MD	cerebro-oculardysplasia muscular dystrophy		conservatorship
		CON A	concanavalin A
CODO	codocytes	conc.	concentrated
COE	court-ordered examination	CONG	congenital
COEPS	cortically originating extrapyramidal symptoms		gallon
		CONJ	conjunctiva
		CONPA-DRI I	cyclophosphamide, vincristine, doxorubicin, and melphalan
COFS	cerebro-oculo-facio-skeletal		
COG	center of gravity	CONPA-DRI II	conpadri I plus high-dose methotrexate
	Central Oncology Group		
	cognitive function tests	CONPA-DRI III	conpadri I plus intensified doxorubicin
COGN	cognition		
COGTT	cortisone-primed oral glucose tolerance test	cont	continuous
			contusions
		CON-TRAL	contralateral
COH	carbohydrate		
	controlled ovarian hyperstimulation	CONTU	contusion
		CONV	conversation
COHb	carboxyhemoglobin	Conv. ex.	convergence excess
Coke	Coca-Cola®	CO-Ox	Co-oximetry
	cocaine	COP	change of plaster
COL	colonoscopy		cicatricial ocular pemphigoid
COLD	chronic obstructive lung disease		
			colloid osmotic pressure
COLD A	cold agglutin titer		
Collyr	eye wash		complaint of pain
col/ml	colonies per milliliter		cycophosphamide, vincristine (Oncovin), and prednisone
colp	colporrhaphy		
COLTRU	*colletotrichum truncatum*		
COM	chronic otitis media		
COMF	comfortable	COP 1	copolymer 1

COPA	cuffed oropharyngeal airway	COWS	**c**old to the **o**pposite and **w**arm to the **s**ame
COP-BLAM	cyclophosphamide, vincristine (Oncovin), prednisone, bleomycin, doxorubicin (Adriamycin), and procarbazine (Matulane)	COX	Coxsackie virus cyclooxygenase cytochrome C oxidase
		COX-2	cyclooxygenase-2
		CP	centric position cerebral palsy Certified Paramedic
COPD	chronic obstructive pulmonary disease		chemical peel chemistry profiles
COPE	chronic obstructive pulmonary emphysema		chest pain chloroquine-primaquine chondromalacia patella
COPP	cyclophosphamide, vincristine, procarbazine, and prednisone		chronic pain chronic pancreatitis cleft palate
COPS	community outpatient service		clinical pathway closing pressure convenience package
COPT	circumoval precipitin test		cor pulmonale
COR	conditioned orientation response coronary		creatine phosphokinase cyclophosphamide and cisplatin (Platinol)
CORA	conditioned orientation reflex audiometry		cystopanendoscopy
CORE	cardiac or respiratory emergency	C_p	concentration of drug plasma
CORT	Certified Operating Room Technician		phosphate clearance
COS	cataract, left eye change of shift	C/P	carbohydrate-to-protein ratio
	Chief of Staff clinically observed seizure	C&P	compensation and pension complete and pushing cystoscopy and pyelography
C_{osm}	Crisis Outpatient Services osmolal clearance		
COSTART	Coding symbols for a thesaurus of adverse reaction terms	CPA	cardiopulmonary arrest carotid photoangiography cerebellar pontile angle
COT	content of thought		chest pain alert
COTA	Certified Occupational Therapy Assistant		conditioned play audiometry
COTE	comprehensive occupational therapy evaluation		costophrenic angle cyclophosphamide cyproterone acetate
COTT CH	cottage cheese	CPAF	chlorpropamide-alcohol flush
COTX	cast off to x-ray		
COU	cardiac observation unit cataracts, both eyes	C_{PAH}	para-amino hippurate clearance
COWA	controlled oral word association	CPAP	continuous positive airway pressure

CPB	cardiopulmonary bypass	CPER	chest pain emergency room
	cisplatin, cyclophosphamide, and carmustine (BiCNU)	CPET	cardiopulmonary exercise testing
	competitive protein binding	CPETU	chest pain evaluation and treatment unit
CPBA	competitive protein-binding assay	CPF	cerebral perfusion pressure
CPBP	cardiopulmonary bypass	CPFT	Certified Pulmonary Function Technologist
CPC	cancer prevention clinic		
	cerebral palsy clinic	CPG	clinical practice guidelines
	chronic passive congestion	CPG2	carboxypeptidase G2
	clinicopathologic conference	CPGN	chronic progressive glomerulonephritis
	coil planet centrifuge	CPH	chronic persistent hepatitis
	continue plan of care		
CPCR	cardiopulmonary-cerebral resuscitation	CPhT	Certified Pharmacy Technician
CPCS	clinical pharmacokinetics consulting service	CPI	constitutionally psychopathia inferior
CPD	cephalopelvic disproportion	CPID	chronic pelvic inflammatory disease
	chorioretinopathy and pituitary dysfunction	CPIP	chronic pulmonary insufficiency of prematurity
	chronic peritoneal dialysis		
	citrate-phosphate-dextrose	CPK	creatine phosphokinase (BB, MB, MM are isoenzymes)
CPDA-1	citrate-phosphate-dextrose-adenine-one	CPK-1	creatine phosphokinase MM fraction
CPDA-2	citrate phosphate dextrose adenine-two	CPK-2	creatine phosphokinase MB fraction
CPDD	calcium pyrophosphate deposition disease	CPK-BB	creatine phosphokinase BB fraction
CPDG2	carboxypeptidase-G2	CPKD	childhood polycystic kidney disease
CPE	cardiogenic pulmonary edema	CPK-MB	creatine phosphokinase of muscle band
	chronic pulmonary emphysema	CPL	criminal procedure law
	Clinical Pastoral Education	CPM	central pontine myelinolysis
	clubbing, pitting, or edema		chlorpheniramine maleate
	complete physical examination		Clinical Practice Model
CPE-C	cyclopentenylcytosine		continue present management
CPEO	chronic progressive external ophthalmoplegia		continuous passive motion
			counts per minute

	cycles per minute	CPRS-	Comprehensive
	cyclophosphamide	OCS	Psychiatric Rating
CPmax	peak serum concentration		Scale, Obsessive-
CPMDI	computerized		Compulsive Subscale
	pharmacokinetic model-	CPS	carbamyl phosphate
	driven drug infusion		synthetase
CPmin	trough serum		cardiopulmonary support
	concentration		chest pain syndrome
CPMM	constant passive motion		child protective services
	machine		Chinese paralytic
CPN	chronic pyelonephritis		syndrome
CPO	continue present orders		chloroquine-
CPOX	chicken pox		pyrimethamine
CPP	central precocious puberty		sulfadoxine
	cerebral perfusion		clinical performance
	pressure		score
	chronic pelvic pain		clinical pharmacokinetic
	coronary perfusion		service
	pressure		coagulase-positive
	cryo-poor plasma		staphylococci
CPPB	continuous positive		complex partial seizures
	pressure breathing		counts per second
CPPD	calcium pyrophosphate		cumulative probability of
	dihydrate		success
	cisplatin	CPs	clinical pathways
CP & PD	chest percussion and	CPS I	carbamyl phosphate
	postural drainage		synthetase I
CPPV	continuous positive	CPSC	Consumer Product Safety
	pressure ventilation		Commission
CPQ	Conner's Parent	CPT	camptothecin
	Questionnaire		carnitine palmitoyl
CPR	cardiopulmonary		transferase
	resuscitation		chest physiotherapy
	computer-based patient		child protection team
	records		chromo-perturbation
	computerized patient		cold pressor test
	record		Continuous Performance
	tablet (French)		Test
CPR-1	all measures except		current perception
	cardiopulmonary		threshold
	resuscitation		Current Procedural
CPR-2	no extraordinary measures		Terminology (coding
	(to resuscitate)		system)
CPR-3	comfort measures only	CPT-11	irinotecan hydrochloride
CPRAM	controlled partial		(Camptosar)
	rebreathing anesthesia	CPTA	Certified Physical
	method		Therapy Assistant
CP/ROMI	chest pain, rule out	CPT/C	current perception
	myocardial infarction		threshold, computerized

CPTH	chronic post-traumatic headache	CRAbs	chelating recombinant antibodies
CPU	children's psychiatric unit	CRADA	Cooperative Research and Development Agreement (with NIH)
	clinical pharmacology unit		
CPUE	chest pain of unknown etiology	CRAG	cerebral radionuclide angiography
CPX	complete physical examination	CrAg	cryptococcal antigen
		CRAMS	circulation, respiration, abdomen, motor, and speech
CPZ	chlorpromazine Compazine® (CPZ is a dangerous abbreviation as it could be either)		
		CRAN	craniotomy
		CRAO	central retinal artery occlusion
CQI	continuous quality improvement	CRAX	crackers
CR	cardiac rehabilitation	CRBBB	complete right bundle branch block
	cardiorespiratory	CRBP	cellular retinol-binding protein
	case reports		
	chief resident	CRBSI	vascular-catheter-related bloodstream infections
	chorioretinal		
	clockwise rotation	CRC	case review committee
	closed reduction		child-resistant container
	colon resection		clinical research center
	complete remission		Clinical Research Coordinator
	contact record		
	controlled release		colorectal cancer
	cosmetic rhinoplasty	CR & C	closed reduction and cast
	creamed	CrCl	creatinine clearance
	cycloplegia retinoscopy	CRD	childhood rheumatic disease
Cr	chromium		
C/R	conscious, rational		chronic renal disease
C & R	convalescence and rehabilitation		chronic respiratory disease
	cystoscopy and retrograde		cone-rod dystrophy
CR₁	first cranial nerve		congenital rubella deafness
CRA	central retinal artery		
	chronic rheumatoid arthritis		crown-rump distance
		CRE	cumulative radiation effect
	cis-retinoic acid (isotretinion, Accutane®)	CREAT	serum creatinine
		CREF	cycloplegic refraction
	Clinical Research Associate	CRELM	screening tests for Congo-Crimean, Rift Valley, Ebola, Lassa, and Marburg fevers
	colorectal anastomosis		
	corticosteroid-resistant asthma	CREP	crepitation
CRABP	cellular retinoic acid binding protein	CREST	calcinosis, Raynaud's disease, esophageal

	dysmotility, sclerodactyly, and telangiectasia	CRP	chronic relapsing pancreatitis
CRF	cardiac risk factors		coronary rehabilitation program
	case report form		C-reactive protein
	chronic renal failure	C&RP	curettage and root planning
	corticotropin-releasing factor	CRPA	C-reactive protein agglutinins
CRFZ	closed reduction of fractured zygoma	CRPD	chronic restrictive pulmonary disease
CRHCa	cancer-related hypercalcemia	CRPF	chloroquine-resistant *Plasmodium falciparum*
CRI	Cardiac Risk Index	CRPS I	complex regional pain syndrome type I
	catheter-related infection		
	chronic renal insufficiency	CRQ	Chronic Respiratory (Disease) Questionnaire
CRIB	Clinical Risk Index for Babies		
CRIE	crossed radioimmuno-electrophoresis	CRR	community rehabilitation residence
CRIF	closed reduction and internal fixation	CRRT	continuous renal replacement therapy
CRIMF	closed reduction/intermaxillary fixation	CRS	Carroll Self-Rating Scale
CRIS	controlled-release infusion system		catheter-related sepsis
			Chinese restaurant syndrome
crit	hematocrit		cocaine-related seizure(s)
CRKL	crackles		colon-rectal surgery
CRL	crown rump length		congenital rubella syndrome
CRM	cream		cryoreductive surgery
	cross-reacting mutant		cytokine-release syndrome
CRM +	cross-reacting material positive	CRST	calcification, Raynaud's phenomenom, scleroderma, and telangiectasia
CRMD	children with retarded mental development		
CRN	crown	CRT	cadaver renal transplant
CRNA	Certified Registered Nurse Anesthetist		capillary refill time
			cathode ray tube
CRNH	Certified Registered Nurse in Hospice		central reaction time
CRNI	Certified Registered Nurse Intravenous		Certified Rehabilitation Therapist
			copper reduction test
CRNP	Certified Registered Nurse Practitioner		cranial radiation therapy
CRO	cathode ray oscilloscope	Cr Tr	crutch training
	contract research organization(s)	CRTT	Certified Respiratory Therapy Technician
CROM	cervical range of motion	CRTX	cast removed take x-ray
CROS	contralateral routing of signals	CRU	cardiac rehabilitation unit

74

clinical research unit
CRV central retinal vein
CRVF congestive right
    ventricular failure
CRVO central retinal vein
    occlusion
CRx chemotherapy
CIIRx Century II Bicarbonate
    Dialysis Machine
CRYO cryoablation
    cryosurgery
CRYST crystals
CS cardioplegia solution
    cat scratch
    cervical spine
    cesarean section
    chest strap
    cholesterol stone
    chlorobenzylidene
    malononitrile
    cigarette smoker
    clinically significant
    clinical stage
    close supervision
    conditionally susceptible
    congenital syphilis
    conjunctiva-sclera
    consciousness
    conscious sedation
    consultation
    consultation service
    coronary sinus
    corticosteroid(s)
    Cushing's syndrome
    cycloserine
    o-chlorobenzylidene
    malononitrile
C&S conjunctiva and sclera
    cough and sneeze
    culture and sensitivity
C/S cesarean section
    culture and sensitivity
CSA compressed spectral
    activity
    controlled substance
    analogue
    corticosteroid-sensitive
    asthma
CsA cyclosporin

CSB caffeine sodium benzoate
    Cheyne-Stokes breathing
    Children's Services Board
CSB I & Chemistry Screening
II   Batteries I and II
CSBF coronary sinus blood flow
CSBO complete small bowel
    obstruction
CSC cornea, sclera, and
    conjunctiva
    cryopreserved stem cells
CSCI continuous subcutaneous
    infusion
CSCR central serous
    chorioretinopathy
CSD cat scratch disease
    celiac sprue disease
C S&D cleaned, sutured, and
    dressed
CSDD Center for the Study of
    Drug Development
CSE combined spinal/epidurals
    cross-section
    echocardiography
C sect. cesarean section
CSF cerebrospinal fluid
    colony-stimulating factors
CSFELP cerebrospinal fluid
    electrophoresis
CSFP cerebrospinal fluid
    pressure
CSGIT continuous-suture graft-
    inclusion technique
C-Sh chair shower
CSH carotid sinus
    hypersensitivity
    chronic subdural
    hematoma
CSI Computerized Severity
    Index
    continuous subcutaneous
    infusion
    craniospinal irradiation
CSICU cardiac surgery intensive
    care unit
CSID congenital sucrase-
    isomaitase deficiency
CSII continuous subcutaneous
    insulin infusion

C

CS IV	clinical stage 4	C_{ss}	concentration of drug at steady-state
CSLU	chronic status leg ulcer		
CSM	carotid sinus massage	CSSD	closed system sterile drainage
	cerebrospinal meningitis		
	cervical spondylotic myelopathy	CST	cardiac stress test
			castration
	circulation, sensation, and movement		central sensory conducting time
	Committee on Safety of Medicines (United Kingdom)		cerebroside sulfotransferase
			Certified Surgical Technologist
CSME	cotton spot macular edema		contraction stress test
CSMN	chronic sensorimotor neuropathy		convulsive shock therapy
			cosyntropin stimulation test
CSN	cystic suppurative necrosis		static compliance
CSNB	congenital stationary night blindness	C_{STAT}	static lung compliance
		CSU	cardiac surgery unit
CSNRT	corrected sinus node recovery time		cardiac surveillance unit
			cardiovascular surgery unit
CSNS	carotid sinus nerve stimulation		casualty staging unit
CSO	Consumer Safety Officer (FDA)		catheter specimen of urine
	copied standing orders	CSW	Clinical Social Worker
CSOM	chronic serous otitis media	CSWSS	continuous spike-waves during slow sleep
	chronic suppurative otitis media	CT	calcitonin
			cardiothoracic
CSP	cellulose sodium phosphate		carpal tunnel
			cellulose triacetate (filter)
	chiral stationary phase		cervical traction
C-spine	cervical spine		chemotherapy
CSR	central supply room		chest tube
	Cheyne-Stokes respiration		circulation time
	corrected sedimentation rate		clinical trial
			clotting time
	corrective septorhinoplasty		coagulation time
			coated tablet
C-S RT	cranio-spinal radiotherapy		compressed tablet
CSS	Canadian Stroke Scale (score)		computed tomography
			Coomb's test
	carotid sinus stimulation		corneal thickness
	Central Sterile Services		corneal transplant
	chemical sensitivity syndrome		corrective therapy
			cytarabine and thioguanine
	chewing, sucking, and swallowing		cytoxic drug

C$_t$	concentration of drug in tissue	CTL	cervical, thoracic, and lumbar
CTA	catamenia (menses)		chronic tonsillitis
	clear to auscultation		cytotoxic T-lymphocytes
C-TAB	cyanide tablet	CTM	Chlor-Trimeton®
CTAP	clear to auscultation and percussion		clinical trials materials
	computed tomography during arterial portography	CT/MPR	computed tomography with multiplanar reconstructions
CTB	ceased to breathe		
	cholera toxin B	CTN	calcitonin
CTC	Cancer Treatment Center	C & T N, BLE	color and temperature normal, both lower extremities
	circular tear capsulotomy		
	clinical trial certificate (United Kingdom's equivalent to the Investigational New Drug Application)	cTNM	clinical-diagnostic staging of cancer
		CTP	comprehensive treatment plan
	Common Toxicity Criteria	CTPN	central total parenteral nutrition
	cyclophosphamide, thiotepa, and carboplatin	CTR	carpal tunnel release
			carpal tunnel repair
CTCL	cutaneous T-cell lymphoma (mycosis fungoides)		cosmetic transdermal reconstruction
		CTRS	Certified Therapeutic Recreation Specialist
CT & DB	cough, turn & deep breath		Conners Teachers Rating Scale
CTD	carpal tunnel decompression	CT-RT	chemo-radiotherapy
	chest tube drainage	CTS	cardiothoracic surgeon
	connective tissue disease		carpal tunnel syndrome
	corneal thickness depth	CTSP	called to see patient
	cumulative trauma disorder	CTW	central terminal of Wilson
		CTX	cerebrotendinous xanthomatosis
CTDW	continues to do well		
CTF	Colorado tick fever		chemotherapy
	continuous tube feeding		cyclophosphamide (Cytoxan®)
C/TG	cholesterol to triglyceride ratio		
		CTXN	contraction
CTGA	complete transposition of the great arteries	CTZ	chemoreceptor trigger zone
			co-trimoxazole (sulfamethoxazole and trimethoprin)
	corrected transposition of the great arteries		
CTH	clot to hold		
CTI	certification of terminal illness	CU	cause undetermined
			cause unknown
CTICU	cardiothoracic intensive care unit		chronic undifferentiated
			color unit

C

	convalescent unit		group B coxsackievirus
	Cuprophan (filter)	CVC	central venous catheter
Cu	copper		chief visual complaint
C_u	urea clear clearance		consonant vowel
CUA	clean urinalysis		consonant
	cost-utility analysis	CVD	cardiovascular disease
CUC	chronic ulcerative colitis		collagen vascular disease
	Clinical Unit Clerk	CVEB	cisplatin, vinblastine,
CUD	cause undetermined		etoposide, and
	controlled unsterile		bleomycin
	delivery	CVENT	controlled ventilation
CUFCM	Century Ultrafiltration	CVF	cardiovascular failure
	Control Machine		central visual field
CUG	cystourethrogram		cervicovaginal fluid
CUP	carcinoma of unknown	CVG	coronary vein graft
	primary (site)	CVHD	chronic valvular heart
CUPS	carcinoma of unknown		disease
	primary site	CVI	carboplatin, etoposide,
CUR	curettage		ifosfamide, and mesna
	cystourethrorectocele		uroprotection
CUS	carotid ultrasound		cerebrovascular
	chronic undifferentiated		insufficiency
	schizophrenia		common variable immuno-
	contact urticaria syndrome		deficiency (disease)
CUSA	Cavitron ultrasonic		continuous venous
	suction aspirator		infusion
CUT	chronic undifferentiated	CVICU	cardiovascular intensive
	type (schizophrenia)		care unit
CUTA	congenital urinary tract	CVID	common variable immune
	anomaly		deficiency
CV	cardiovascular	CVINT	cardiovascular
	cell volume		intermediate
	cisplatin and etoposide	CVL	central venous line
	coefficient of variation		clinical vascular
	color vision		laboratory
	common ventricle	CVM	Center for Veterinary
	consonant vowel		Medicine
	contrast venography	CVMT	cervical-vaginal, motion
	curriculum vitae		tenderness
C/V	cervical/vaginal	CVN	central venous nutrient
CVA	cerebrovascular accident	CVNSR	cardiovascular normal
	costovertebral angle		sinus rhythm
CVAD	central venous access	CVO	central vein occlusion
	device		conjugate diameter of
CVAH	congenital virilizing		pelvic inlet
	adrenal hyperplasia	CvO_2	mixed venous oxygen
CVAT	costovertebral angle		content
	tenderness	CVOD	cerebrovascular
CVB	chronic villi biopsy		obstructive disease

CVOR	cardiovascular operating room	CWL	Caldwell-Luc
CVP	central venous pressure	CWMS	color, warmth, movement, and sensation
	cyclophosphamide, vincristine, and prednisone	CWP	centimeters of water pressure
			childbirth without pain
CVPP	lomustine, vinblastine, procarbazine, and prednisone		coal worker's pneumoconiosis
			cold wet packs
CVR	cerebral vascular resistance	cWPW	concealed Wolff-Parkinson-White syndrome
	cerebrovascular resuscitation	CWR	clockwise rotation
	coronary vascular reserve	CWS	comfortable walking speed
CVRI	coronary vascular resistance index		cotton wool spots
CVS	cardiovascular surgery	CWT	compensated work training
	cardiovascular system	CWV	closed wound vacuum
	challenge virus standard	CX	cancel
	chorionic villi sampling		cervix
	clean voided specimen		chronic
	continuing vegetative state		culture
CVSCU	cardiovascular special care unit		cylinder axis
			cystectomy
CVST	cardiovascular stress test	CXA	circumflex artery
	cerebral venous sinus thrombosis	CxBx	cervical biopsy
		CxMT	cervical motion tenderness
CVSU	cardiovascular specialty unit	CXR	chest x-ray
CVT	calf vein thrombosis	CXTX	cervical traction
CVTC	central venous tunneled catheter	CY	cyclophosphamide
		C&Y	Children with Youth (program)
CVU	clean voided urine	CYA	cover your ass
CVUG	cysto-void urethrogram	CyA	cyclosporine
CVVH	continuous venovenous hemofiltration	CyADIC	cyclophosphamide, doxorubicin (Adriamycin), and dacarbazine
CW	careful watch		
	case worker		
	chest wall	Cyclo C	cyclocytidine HCl
	clockwise	CYL	cylinder
	compare with	CYP	cytochrome P-450
C/W	consistent with	CYRO	cryoprecipitate
	crutch walking	CYSTA	cystathionine
CWAF	Chemical Withdrawal Assessment Flowsheet	CYSTO	cystogram
			cystoscopy
CWAP	continuous wave arthroscopy pump	CYT	cyclophosphamide
		CYVA	cyclophosphamide,
CWD	cell wall defective	DIC	vincristine,
CWE	cotton wool exudates		

C

	Adriamycin®, and dacarbazine	**D**	
CZE	capillary zone electrophoresis		
CZI	crystalline zinc insulin (regular insulin)		
CZN	chlorzotocin	D	daughter
CZP	clonazepam		day

D	daughter
	day
	dead
	decay
	depression
	dextrose
	dextro
	diarrhea
	diastole
	dilated
	diminished
	Dinamap (blood pressure monitor)
	diopter
	distal
	distance
	divorced
D+	note has been dictated/ look for report
D−	note not dictated, save chart for doctor
$D_{0(2/7/99)}$	Day zero (the day treatment begins, February 7th, 1999)
D_1	day one (first day of treatment)
D-1 to D-12	dorsal vertebrae 1 to 12 dorsal nerves 1-12
D_1	first diagonal branch (coronary artery)
D_2	second diagonal branch (coronary artery)
	ergocalciferol
2/d	twice a day (this is a dangerous abbreviation)
2-D	two-dimensional
3-D	three-dimensional
D_3	cholecalciferol
D-3+7	cytarabine and daunorubicin
4D	4 prism diopters
5xD	five times a day (this is a dangerous abbreviation)

D50	50% dextrose injection	DAH	diffuse alveolar hemorrhage
D5/.45	dextrose 5% in 0.45% sodium chloride injection		disordered action of the heart
DA	dark adaptation (test)	DAI	diffuse axonal injury
	Debtors Anonymous	DAL	diffuse aggressive lymphomas
	degenerative arthritis		
	delivery awareness		drug analysis laboratory
	Dental Assistant	DALE	disability-adjusted life expectancy
	diagnostic arthroscopy		
	diastolic augmentation	DALM	dysplasia-associated lesion or mass
	direct admission		
	direct agglutination	DALY	disability-adjusted life year(s)
	diversional activity		
	dopamine	DAM	diacetylmonoxine
	drug addict	DAMA	discharged against medical advice
	drug aerosol		
Da	daltons	DANA	drug induced antinuclear antibodies
D/A	discharge and advise		
DAA	dead after arrival	DAo	descending aorta
	dissection aortic aneurysm	DAOM	depressor anguli oris muscle
DA/A	drug/alcohol addiction		
DAB	days after birth	DAP	dapsone
	diamino benzidine		diabetes-associated peptide
DABA	Diplomate of the American Board of Anesthesiology		diastolic augmentation pressure
			distending airway pressure
DAC	day activity center		Draw-A-Person
	disabled adult child		
	Division of Ambulatory Care	DAPT	Draw-A-Person Test
DACL	Depression Adjective Checklists	DAR	daily affective rhythm
			data, action, response
DACS	density-adjusted cell sorting	DARE	data, action, response, and evaluation
DACT	dactinomycin	DARP	drug abuse rehabilitation program
DAD	diffuse alveolar damage		
	diode array detector		drug abuse reporting program
	dispense as directed		
	drug administration device	D/ART	depression/awareness, recognition and treatment
	father		
DAE	diving air embolism	DAS	day of admission surgery
DAF	decay-accelerating factor		developmental apraxia of speech
	delayed auditory feedback		
DAFE	Dial-A-Flow Extension®		died at scene
DAFM	double aerosol face mask	DAs	daily activities
DAG	diacylglycerol	DASE	dobutamine-atropine stress echocardiography
	dianhydrogalactitol		

D

81

DAST	Drug Abuse Screening Test	DBPT	dacarbazine (DTIC), carmustine (BCNU), cisplatin (Platinol), and tamoxifen
DAT	daunorubicin, cytaribine, (ara-C), and thioguanine		
	definitely abnormal tracing (electrocardiogram)	DBQ	debrisoquin
		DBS	deep brain stimulation
	dementia of the Alzheimer type		desirable body weight diminished breath sounds
	diet as tolerated	DBW	dry body weight
	diphtheria antitoxin	DBZ	dibenzamine
	direct agglutination test	DC	daunorubicin and cytarabine
	direct antiglobulin test		
DAU	daughter		daycare
	drug abuse urine		decrease
DAUNO	daunorubicin		dextrocardia
DAVA	vindesine sulfate		diagonal conjugate
DAV SEP	deviated septum		direct Coombs (test)
DAW	dispense as written		discharge
DAWN	Drug Abuse Warning Network		Doctor of Chiropractic
		D&C	dilation and curettage
dB	decibel		direct and consensual
DB	date of birth	d/c	discontinue
	deep breathe	DC65®	Darvon Compound 65®
	demonstration bath	DCA	directional coronary atherectomy
	dermabrasion		
	diaphragmatic breathing		disk/condyle adhesion
	direct bilirubin		double cup arthroplasty
	double blind		sodium dichloroacetate
DB & C	deep breathing and coughing	DCAG	double coronary artery graft
DBD	milolactol (dibromodulicitol)	DC-ART	disease controlling anti-rheumatic therapy
DBE	deep breathing exercise	DC&B	dilation, currettage, and biopsy
DBED	penicillin G benzathine		
dBEMCL	decibel effective masking contralateral	DCBE	double contrast barium enema
D₅BES	dextrose in balanced electrolyte solution	DCC	day care center
		DCCF	dural carotid-cavernous fistula
DBI®	phenformin HCl		
DBIL	direct bilirubin	DCCT	Diabetes Control and Complications Trial (questionnaire)
DBL	double beta-lactam		
DBMT	displacement bone marrow transplantation	DC'd	discontinued
DBP	D-binding protein	DCE	delayed contrast-enhancement
	diastolic blood pressure		
	dibutyl phthalate		designated compensable event
DBPCFC	double-blind, placebo-controlled food challenge	DCF	data collection form
			Denomination Commune

	Francaise (French-approved nonproprietary name)	DCU	day care unit
		DCUS	duplex color ultrasonography
	pentostatin (Nipent; 2' deoxycoformycin)	DCW	direct care worker
DCFS	Department of Children and Family Services	DCYS	Department of Children and Youth Services
DCG	diagnostic cardiogram	DD	delivery date
DCH	delayed cutaneous hypersensitivity		dependent drainage
			Descemet's detachment
DCIA	deep circumflex iliac artery (flap)		detrusor dyssynergia
			developmentally delayed
DCIS	ductal carcinoma *in situ*		developmental disabilities
DCLHb	diaspirin cross-linked hemoglobin		developmentally disabled
			dialysis dementia
			died of the disease
DCM	dilated cardiomyopathy		differential diagnosis
DCMXT	dichloromethotrexate		discharge diagnosis
DCN	Darvocet N®		disk diameter
DCNU	chlorozotocin		Doctor of Divinity
DCO	diffusing capacity of carbon monoxide		double dose (used by Radiology)
DCP	dynamic compression plate		down drain
			dry dressing
DCP®	calcium phosphate, dibasic		dual disorder
			Duchenne's dystrophy
DCPM	daunorubicin, cytarabine, prednisolone, and mercaptopurine		due date
		D/D	diarrhea/dehydration
		D → D	discharge to duty
DCPN	direction-changing positional nystagmus	D & D	debridement and dressing
			diarrhea and dehydration
DCR	dacryocystorhinostomy		drilling and drainage
	delayed cutaneous reaction	DDA	dideoxyadenosine
		DDAVP®	desmopressin acetate
DCRF	data case report forms	DDC	zalcitabine (dideoxy-cytidine; Hivid)
3DCRT	3 dimensional conformal radiation therapy	DDD	defined daily doses
			degenerative disk disease
DCS	decompression sickness		dense deposit disease
	dorsal column stimulator		fully automatic pacing
DCSA	double contrast shoulder arthrography	DDDR	rate-adaptive DDD pacemaker device
DCT	daunorubicin, cytarabine, and thioguanine	DDE	dichlorodiphenylethylene
	deep chest therapy	DDGB	double-dose gallbladder (test)
	direct (antiglobulin) Coombs test	DDH	developmental dysplasia of the hip
DCTM	delay computer tomographic myelography	DDHT	double dissociated hypertropia

DDI	didanosine (dideoxyinosine; Videx)	DED	diabetic eye disease
			died in emergency department
	dressing dry, intact	DEEDS	drugs, exercise, education, diet, and self-monitoring
DDIs	drug-drug interactions		
DDis	developmental disorder	DEEG	depth electroencephalogram
DDNS	digestive disease and nutrition service		deteriorating electroencephalogram
DDP	cisplatin	DEET	diethyltoluamide
DDRA	dead despite resuscitation attempt	DEF	decayed, extracted, or filled
DDS	dialysis disequilibrium syndrome		defecation
			deficiency
	Doctor of Dental Surgery	DEFT	defendant
	double decidual sac (sign)	DEG	diethylene glycol
	4, 4-diaminodiphenyl-sulfone (dapsone)	degen	degenerative
		DEHP	diethylhexyl phthalate
DDST	Denver Development Screening Test	DEL	delivered
			delivery
DDT	chlorophenothane		deltoid
DDTP	drug dependence treatment program	DEM	drug evaluation matrix
		DEP ST SEG	depressed ST segment
DDx	differential diagnosis		
DE	dermal epidermal (junction)	DER	disulfiram-ethanol reaction
	digitalis effect	DERM	dermatology
D_5E_{48}	5% Dextrose and Electrolyte 48	DES	desflurane
			diethylstilbestrol
D_5E_{75}	5% Dextrose and Electrolyte 75		diffuse esophageal spasm
			disequilibrium syndrome
2DE	two-dimensional echocardiography		Dissociative Experience Scale
D&E	dilation and evacuation		dry eye syndrome
DEA#	Drug Enforcement Administration number (physician's federal narcotic number)	DESAT	desaturation
		DESF	desflurane (Suprane)
		DESI	Drug Efficacy Study Implementation
DEAE	diethylaminoethyl	DET	diethyltryptamine
DEB	dystrophic epidermolysis bullosa		dipyridamole echocardiography test
DEC	deciduous (primary teeth)	DETOX	detoxification
	decrease	DEV	deviation
	diethylcarbamazine		duck embryo vaccine
DECA	nandrolone decanoate	DEVR	dominant exudative vitreoretinopathy
DECAFS	Department of Children and Family Services	DEX	dexamethasone
			dexter (right)
DECEL	deceleration		dexverapamil
decub	decubitus		

DEXA	dual-energy x-ray absorptiometry	DFS	disease-free survival Division of Family Services Doppler flow studies
DF	day frequency (of voiding)		
	decayed and filled	DFU	dead fetus in uterus
	deferred	DFV	diarrhea, fever, and vomiting
	defibrotide		
	degree of freedom	DFW	Dexide face wash
	dengue fever	DFWO	dorsiflexory wedge osteotomy
	dexfenfluramine		
	diabetic father	DG	diagnosis
	diastolic filling		dorsal glides
	dietary fiber		downward gaze
	dorsiflexion	DGE	delayed gastric emptying
	drug free	DGGE	denaturing gradient gel electrophoresis
	dye free		
DFA	delayed feedback audiometry	DGI	disseminated gonococcal infection
	diet for age	DGL	deglycyrrhizinated licorice
	difficulty falling asleep	DGR	duodenogastric reflux
	direct fluorescent antibody	DGM	ductal glandular mastectomy
	distal forearm	DH	delayed hypersensitivity
DFD	defined formula diets		Dental Hygienist
	degenerative facet disease		dermatitis herpetiformis
DFE	dilated fundus examination		developmental history
			diaphragmatic hernia
	distal femoral epiphysis	D+H	delusions and hallucinations
DFG	direct forward gaze		
DFI	disease-free interval	DHA	dihydroxyacetone
DFLE	disability-free life expectancy		docosahexaenoic acid
DFM	decreased fetal movement	DHAC	dihydro-5-azacytidine
	deep finger massage	DHAD	mitoxanthrone HCl
	deep friction massage	DHANP	Diplomate of the Homeopathic Academy of Naturopathic Physicians
DFMC	daily fetal movement count		
DFMO	eflornithine (difluoro-methylorithine)		
		DHAP	dexamethasone, high-dose cytarabine, (ara-A) cisplatin (Platinol AQ)
DFMR	daily fetal movement record		
		DHBV	duck hepatitis B virus
DFO	deferoxamine (Desferal)	DHCA	deep hypothermia circulatory arrest
DFOM	deferoxamine (Desferal)		
DFP	diastolic filling period	DHCC	dihydroxycholecalciferol
	isoflurophate (diisopropyl fluorophosphate)	DHD	dissociated horizontal deviation
DFR	diabetic floor routine		
DFRC	deglycerolized frozen red cells	DHE 45®	dihydroergotamine mesylate

85

DHEA	dehydroepiandrosterone			confusion, **i**nfection,
DHEAS	dehydroepiandrosterone sulfate			(**u**rinary), **a**trophic urethritis/vaginitis,
DHF	dengue hemorrhagic fever			**ph**armaceuticals, **p**sychological,
DHFR	dihydrofolate reductase			**e**xcessive excretion
DHHS	Department of Health and Human Services			(e.g., CHF, hyperglycemia)
DHI	dynamic hyperinflation			**r**estricted mobility, and
DHIC	detrusor hyperactivity with impaired			stool impaction
	contractility		DIAS	diastolic
DHL	diffuse histiocytic		DIAS BP	diastolic blood pressure
	lymphoma		Diath SW	diathermy short wave
DHP	dihydropyridine		DIAZ	diazepam
DHP-1	dehydropeptidase-1		DIB	disability insurance
DHPG	ganciclovir			benefits
DHPR	dihydropteridine reductase		DIBC	drug-induced blood
DHR	delayed hypersensitivity			cytopenias
	reaction		DIBS	dead-in-bed syndrome
DHS	Department of Human Services		DIC	dacarbazine
	duration of hospital stay			diagnostic imaging center
	dynamic hip screw			differential interference
DHST	delayed hypersensitivity test			contrast
DHT	dihydrotachysterol			disseminated intravascular coagulation
	dihydrotestosterone			drug information center
	dissociated hypertropia		DICC	dynamic infusion
	Dobhoff tube			cavernosometry and
DHTF	Dobhoff tube			cavernosography
	feeding		DICE	dexamethasone,
DI	(Beck) Depression Inventory			ifosfamide, cisplatin, and etopside, with
	date of injury			mesna
	Debrix Index		DICLOX	dicloxacillin
	detrusor instability		DICP	demyelinated
	diabetes insipidus			inflammatory chronic
	diagnostic imaging			polyneuropathy
	dorsal interossei		DICT	dose-intensive
	drug interactions			chemotherapy
D&I	debridement and irrigation		DID	delayed ischemia deficit
	dry and intact			dissociative identity
DIA	drug-induced			disorder
	agranulocytosis			drug-induced disease
	drug-induced amenorrhea		di,di	dichorionic, diamniotic
diag.	diagnosis		DIE	died in emergency
DIAP-	(causes of transient			department
PERS	incontinence) **d**elirium/		DIED	died in emergency
				department

DIF	differentiation-inducing factor	DIR	directions
DIFF	differential blood count	DIRD	drug-induced renal disease
DIG	digoxin (this is a dangerous abbreviation)	DIS	Diagnostic Interview Schedule (questionnaire)
DIH	died in hospital		digital imaging spectrophotometer
DIJOA	dominantly inherited juvenile optic atrophy		dislocation
DIL	daughter-in-law	DISC	disabled infectious single cycle (virus)
	dilute		dynamic integrated stabilization chair
	drug-induced lupus		
DILC	dose-intensity limiting criterium	disch.	discharge
DILD	diffuse infiltrative lung disease	DISCUS	Dyskinesia Indentification System Condensed User Scale
	drug-induced liver disease	DISH	diffuse idiopathic skeletal hyperostosis
DILE	drug induced lupus erythematosus	DISI	dorsal intercalated segmental (segment) instability
DILS	drug-induced lupus syndrome	DISIDA	diisopropyl imino diacetic acid
DIM	diminish		
D$_5$IMB	Ionosol MB with 5% dextrose injection	D$_5$ISOM	5% Dextrose and Isolyte M
DIMD	drug induced movement disorders	D$_5$ISOP	5% Dextrose and Isolyte P
DIMOAD	diabetes insipidus, diabetes mellitus, optic atrophy, and deafness	DISR	drug-induced skin reactions
DIMS	disorders of initiating and maintaining sleep	DIST	distal
			distilled
DIND	delayed ischemic neurologic deficit	DIT	diiodotyrosine
			drug-induced thrombocytopenia
DIOS	distal ileal obstruction syndrome	DIU	death in utero
	distal intestinal obstruction syndrome	DIV	double inlet ventricle
		DIVA	digital intravenous angiography
DIP	desquamative interstitial pneumonia	Div ex	divergence excess
	diplopia	DIVP	dilute intravenous Pitocin
	distal interphalangeal	DJD	degenerative joint disease
	drip infusion pyelogram	DK	dark
	drug-induced parkinsonism		diabetic ketoacidosis
			diseased kidney
DIPC	dynamic infusion pharmacocavemosometry	DKA	diabetic ketoacidosis
			didn't keep appointment
DIPJ	distal interphalangeal joint	DKB	deep knee bends
		DKC	double knee to chest

dl	deciliter (100 mL)	DM	dehydrated and malnourished
DL	danger list		dermatomyositis
	deciliter		dextromethorphan
	diagnostic laparoscopy		diabetes mellitus
	direct laryngoscopy		diabetic mother
	drug level		diastolic murmur
D_L	maximal diffusing capacity	DM-1	diabetes mellitus type 1
DLB	Dementia with Lewy bodies	DM-2	diabetes mellitus type 2
		DMAC	*Mycobacterium avium-intracellulare* complex
	direct laryngoscopy and bronchoscopy	DMAD	disease-modifying antirheumatic drug
DLC	double lumen catheter		
DLCL	diffuse large cell lymphoma	DMAIC	disseminated *Mycobacterium avium-intracellulare* complex
DLCO sb	diffusion capacity of carbon monoxide, single breath	DMARD	disease modifying antirheumatic drug
DLD	date of last drink	DMAS	Drug Management and Authorization Section
DLE	discoid lupus erythematosus	DMAT	disaster medical assistance team
	disseminated lupus erythematosis	DMBA	dimethylbenzanthracene
DLF	digitalis-like factor	DMC	dactinomycin, methotrexate, and cyclophosphamide
DLI	donor leukocyte infusions		
DLIF	digoxin-like immunoreactive factors		diabetes management center
DLIS	digoxin-like immunoreactive substance	DMD	disciform macular degeneration
			Doctor of Dental Medicine
DLMP	date of last menstrual period		Duchenne's muscular dystrophy
DLNG	dl-norgestrel		
DLNMP	date of last normal menstrual period	DMD w/ SRNM	disciform macular degeneration with subretinal neovascular membrane
DLP	dislocation of patella		
DLPD	diffuse lymphocytic poorly differentiated	DME	durable medical equipment
D5LR	dextrose 5% in lactated Ringer's injection	DMEM	Dulbecco's Modified Eagle Medium
DLS	daily living skills	DMF	decayed, missing, or filled
	digitalis-like substances		dimethylformamide
DLSC	double lumen subclavian catheter		Drug Master File
DLT	dose-limiting toxicity	DMFS	decayed, missing, or filled surfaces
	double-lung transplant	DMH	Department of Mental Health
DLU	diffused lung uptake		
DLV	delavirdine (Rescriptor)		

DMI	desipramine	DNCB	dinitrochlorobenzene
	diaphragmatic myocardial infarction	DNC	did not come
		DND	died a natural death
DM Isch	diaphragmatic myocardial ischemia	DNEPTE	did not exist prior to enlistment
DMKA	diabetes mellitus ketoacidosis	DNET	dysembryoplastic neuroepithelial tumor
DMO	dimethadone	DNFC	does not follow commands
DMOOC	diabetes mellitus out of control	DNI	do not intubate
DMP	dimethyl phthalate	DNIC	diffuse noxious inhibitory control
DMPA	depot-medroxypro-gesterone acetate	DNIF	duties not including flying
D-MRI	dynamic magnetic resonance imaging	DNKA	did not keep appointment
		DNN	did not nurse
DMS	dimethylsulfide	DNP	did not pay
DMSA	succimer (dimercaptosuccinic acid)		dinitrophenylhydrazine
			do not publish
		DNR	daunorubicin
DMSO	dimethyl sulfoxide		did not respond
DMT	dimethyltryptamine		do not report
DMV	disk, macula, and vessels		do not resuscitate
			dorsal nerve root
	Doctor of Veterinary Medicine	DNS	deviated nasal septum
			doctor did not see patient
DMVP	disk, macula, vessel, periphery		do not show
			dysplastic nevus syndrome
DMX	diathermy, massage, and exercise	D_5 1/4 NS	dextrose 5% in 1/4 normal saline (0.225% sodium chloride) injection
DN	denuded		
	diabetic nephropathy	D_5NS	5% dextrose in normal saline (0.9% sodium chloride) injection
	dicrotic notch		
	down		
	dysplastic nevus (nevi)	DNT	did not test
D & N	distance and near (vision)	DO	diet order
D5NS	dextrose 5% in 0.9% sodium chloride injection		distocclusal
			Doctor of Osteopathy
D_5 1/2NS	dextrose 5% in 0.45% sodium chloride injection		doctor's order
		D/O	disorder
		✔DO	check doctor's order
DNA	deoxyribonucleic acid	DO_2	oxygen delivery
	did not answer	DOA	date of admission
	did not attend		dead on arrival
	does not apply		dominant optic atrophy
DNA ds	deoxyribonucleic acid double strand		driver of automobile
			duration of action
DNA ss	deoxyribonucleic acid single strand	DOA-DRA	dead on arrival despite resuscitative attempts

89

DOB	dangle out of bed	DORx	date of treatment
	date of birth	DOS	date of surgery
	Dobrava hantavirus		doctor's order sheet
	dobutamine	DOSA	day of surgery
	doctor's order book		admission
DOC	date of conception	DOSAK	Central Tumor Registry
	diabetes out of control		operated by the
	died of other causes		German-Austrian-Swiss
	diet of choice		Association for Head
	drug of choice		and Neck Tumors
DOCA	desoxycorticosterone	DOSS	docusate sodium (dioctyl
	acetate		sodium sulfosuccinate)
DOCP	desoxycorticosterone	DOT	date of transcription
	pivalate		date of transfer
DOD	date of death		died on table
	dead of disease		directly observed therapy
	Department of Defense		Doppler ophthalmic test
	drug overdose	DOTS	directly observed
DODD	demand oxygen delivery		treatment, short course
	device	DOV	date of visit
DOE	date of examination		distribution of ventilation
	dyspnea on exertion	DOX	doxepin
DOES	disorders of excessive		doxorubicin
	somnolence	doz	dozen
DOH	Department of Health	DP	dental prosthesis
DOI	date of implant		diastolic pressure
	(pacemaker)		disability pension
	date of injury		discharge planning
DO_2I	oxygen delivery index		dorsalis pedis (pulse)
DOJ	Department of Justice	DPA	Department of Public
DOL	days of life		Assistance
DOL #2	second day of life		dipropylacetic acid
DOLV	double outlet left		dual photon
	ventricle		absorptiometry
DOM	Doctor of Oriental		durable power of attorney
	Medicine	DPAP	diastolic pulmonary artery
	domiciliary		pressure
	domiciliary care	DPB	days postburn
DON	Director of Nursing	DPBS	Dulbecco's phosphate-
DOOC	diabetes out of control		buffered saline
DOP	dopamine	DPC	delayed primary closure
DOPS	diffuse obstructive		discharge planning
	pulmonary syndrome		coordinator
	dihydroxyphenylserine		distal palmar crease
	Director of Pharmacy	DPDL	diffuse poorly
	Service(s)		differentiated
DOR	date of release		lymphocytic lymphoma
DORV	double-outlet right	2,3-DPG	2,3-diphosphoglyceric
	ventricle		acid

			tetanus, poliomyelitis, and measles
DPH	Department of Public Health		
	diphenhydramine	DPU	delayed pressure urticaria
	Doctor of Public Health phenytoin (diphenylhydantoin)	DPUD	duodenal peptic ulcer disease
DPI	dietary protein intake	DPVSs	dilated perivascular spaces
	dry powder inhaler	DPXA	dual-photon x-ray absorptiometry
DPIL	dextrose (percentage), protein (grams per kilogram) Intralipid® (grams per kilogram)	D/Q	deep quiet
		D&Q	deep and quiet
		DQOL	diabetes quality of life
DPL	diagnostic peritoneal lavage	Dr	doctor
		DR	delivery room
D5PLM	dextrose 5% and Plasmalyte M® injection		diabetic retinopathy
			diagnostic radiology
			dining room
DPM	distintegrations per minute (dpm)		diurnal rhythm
		DRA	drug-related admissions
	Doctor of Podiatric Medicine	DRAPE	drug-related adverse patient event
	drops per minute	DRE	digital rectal examination
DPN	¹¹C-diprenorphine	DRESS	depth resolved surface coil spectroscopy
	diabetic peripheral neuropathy		
		DREZ	dorsal root entry zone
DPOA	durable power of attorney	DRG	diagnosis-related groups
DPOAHC	durable power of attorney for health care		dorsal root ganglia
		DRGE	drainage
DPP	dorsalis pedal pulse	DRI	Discharge Readiness Index
	duration of positive pressure		dopamine reuptake inhibitor
DPPC	colfosceril palmitate (dipalmitoylphosphati-dylcholine)	DRM	drug-related morbidity
		DRN	drug-related neutropenia
		DRP	drug-related problem
DPR	diagnostic procedure room	DRPLA	dentatorubral-pallidolluysian atrophy
		DRR	drug regimen review
DPS	disintegration per second	DRS	Disability Rating Scale
DPSS	Department of Public Social Service		Duane's retraction syndrome
DPsy	Doctor of Psychology	DRSG	dressing
DPT	Demerol®, Phenergan®, and Thorazine® (this is a dangerous abbreviation)	DRSI	disease-related symptom improvement
		DRSP	drug-resistant *Streptococcus pneumoniae*
	diphtheria, pertussis, and tetanus (immunization)		
	Driver Performance Test	DRT	drug-related thrombocytopenia
DPTPM	diphtheria, pertussis,		

DRUB	drug screen-blood	DSIAR	double-stapled ileoanal reservoir
DRUJ	distal or radial ulnar joint	DSM	disease state management
DS	deep sleep		drink skim milk
	Dextrostix®	DSM III	Diagnostic & Statistical Manual, 3rd edition
	discharge summary		
	disoriented	DSM-IV	Diagnostic and Statistical Manual of Mental Disorders, 4th edition
	double strength		
	Down syndrome		
	drug screen	DSO	distal-lateral subungual onychomycosis
D/S	5% dextrose and 0.9% sodium chloride (saline) injection		
		DSP	digital signal processor
		D-SPINE	dorsal spine
D&S	diagnostic and surgical	DSPS	delayed sleep phase syndrome
	dilation and suction		
D5S	dextrose 5% in 0.9% sodium chloride (saline) injection	DSRF	drainage subretinal fluid
		DSS	dengue shock syndrome
			Department of Social Services
D$_5$-1/2S	5% dextrose in 0.45% sodium chloride (saline) injection		
			Disability Status Scale
			discharge summary sheet
DSA	digital subtraction angiography (angiocardiography)		disease-specific survival
			distal splenorenal shunt
			docusate sodium
DSAP	disseminated superficial actinic porokeratosis	DSSN	distal symmetric sensory neuropathy
DSB	drug-seeking behavior		
DSC	Down syndrome child	DSST	Digit-Symbol Substitution Test
DSD	discharge summary dictated		
		DST	daylight saving time
	dry sterile dressing		dexamethasone suppression test
DSDB	direct self-destructive behavior		
			digit substitution test
DSF	doxorubicin, streptozocin, and fluorouracil		donor-specific (blood) transfusion
DSG	desogestrel	DSU	day stay unit
	dressing		day surgery unit
DSG	deoxyspergualin	DSUH	direct suggestion under hypnosis
DSHEA	Dietary Supplement Health and Education Act of 1994		
		DSV	digital subtraction ventriculography
DSHR	delayed skin hypersensitivity reaction	DSWI	deep sternal wound infection
			deep surgical wound infection
DSHS	Department of Social and Health Services		
		DT	delirium tremens
DSI	deep shock insulin		dietary thermogenesis
	Depression Status Inventory		dietetic technician
			diphtheria and tetanus

	toxoids, pediatric strength	DTUS	diathermy, traction, and ultrasound
	discharge tomorrow	DVG	double vein graft
D/T	date/time	DTV	due to void
	due to	DTwP	diphtheria and tetanus toxoids with whole-cell pertussis vaccine
d/t	due to		
d4T	stavudine (Zerit)		
D & T	diagnosis and treatment	DTX	detoxification
	dictated and typed	DU	decubitus ulcer
DTaP	diphtheria and tetanus toxoids with acellular pertussis vaccine		developmental unit
			diabetic urine
			diagnosis undetermined
DTBC	tubocurarine (D-tubocurarine)		duodenal ulcer
			duroxide uptake
DTBE	Division of Tuberculosis Elimination	DUB	Dubowitz (score)
			dysfunctional uterine bleeding
DTC	day treatment center		
	diticarb (diethyldiothio-carbamate)	DUD	dihydrouracil dehydrogenase
	tubocurarine (D-tubocurarine)	DUE	drug use evaluation
		D&UE	dilation and uterine evacuation
DTD #30	dispense 30 such doses		
DTF	deep transverse friction	DUF	Doppler ultrasonic flowmeter
DTH	delayed-type hypersensitivity		
		DUI	driving under the influence
DTIC	dacarbazine		
D TIME	dream time	DUID	driving under the influence of drugs
DTM	deep tissue massage		
	dermatophyte test medium	DUII	driving under the influence of intoxicants
DTO	danger to others		
	deodorized tincture of opium (warning: this is *NOT* paregoric)	DUIL	driving under the influence of liquor
		DUKM	dialysate urea kinetic modeling
DTOGV	dextral-transposition of great vessels		
		DUM	drug use monitoring
DTP	distal tingling on percussion (+Tinel's sign)	DUN	dialysate urea nitrogen
		DUNHL	diffuse undifferentiated non-Hodgkins lymphoma
DTPA	pentetic acid (diethylenetriaminepen-taacetic acid)		
		DUO	Duotube®
		DUR	drug utilization review
DTR	deep tendon reflexes		duration
	Dietetic Technician Registered	DUS	digital ultrasound
			distal urethral stenosis
DTs	delirium tremens		
DTS	danger to self		Doppler ultrasound stethoscope
	donor specific transfusion		
DTT	diphtheria tetanus toxoid	3DUS	three-dimensional ultrasound
	dithiothreitol		

DUSN	diffuse unilateral subacute neuroretinitis		detention warrant
			dextrose in water
DV	distance vision		diffusion-weighted (imaging)
	double vision		distilled water
D&V	diarrhea and vomiting		doing well
	disks and vessels		double wrap
DVA	Department of Veterans Affairs	D/W	dextrose in water
			discussed with
	distance visual acuity	D_5W	5% dextrose (in water) injection
	vindesine		
DVC	direct visualization of vocal cords	D10W	10% dextrose (in water) injection
D V® Cream	dienestrol vaginal cream	D20W	20% dextrose (in water) injection
DVD	dissociated vertical deviation	D50W	50% dextrose (in water) injection
	double vessel disease	D70W	70% dextrose (in water) injection
DVI	atrioventricular sequential pacing	5 DW	5% dextrose (in water) injection
	digital vascular imaging	DWDL	diffuse well differentiated lymphocytic lymphoma
DVIU	direct vision internal urethrotomy		
DVPX	divalproex sodium (Depakote)	DWI	diffusion-weighted (magnetic resonance) imaging
DVM	Doctor of Veterinary Medicine		driving while intoxicated
			driving while impaired
DVMP	disks, vessels, and macula periphery	DWMRI	diffusion-weighted magnetic resonance imaging
DVP	cyclophosphamide, vincristine, and prednisone		
		DWRT	delayed work recall test
DVP-Asp	daunorubicin, vincristine, prednisone, and asparaginase	DWSCL	daily wear soft contact lens
DVPA	daunorubicin, vincristine, prednisone, and asparaginase	Dx	diagnosis
			disease
DVR	Division of Vocational Rehabilitation	DXA	dual-energy x-ray absorptiometry
	double valve replacement	DxLS	diagnosis responsible for length of stay
DVSA	digital venous subtraction angiography	DXM	dexamethasone
DVT	deep vein thrombosis	DXR	delayed xenograft rejection
DVTS	deep venous thromboscintigram	DXT	deep x-ray therapy
DVVC	direct visualization of vocal cords	DXRT	deep x-ray therapy
		DXS	Dextrostix®
DW	daily weight	DY	dusky (infant color)
	deionized water		dysprosium

DYF	drag your feet (author's note: see you in court)		**E**
DYFS	Division of Youth and Family Services		
DZ	diazepam		
	disease		
	dizygotic	E	edema
	dozen		effective
DZP	diazepam		eloper
DZT	dizygotic twins		enema
			engorged
			eosinophil
			Escherichia
			esophoria for distance
			evaluation
			evening
			expired
			eye
		E′	elbow
			esophoria for near
		E_1	estrone
		E2	estradiol
		E3	estriol
		4E	4 plus edema
		E20	Enfamil 20®
		E → A	say E,E,E, comes out as A,A,A upon auscultation of lung showing consolidation
		EA	early amniocentesis
			elbow aspiration
			electroacoustic analysis
			enteral alimentation
			esophageal atresia
		E&A	evaluate and advise
		EAA	electrothermal atomic absorption
			essential amino acids
			excitatory amino acid
		EAB	elective abortion
			Ethical Advisory Board
		EAC	erythema annulare centrifugum
			external auditory canal
		EACA	aminocaproic acid (epsilon-aminocaproic acid)
		EADs	early after-depolarizations

EAE	experimental autoimmune encephalomyelitis	EBF	erythroblastosis fetalis
		EBL	estimated blood loss
EAEC	enteroaggregative *Escherichia coli*	EBL-1	European bat lyssavirus 1
		EBM	evidence-based medicine
EAggEC	enteroaggregative *Escherichia coli*		expressed breast milk
		EBMT	European Bone Marrow Transplant (registry group)
EAHF	eczema, allergy, and hay fever		
EAL	electronic artificial larynx	EBNA	Epstein-Barr (virus) nuclear antigen
EAM	external auditory meatus		
EAP	Employment (employee) Assistance Programs	EBO	evidence-based outcomes
	erythrocyte acid phosphatase	EBP	epidural blood patch
		EBR	external beam radiotherapy
	etoposide, doxorubicin (Adriamycin), and cisplatin (Platinol)	EBRs	evidence-based recommendations
EARLIES	early decelerations	EBRT	external beam radiation therapy
EART	extended abdominal radiation therapy	EBS	epidermolysis bullosa
EAR OX	ear oximetry	EBSB	equal breath sounds bilaterally
EAS	external anal sphincter		
EAST	external rotation, abduction stress test	EBV	Epstein-Barr virus
		EBVCA	Epstein-Barr viral capsid antigen
EAT	Eating Attitudes Test		
	ectopic atrial tachycardia	EBVEA	Epstein-Barr virus, early antigen
EAU	experimental autoimmune uveitis	EBVNA	Epstein-Barr virus, nuclear antigen
EB	epidermolysis bullosa	EC	ejection click
	Epstein-Barr (virus)		endocervical
EBA	epidermolysis bullosa acquisita		enteric coated
			Escherichia coli
EBB	electron beam boosts		etopside and carboplatin
	equal breath bilaterally		European Community
EBBS	equal bilateral breath sounds		extracellular
			eye care
EBC	esophageal balloon catheter		eyes closed
		E & C	education and counseling
EBCT	electron-beam computed tomography	ECA	enteric coated aspirin (tablets)
EBD	endocardial border delineation		Epidemiological Catchment Area
	endoscopic balloon dilation		ethacrynic acid
	evidence based decision (making)		external carotid artery
		ECASA	enteric coated aspirin (tablets)
EBE	equal bilateral expansion		
EBEA	Epstein-Barr (virus) early antigen	ECBD	exploration of common bile duct

ECC	edema, clubbing, and cyanosis	EC/IC	extracranial/intracranial
	embryonal cell cancer	ECID	European Centre for Infectious Disease
	emergency cardiac care	ECK1	*Escherichia coli* K1
	endocervical curettage	ECL	electrochemiluminescence
	estimated creatinine clearance		enterochromaffin-like
			extend of cerebral lesion
	external cardiac compression		extracapillary lesions
	extracorporeal circulation	ECM	erythema chronicum migrans
ECCE	extracapsular cataract extraction		extracellular mass
			extracellular matrix
ECCP	extracorporeal photophoresis	ECM/ BCM	extracellular mass, body cell mass ratio
ECD	endocardial cushion defect	ECMO	extracorporeal membrane oxygenation (oxygenator)
	equivalent current dipole		
ECDB	encourage to cough and deep breathe	ECN	extended care nursery
		ecNOS	endothelial constitutive nitric oxide synthetase
ECE	extracapsular extension		
ECEMG	evoked compound electromyography	ECochG	electrocochleography
		ECOG	Eastern Cooperative Oncology Group
ECF	epirubicin, cisplatin, and fluorouracil		
		ECoG	electrocochleography
	extended care facility		electrocorticogram
	extracellular fluid	E coli	*Escherichia coli*
ECF-A	eosinophil chemotactic factors of anaphylaxis	ECP	emergency contraceptive pills
ECG	electrocardiogram		extracorporeal photochemotherapy
ECHINO	echinocyte		
ECHO	echocardiogram		extracorporeal photopheresis
	enterocytopathogenic human orphan (virus)	ECPD	external counterpressure device
	etoposide, cyclophosphamide, doxorubicin (hydroxydaunomycin), and vincristine (Oncovin)	ECR	emergency chemical restraint
			extensor carpi radialis
		ECRB	extensor carpi radialis brevis
ECHO/ RV	echocardiography/ radionuclide ventriculography	ECRL	extensor carpi radialis longus
		ECS	electrocerebral silence
ECI	extracorporeal irradiation	ECT	electroconvulsive therapy
ECIB	extracorporeal irradiation of blood		emission computed tomography
ECIC	external carotid and internal carotid		enhanced computed tomography
	extracranial to intracranial (anastamosis)	ECU	electrocautery unit
			emotional care units

E

	environmental control unit	EDENT	edentulous
	extensor carpi ulnaris	EDF	elongation, derotation, and flexion
ECV	external cephalic version		
ECVE	extracellular volume expansion	EDH	epidural hematoma
		EDHF	endothelium-derived hyperpolarizing factor
ECW	extracellular water		
ED	education	EDI	Eating Disorders Inventory
	effective dose		
	elbow disarticulation	EDITAR	extended-duration topical arthropod repellent
	emergency department		
	emotional disorder	EDL	extensor digitorum longus
	epidural	ED/LD	emotionally disturbed and learning disabled
	erectile dysfunction		
	ethynodiol diacetate	EDLF	endogenous digitalis-like factors
	every day (this is a dangerous abbreviation)	EDLS	endogenous digitalis-like substance
	extensive disease		
ED$_{50}$	median effective dose	EDM	early diastolic murmur
EDA	elbow disarticulation		esophageal Doppler monitor
EDAM	edatrexate		
EDAP	Emergency Department Approved for Pediatrics	EDNO	endothelium-related nitric oxide
EDAS	encephalodural arterio-synangiosis	EDP	emergency department physician
EDAT	Emergency Department Alert Team		end-diastolic pressure
		EDQ	extensor digiti quinti (tendon)
EDAX	energy-dispersive analysis of x-rays		
		EDQV	extensor digiti quinti five
EDB	ethylene dibromide	EDR	edrophonium
	extensor digitorum brevis	EDRF	endothelium derived relaxing factor (nitric oxide)
EDC	effective dynamic compliance		
		EDS	Ehlers-Danlos syndrome
	electrodesiccation and curettage		excessive daytime somnolence
	end diastolic counts		
	estimated date of conception	EDSS	Expanded Disability Status Scale (Score)
		EDT	exposure duration threshold
	estimated date of confinement		
	extensor digitorium communis	EDTA	edetic acid (ethylenedi-aminetetraacetic acid)
EDCF	endothelium-derived constricting factor	EDTU	emergency diagnostic and treatment unit
EDCP	eccentric dynamic compression plates	EDU	eating disorder unit
		EDV	end-diastolic volume
EDD	esophageal detector device		epidermal dysplastic verruciformis
	expected date of delivery	EDW	estimated dry weight
		EDX	edatrexate

EE	emetic episodes	EFHBM	eosinophilic fibrohistiocytic lesion of bone marrow
	end to end		
	equine encephalitis	EFM	electronic fetal monitor(ing)
	ethinyl estradiol		
	external ear		external fetal monitoring
E & E	eyes and ears	EFMM	external fetal maternal monitor
EEA	electroencephalic audiometry		
	elemental enteral alimentation	EFMT	electric field mediated transfer
	end-to-end anastomosis	EFN	effusion
	energy expended with activity	EFW	estimated fetal weight
		EF/WM	ejection fraction/wall motion
EEC Syn-drome	ectrodactyly-ectodermal dysplasia, cleft syndrome	*e.g.*	for example
		EGA	esophageal gastric (tube) airway
EEE	eastern equine encephalomyelitis		estimated gestational age
	edema, erythema, and exudate	EGBUS	external genitalia, Bartholin, urethral, and Skene's glands
	external eye examination		
EEG	electroencephalogram	EGC	early gastric carcinoma
EEN	estimated energy needs	EGCG	epigallocatechin gallate
EENT	eyes, ears, nose, and throat	EGFR	epidermal growth factor receptor
EEP	end expiratory pressure	EGD	esophagogastroduodenoscopy
EER	extended endocardial resection	EGDT	esophagogastric devascularization and transection
EES®	erythromycin ethylsuccinate	EGF	epidermal growth factor
EET	early exercise testing	EGF-R	epidermal growth factor receptor
EEV	encircling endocardial ventriculotomy	EGG	electrogastrography
EF	eccentric fixation	EGJ	esophagogastric junction
	ejection fraction	EGL	eosinophilic granuloma of the lung
	endurance factor		
	erythroblastosis fetalis	EGS	ethylene glycol succinate
	extended-field (radiotherapy)	EGSs	external guide sequences
		EGTA	esophageal gastric tube airway
EFA	essential fatty acid		
EFAD	essential fatty acid deficiency		ethyleneglycoltetracetic acid
EFBW	estimate fetal body weight	EH	educationally handicapped
			enlarged heart
EFD	episode free day		essential hypertension
EFE	endocardial fibroelastosis		extramedullary hematopoiesis
EFF	effacement		
EFR	effective filtration rate	EHB	elevate head of bed
EFS	event-free survival		extensor hallucis brevis

E

EHBA	extrahepatic biliary atresia		end-inspiratory pressure
			extensor indicis proprius
EHBF	extrahepatic blood flow		
EHC	enterohepatic circulation	eIPV	enhanced inactivated polio vaccine
EHDA	etidronate sodium		
EHDP	etidronate disodium	EIR	entomological inoculation rate
EHE	epithelioid hemangioen-dothelioma		
		EIS	endoscopic injection scleropathy
EHEC	enterohemorrhagic *Escherichia coli*		
		EITB	enzyme-linked immunoelectrotransfer blot
EHF	epidemic hemorrhagic fever		
		EIV	external iliac vein
	extremely high frequency	EJ	ejection
EHH	esophageal hiatal hernia		elbow jerk
EHL	electrohydraulic lithotripsy		external jugular
		EJB	ectopic junctional beat
	extensor hallucis longus	EJN	extended jaundice of newborn
EHN	ethotoin		
EHO	extrahepatic obstruction	EJV	external jugular vein
EHPH	extrahepatic portal hypertension	EK	Ektachem 400 (analysis for potassium, carbon dioxide, chloride, glucose, and blood urea nitrogen)
EHS	employee health service		
EHT	electrohydrothermosation		
EI	environmental illness		
	enzyme immunoassay		
E/I	expiratory to inspiratory (ratio)		erythrokinase
		EKC	epidemic keratoconjunctivitis
E & I	endocrine and infertility		
EIA	enzyme immunoassay	EKG	electrocardiogram
	exercise induced asthma	EKO	echoencephalogram
EIAB	extracranial-intracranial arterial bypass	EKY	electrokymogram
		EL	exercise limit
EIB	exercise induced bronchospasm	E-L	external lids
		ELA	Establishment License Application
EIC	extensive intraductal component		
		ELAD	extracorporeal liver-assist device
EICA	extra-intracranial artery (bypass)		
		ELAFF	extended lateral arm free flap
EID	electroimmunodiffusion		
	electronic infusion device	ELAM	endothelial leukocyte adhesion molecule
EIDC	extreme intervertebral disk collapse		
		ELB	early light breakfast
EIEC	enteroinvasive *Escherichia coli*		elbow
		ELBW	extremely low birth weight (less then 1000 g)
EIL	elective induction of labor		
EIOA	excessive intake of alcohol		
		ELC	earlobe creases
EIP	elective interruption of pregnancy	ELCA	excimer laser coronary angioplasty

ELEC	elective		dactinomycin
ELF	elective low forceps		(actinomycin-D),
	endoscopic laser		cyclophosphamide, and
	foraminotomy		vincristine (Oncovin)
	epithelial lining fluid	EMB	endometrial biopsy
	etoposide, leucovorin, and		endomyocardial biopsy
	fluorouracil		ethambutol (Myambutol)
ELH	endolymphatic hydrops		Explanation of Medicare
ELI	endomyocardial		Benefits
	lymphocytic infiltrates	EMC	encephalomyocarditis
ELIG	eligible		endometrial currettage
ELISA	enzyme-linked		essential mixed
	immunosorbent assay		cryoglobulinemia
Elix	elixir	EMD	electromechanical
ELLIP	ellipotocytosis		dissociation
ELND	elective lymph node	EMDR	eye movement
	dissection		desensitization and
ELOP	estimated length of		reprocessing
	program	EME	extreme medical
ELOS	estimated length of stay		emergency
ELP	electrophoresis	EMEA	European Medicines
ELPS	excessive lateral pressure		Evaluations Agency
	syndrome	EMF	elective mid forceps
ELS	Eaton-Lambert syndrome		electromagnetic field(s)
ELSI	ethical, legal, and social		electromagnetic flow
	implications		endomyocardial fibrosis
ELSS	emergency life support		erythrocyte maturation
	system		factor
ELT	endoscopic laser therapy		evaporated milk formula
	euglobulin lysis time	EMG	electromyograph
ELVIS™	Enzyme Linked Virus		emergency
	Inducible System		essential monoclonal
EM	early memory		gammopathy
	ejection murmur	EMI	elderly and mentally
	electron microscope		infirm
	emergency medicine	EMIC	emergency maternity and
	emmetropia		infant care
	erythema migrans	E-MICR	electron microscopy
	erythema multiforme	EMIT	enzyme-multiplied
	esophageal manometry		immunoassay technique
	estramustine (Emcyt)		(test)
	extensive metabolizers	EMLA®	eutectic mixture of local
	external monitor		anesthetics (lidocaine
E & M	Evaluation and		and prilocaine in an
	Management (coding		emulsion base)
	system)	EMLB	erythromycin lactobionate
EMA	early morning awakening	EMMV	extended mandatory
	endomysial antibody		minute ventilation
EMA-CO	etoposide, methotrexate,	EMo	ear mold

E

EMP	electromolecular propulsion		erythema nodosum
	estramustine phosphate	E/N	eggnog
EMR	educable mentally retarded	E 50% N	extension 50% of normal
		ENA	extractable nuclear antigen
	electrical muscle stimulation	ENB	esthesioneuroblastoma
		ENC	encourage
	electronic medical record	ENDO	endodontia
	emergency mechanical restraint		endodontics
			endoscopy
	empty, measure, and record		endotracheal
		ENF	Enfamil®
	endoscopic mucosal resection	ENF c Fe	Enfamil® with iron
		ENG	electronystagmogram
	eye movement recording		engorged
EMS	early morning specimen	ENL	enlarged
	early morning stiffness		erythema nodosum leprosum
	electrical muscle stimulation	ENMG	electroneuromyography
	emergency medical services	ENOG	electroneurography
		ENP	extractable nucleoprotein
	eosinophilia myalgia syndrome	ENS	exogenous natural surfactant
EMSU	early morning specimen of urine	ENT	ears, nose, throat
		ENVD	elevated new vessels on the disk
EMT	emergency medical technician	ENVE	elevated new vessels elsewhere
	estramustine (Emcyt)	ENVT	environment
EMTA	Emergency Medical Technician, Advanced	EO	elbow orthosis
			embolic occlusion
EMTC	emergency medical trauma center		eosinophilia
			ethylene oxide
EMT-D	emergency medical technician-defibrillation		eyes open
EMTP	Emergency Medical Technician, Paramedic	EOA	erosive osteoarthritis
			esophageal obturator airway
EMU	early morning urine		examine, opinion, and advice
	electromagnetic unit		
	epilepsy monitoring unit		external oblique aponeurosis
EMV	equine morbilli virus	EOAE	evoked otoacoustic emissions
	eye, motor, verbal (grading for Glasgow Coma Scale)	EOB	edge of bed
			end of bed
EMVC	early mitral valve closure		explanation of benefits
EMW	electromagnetic waves	EOC	enema of choice
EN	enema		epithelial ovarian cancer
	enteral nutrition	EOD	end organ damage

	every other day (this is a dangerous abbreviation)	E-Panel	electrolyte panel (potassium, sodium, carbon dioxide, and chloride)
	extent of disease		
EOE	extraosseous Ewing's sarcoma	EPAP	expiratory positive airway pressure
EOFAD	early-onset form of familial Alzheimer's disease	EPB	extensor pollicis brevis
		EPC	erosive prephloric changes
E of I	evidence of insurability		external pneumatic compression
EOG	electro-oculogram		
	Ethrane, oxygen, and gas (nitrous oxide)	EPD	electrode placement device
EOL	end of file		equilibrium peritoneal dialysis
EOM	error of measurement		
	external otitis media	EPEC	enteropathogen *Escherichia coli*
	extraocular movement		
	extraocular muscles	EPEG	etoposide (VePesid)
EOMI	extraocular muscles intact	EPEs	extrapyramidal effects
		EPF	Enfamil Premature Formula®
EOO	external oculomotor ophthalmoplegia		
		EPG	electronic pupillography
EOP1	end-of-phase 1	EPI	echoplanar imaging
EOP2	end-of-phase 2		epinephrine
EOR	emergency operating room		epirubicin
			epitheloid cells
	end of range		exercise pressure index
EORA	elderly onset rheumatoid arthritis		exocrine pancreatic insufficiency
EORTC	European Organization for Research on the Treatment of Cancer	EPIC	etoposide, ifosfamide, and cisplatin (Platinol AQ)
EOS	end of study	EPID	epidural
	eosinophil	epiDX	epirubicin (4'-epidoxorubicin)
EP	ectopic pregnancy		
	electrophysiologic	EPIG	epigastric
	elopement precaution	EPIS	epileptic postictal sleep
	endogenous pyrogen		episiotomy
	Episcopal	epith.	epithelial
	esophageal pressure	EPL	effective patent life
	etoposide and cisplatin (Platinol AQ)		extensor pollicis longus (tendon)
	evoked potentials	EPM	electronic pacemaker
E&P	estrogen and progesterone	EPMR	electronic patient medical record
EPA	eicosapentaenoic acid		
	Environmental Protection Agency	EPN	estimated protein needs
		EPO	epoetin alfa (erythropoietin; Epogen)
EPAB	extracorporeal pneumoperititoneal access bubble		
			evening primrose oil

	exclusive provider organization		evoked response audiometry
EPOCH	etoposide, prednisone, vincristine (Oncovin), cyclophosphamide, doxorubicin (hydroxydaunorubicin)	%ERAD	eradication rates
		ERBD	endoscopic retrograde biliary drainage
		ER by ICA	estrogen receptor immunocytochemistry assay
EPP	erythropoietic protoporphyria		
EPR	electron paramagnetic (spin) resonance	ERC	endoscopic retrograde cholangiography
	electrophrenic respiration	ERCP	endoscopic retrograde cholangiopancreatography
	emergency physical restraint	ERCT	emergency room computerized tomography
	epirubicin		
	estimated protein requirement	ERD	early retirement with disability
EPS	electrophysiologic study	ERE	external rotation in extension
	expressed prostatic secretions	ERF	external rotation in flexion
	extrapulmonary shunt		
	extrapyramidal syndrome (symptom)	ERFC	erythrocyte rosette forming cells
EPSA	evoked potential signal averaging	ERG	electroretinogram
		ERL	effective refractory length
EPSCCA	extrapulmonary small cell carcinoma	ERLND	elective regional lymph node dissection
EPSDT	early periodic screening, diagnosis, and treatment	ERMS	exacerbating-remitting multiple sclerosis
EPSE	extrapyramidal side effects	ERNA	equilibrium radionuclide angiocardiography
EPSP	excitatory postsynaptic potential	ERP	effective refractory period
EPSS	E point septal separation		emergency room physician
EPT	electroporation therapy		endocardial resection procedure
	endpoint temperature		
EPT®	early pregnancy test		endoscopic retrograde pancreatography
EPTE	existed prior to enlistment		event-related potentials
EPTS	existed prior to service		
ER	emergency room		estrogen receptor protein
	estrogen receptors	ERPF	effective renal plasma flow
	extended release		
	extended external rotation	ER/PR	estrogen receptor/ progesterone receptor
	external resistance		
E & R	equal and reactive	ERS	endoscopic retrograde sphincterotomy
	examination and report		evacuation of retained secundines (afterbirth)
ER+	estrogen receptor-positive		
ERA	estrogen receptor assay		

ERSR	Electronic Regulatory Submission and Review	ESI-MS	electrospray ionization-mass spectrometry
ERT	estrogen replacement therapy	ESL	English as a second language
	external radiotherapy	ESLD	end-stage liver disease
ERTD	emergency room triage documentation		end-stage lung disease
		ESM	ejection systolic murmur
ERUS	endorectal ultrasound		endolymphatic stromal myosis
ERV	expiratory reserve volume		
ERYTH	erythromycin		ethosuximide
ES	electrical stimulation	ESN	educationally subnormal
	Eleutherococcus senticosus (Siberian Ginseng)	ESN(M)	educationally subnormal-moderate
		ESN(S)	educationally subnormal-severe
	emergency service	ESO	esophagus
	endoscopic sclerotherapy		esotropia
	endoscopic sphincterotomy	ESO/D	esotropia at distance
		ESO/N	estropia at near
	end-to-side	ESP	endometritis, salpingitis, and peritonitis
	Ewing's sarcoma		
	ex-smoker		end systolic pressure
	extra strength		especially
ESA	end-to-side anastomosis		extrasensory perception
	ethmoid sinus adenocarcinoma	ESR	erythrocyte sedimentation rate
ESADDI	estimated safe and adequate daily dietary intake	ESRD	end-stage renal disease
		ESRF	end-stage renal failure
ESAP	evoked sensory (nerve) action potential	ESS	emotional, spiritual, and social
ESAT	extrasystolic atrial tachycardia		endoscopic sinus surgery
			Epworth Sleepiness Scale
ESC	end systolic counts		essential
ESCS	electrical spinal cord stimulation		euthyroid sick syndrome
		EST	Eastern Standard Time
ESD	Emergency Services Department		endoscopic spincterotomy
			electroshock therapy
	esophagus, stomach, and duodenum		electrostimulation therapy
			established patient
ESF	external skeletal fixation		estimated
ESFT	Ewing's sarcoma family of tumors		exercise stress test
		E-stim	electrical stimulation
ESHAP	etopside, methylprednisolone (Solu-Medrol), high-dose cytarabine (ara-C), and cisplatin (Platinol AQ)	ESU	electrosurgical unit
		ESWL	extracorporeal shock wave lithotripsy
		ET	ejection time
			embryo transfer
			endometrial thickness
ESI	epidural steroid injection		endothelin

	endotoxin	ETO	estimated time of
	endotracheal		ovulation
	endotracheal tube		ethylene oxide
	enterostomal therapy		etoposide (VePesid)
	(therapist)		eustachian tube
	esotropia		obstruction
	essential thrombocythemia	ETOH	alcohol
	essential tremor		alcoholic
	eustachian tube	ETOP	elective termination of
	Ewing's tumor		pregnancy
	exchange transfusion	ETP	elective termination of
	exercise treadmill		pregnancy
et	and	ETS	elevated toilet seat
ET'	esotropia at near		endoscopic transthoracic
E(T)	intermittent esotropia at		sympathectomy
	infinity		endotracheal suction
E(T')	intermittent esotropia at		end-to-side
	near		environmental tobacco
ET @ 20'	esotropia at 6 meters		smoke
	(infinity)		erythromycin topical
ETA	endotracheal airway		solution
	ethionamide	ETT	endotracheal tube
et al	and others		esophageal transit time
ETC	and so forth		exercise tolerance test
	Emergency and Trauma		exercise treadmill test
	Center		extrathyroidal thyroxine
	estimated time of	ETT-Tl	exercise treadmill test
	conception		with thallium
ETCO$_2$	end tidal carbon dioxide	ETU	emergency and trauma
ETD	eustachian tube		unit
	dysfunction		emergency treatment unit
ETDLA	esophageal-tracheal	ETX	edatrexate
	double lumen airway	EU	Ehrlich units
ETE	end-to-end		equivalent units
ETEC	enterotoxigenic		esophageal ulcer
	Escherichia coli		etiology unknown
ETF	eustachian tubal		European Union
	function		excretory urography
ETH	elixir terpin hydrate	EUA	examine under anesthesia
	ethanol	EUCD	emotionally unstable
	Ethrane		character disorder
ETHc̄C	elixir terpin hydrate with	EUD	external urinary device
	codeine	EUG	extrauterine gestation
ETI	ejective time index	EUL	extra uterine life
	endotracheal intubation	EUM	external urethral meatus
ETKTM	every test known to	EUP	Experimental Use Permit
	man		extrauterine pregnancy
ETLE	extratemporal lobe	EUS	endoscopic
	epilepsy		ultrasonography

	external urethral sphincter		exercise
		exam.	examination
EV	epidermodysplasia verruciformis	EXEF	exercise ejection fraction
	esophageal varices	EXGBUS	external genitalia, Bartholin (glands), urethral (glands), and Skene (glands)
	etoposide and vincristine		
eV	electron volt (unit of radiation energy)		
EVA	Entry and Validation Application	EXH VT	exhaled tidal volume
		EXL	elixir
	ethylene vinyl acetate	EXOPH	exophthalmos
	etoposide, vinblastine, and doxorubicin (Adriamycin)	EXP	experienced
			expired
			exploration
EVAC	evacuation		expose
EVAc	ethylene-vinyl acetate copolymer	expect	expectorant
		exp. lap.	exploratory laparotomy
eval	evaluate	EXT	extension
EWB	emotional well-being		external
EXC	excision		extract
EVD	external ventricular (ventriculostomy) drain		extraction
			extremities
			extremity
EVE	evening	Ext mon	external monitor
EXEC 22	Executive 22 chemistry profile (see SMA-23)	extrav	extravasation
		ext. rot.	external rotation
EVER	eversion	EXTUB	extubation
EVG	endovascular grafting	EX U	excretory urogram
EVL	endoscopic variceal ligation	EZ	Edmonston-Zagreb (vaccine)
EVS	endoscopic variceal sclerosis	EZ-HT	Edmonston-Zagreb high-titer (vaccine)
EW	expiratory wheeze		
	elsewhere		
EWB	estrogen withdrawal bleeding		
EWCL	extended wear contact lens		
EWHO	elbow-wrist-hand orthosis		
EWL	estimated weight loss		
EWSCLs	extended-wear soft contact lenses		
EWT	erupted wisdom teeth		
ex	examined		
	example		
	excision		

E

F

F	facial	FAAN	Fellow of the American Academy of Nursing
	Fahrenheit	FAAP	Fellow of the American Academy of Pediatrics
	fair	FAB	digoxin immune Fab (Digibind®)
	false		French-American-British Cooperative group
	fasting		functional arm brace
	father	FABER	flexion, abduction, and external rotation
	feces	FABF	femoral artery blood flow
	female	FAC	fluorouracil doxorubicin (Adriamycin), and cyclophosphamide
	finger		
	firm		
	flow		fractional area concentration
	fluoride		functional aerobic capacity
	French		
	fundi	FACA	Fellow of the American College of Anaesthetists
	fundus		
F/	full upper denture	FACAG	Fellow of the American College of Angiology
/F	full lower denture		
(F)	final	FACAL	Fellow of the American College of Allergists
°F	degrees Fahrenheit		
F=	firm and equal	FACAN	Fellow of the American College of Anesthesiologists
F_1	offspring from the first generation		
F_2	offspring from the second generation	FACAS	Fellow of the American College of Abdominal Surgeons
F_3	Fluothane		
14 F	14-hour fast required	FACC	Fellow of the American College of Cardiology
F II–F XIII	factor 2 through 13		
FA	fatty acid	FACCP	Fellow of the American College of Chest Physicians
	femoral artery		
	fetus active		
	first aid	FACCPC	Fellow of the American College of Clinical Pharmacology & Chemotherapy
	fluorescein angiogram		
	fluorescent antibody		
	folic acid		
	forearm	FACD	Fellow of the American College of Dentists
	functional activities		
FAA	febrile antigen agglutination	FACEM	Fellow of the American College of Emergency Medicine
	folic acid antagonist		
FAAP	family assessment adjustment pass	FACEP	Fellow of the American College of Emergency Physicians
FAA SOL	formalin, acetic, and alcohol solution	FACGE	Fellow of the American

	College of Gastroenterology	FAGA	full-term appropriate for gestational age
FACH	forceps to after-coming head	FAH	fumarylacetoacetase hydrolase
FACLM	Fellow of the American College of Legal Medicine	FAI	Functional Assessment Inventory
FACN	Fellow of the American College of Nutrition	FAK	focal adhesion kinase
		FAL	femoral arterial line
		FALL	fallopian
FACNP	Fellow of the American College of Neuro-psychopharmacology	FALS	familial amyotrophic lateral sclerosis
		FAM	family
FACOG	Fellow of the American College of Obstetricians & Gynecologists		fluorouracil, doxorubicin (Adriamycin®), and mitomycin
FACOS	Fellow of the American College of Orthopedic Surgeons	FAMA	fluorescent antibody to membrane antigen
		FAME	fluorouracil, doxorubicin (Adriamycin), and semustin (methyl CCNU)
FACP	Fellow of the American College of Physicians
FACPRM	Fellow of the American College of Preventive Medicine
FACR	Fellow of the American College of Radiologists	FAM-S	fluorouracil, doxorubicin (Adriamycin), mitomycin, and streptozotocin
FACS	Fellow of the American College of Surgeons fluorescent-activated cell sorter	FAMTX	fluorouracil, doxorubicin (Adriamycin), and methotrexate
FACSM	Fellow of the American College of Sports Medicine	FANA	fluorescent antinuclear antibody
		FANG	fluorescent angiography
FACT	focused appendix computed tomography	FANSS&M	fundus anterior, normal size and shape and mobile
FACT-An	Functional Assessment of Cancer Therapy–Anemia	FAP	familial adenomatous polyposis familial amyloid polyneuropathy femoral artery pressure fibrillating action potential
FACT-B	....–Breast
FACT-F	....–Fatigue
FACT-L	....–Lung
FAD	familial Alzheimer's disease
	Family Assessment Device	FAQ	frequently asked question(s)
	fetal abdominal diameter	F-ara-A	fludarabine phosphate
	fetal activity determination	FAS	fetal alcohol syndrome
	flavin adenine dinucleotide	FASC	fasciculations
		FASHP	Fellow of the American Society of Health-System Pharmacists
FAE	fetal alcohol effect

F

FAST	fetal acoustic stimulation testing		fever, chills
	fluorescent allergosorbent technique		financial class
			finger clubbing
FAT	Fetal Activity Test		finger counting
	fluorescent antibody test		flexion contractor
	food awareness training		flucytosine (Ancobon)
FAV	facio-auricular vertebral		foam cuffed (tracheal or endotracheal tube)
FAZ	foveal avascular zone		Foley catheter
FB	fasting blood (sugar)		follows commands
	finger breadth		foster care
	flexible bronchoscope		functional capacity
	foreign body		functional class
F/B	followed by	5FC	flucytosine (this is a dangerous abbreviation as it can look like 5FU)
	forward/backward		
	forward bending		
FBC	full (complete) blood count	F + C	flare and cells
		F & C	foam and condom
FBCOD	foreign body, cornea, right eye	F. cath.	Foley catheter
		FCBD	fibrocystic breast disease
FBCOS	foreign body, cornea, left eye	FCC	familial colonic cancer
			family centered care
FBD	fibrocystic breast disease		femoral cerebral catheter
	functional bowel disease		follicular center cells
FBF	forearm blood flow		fracture compound comminuted
FBG	fasting blood glucose		
	foreign-body-type granulomata	FCCA	Final Comprehensive Consensus Assessment
FBH	hydroxybutyric dehydrogenase	FCCC	fracture complete, compound, and comminuted
FBI	flossing, brushing, and irrigation		
	full bony impaction	FCCL	follicular center cell lymphoma
FBL	fecal blood loss	FCCU	family centered care unit
FBM	felbamate (Felbatol)		
	fetal breathing motion	FCD	feces collection device
	foreign body, metallic		fibrocystic disease
FBRCM	fingerbreadth below right costal margin	FCDB	fibrocystic disease of the breast
FBS	failed back syndrome	FCE	fluorouracil, cisplatin, and etoposide
	fasting blood sugar		
	fetal bovine serum		functional capacity evaluation
	foreign body sensation (eye)	FCFD	fluorescence capillary-fill device
FBU	fingers below umbilicus		
FBW	fasting blood work	FCH	familial combined hyperlipidemia
FC	family conference		
	febrile convulsion		fibrosing cholestatic hepatitis
	female child		

FCHL	familial combined hyperlipemia		fluorine-18-labeled deoxyglucose ([18]fluorodeoxyglucose)
FCL	fibular collateral ligament		
F-CL	fluorouracil and calcium leucovorin	FDGB	fall down, go boom
		FDG-PET	positron emission tomography with [18]fluorodeoxyglucose
FCM	flow cytometry		
FCMC	family centered maternity care		
		FDGS	feedings
FCMD	Fukiyama's congenital muscular dystrophy	FDIU	fetal death in utero
		FDL	flexor digitorum longus
FCMN	family centered maternity nursing	FDLMP	first day of last menstrual period
F/C/N/V	fever, cough, nausea, and vomiting	FDM	fetus of diabetic mother
			flexor digiti minimi
FCOU	finger count, both eyes	FDP	fibrin-degradation products
FCP	formocresol pulpotomu		
FCR	flexor carpi radialis		fixed-dose procedure
	fractional catabolic rate		flexor digitorum profundus
FCRB	flexor carpi radialis brevis		
FCRT	fetal cardiac reactivity test	FDQB	flexor digiti quinti brevis
FCS	fever, chills, and sweating	FDR	first-dose reaction
FCSNVD	fever, chills, sweating, nausea, vomiting, and diarrhea	FDS	flexor digitorum superficialis
			for duration of stay
FCU	flexor carpi ulnaris (tendon)	FDT	fronto-dextra transversa (right frontotransverse)
FCV	feline calicivirus	Fe	female
FD	familial dysautonomia		iron
	fetal demise	FEB	febrile
	fetal distress	FEC	fluorouracil, etoposide, and cisplatin
	focal distance		
	forceps delivery		forced expiratory capacity
	free drain	FECG	fetal electrocardiogram
	full denture	FeCh	ferrochelatase
	fully dilated	FECP	free erythrocyte coproporphyrin
F & D	fixed and dilated		
FDA	Food and Drug Administration	FECT	fibroelastic connective tissue
	fronto-dextra anterior	FED	fish eye disease
FDB	first-degree burn	FEES	fiberoptic endoscopic evaluation of swallowing
	flexor digitorum brevis		
FDBL	fecal daily blood loss		
FDCA	Food, Drug, and Cosmetic Act	FEF	forced expiratory flow rate
FDCs	follicular dendritic cells	$FEF_{25\%-75\%}$	forced expiratory flow during the middle half of the forced vital capacity
FDE	fixed-drug eruption		
FDF	flexor digitorum profundus (tendon)		
		FEF_{x-y}	forced expiratory flow
FDG	feeding		

	between two designated volume points in the forced vital capacity		in one second as percent of forced vital capacity
FEHBP	Federal Employee Health Benefits Plan	FEVR	familial exudative vitreoretinopathy
FEL	familial erythrophagocytic lymphohistiocytosis	FF	fat free
			fecal frequency
FeLV	feline leukemia virus		filtration fraction
FEM	femoral		finger to finger
FEM-FEM	femoral femoral (bypass)		flat feet
FEM-POP	femoral popliteal (bypass)		force fluids
FEM-TIB	femoral tibial (bypass)		forward flexion
FERGs	focal electroretinograms		foster father
FEN	fluid, electrolytes, and nutrition		fundus firm
			further flexion
FENa	fractional extraction of sodium	F/F	face to face
		F&F	fixes and follows
FEN-PHEN	fenfluramine and phentermine	F→F	finger to finger
		FF1/U	fundus firm 1 cm above umbilicus
FENS	field-electrical neural stimulation	FF2/U	fundus firm 2 cm above umbilicus
FEOM	full extraocular movements	FF@u	fundus firm at umbilicus
FEP	free erythrocyte porphyrins	FFA	free fatty acid
			fundus fluorescein angiogram
	free erythrocyte protoporphorin	FFAT	Free Floating Anxiety Test
FER	flexion, extension, and rotation	FFB	flexible fiberoptic bronchoscopy
FES	fat embolism syndrome	FFD	fat-free diet
	forced expiratory spirogram		focal-film distance
	functional electrical stimulation	FFDM	freedom from distant metastases
FeSO₄	ferrous sulfate	FFE	free-flow electrophoresis
FESS	functional endonasal sinus surgery	FFI	fast food intake
			fatal familial insomnia
	functional endoscopic sinus surgery	FFM	fat-free mass
			five finger movement
FET	fixed erythrocyte turnover		freedom from metastases
FETI	fluorescence (fluorescent) energy transfer immunoassay	FFP	free from progression
			fresh frozen plasma
		FFROM	full, free range of motion
FEUO	for external use only	FFS	failure-free survival
FEV	familial exudative vitreoretinopathy		fee-for-service
			Fight For Sight
FEV₁	forced expiratory volume in one second		flexible fiberoptic sigmoidoscopy
FEV₁%VC	forced expiratory volume	FFT	fast-Fourier transforms

	flicker fusion threshold	FHVP	free hepatic vein pressure
FFTP	first full-term pregnancy	FHx	family history
FFU/1	fundus firm 1 cm below umbilicus	FIA	familial intracranial aneurysms
FFU/2	fundus firm 2 cm below umbilicus		Family Independence Agency (formerly Department of Social Services)
FG	fibrin glue		
FGC	full gold crown		
FGF	fibroblast growth factor	FIAC	fiacitabine
FGP	fundic gland polyps	FIAU	fialuridine
FGS	fibrogastroscopy	FIB	fibrillation
	focal glomerulosclerosis		fibula
FH	familial hypercholester-olemia	FICA	Federal Insurance Contributions Act (Social Security)
	family history		
	favorable histology	FiCO$_2$	fraction of inspired carbon dioxide
	fetal head		
	fetal heart	FICS	Fellow of the International College of Surgeons
	fundal height		
FH+	family history positive		
FH−	family history negative	FID	father in delivery
FHA	filamentous hemagglutinin		free induction decay
FHB	flexor hallucis brevis	FIF	forced inspiratory flow
FHC	familial hypertrophic cardiomyopathy	FIGLU	formiminoglutamic acid
	family health center	FIGO	International Federation of Gynecology and Obstetrics
FHCIC	Fuchs' heterochromic iridocyclitis		
FHD	family history of diabetes	FIL	father-in-law
FHF	fulminant hepatic failure		Filipino
FHH	familial hypocalciuric hypercalcemia	FIM	functional independence measure
	fetal heart heard	FIN	flexible intramedullary nail
FHI	frontal horn index		
	Fuch's heterochromic iridocyclitis	FIND	follow-up intervention for normal development
FHL	flexor hallucis longus	FiO$_2$	fraction of inspired oxygen
FHM	familial hemiplegic migraine	FIP	feline infectious peritonitis
FHN	family history negative		
FHNH	fetal heart not heard		flatus in progress
FHO	family history of obesity	FIRI	fasting insulin resistance index
FHP	family history positive		
FHR	fetal heart rate	FISH	fluorescent (fluorescence) in situ hybridization
FHRB	fetal heart rate baseline		
FHRV	fetal heart rate variability	FISP	fast imaging with steady state precision
FHS	fetal heart sounds		
	fetal hydantoin syndrome	FITC	fluorescein isothiocyanate conjugated
FHT	fetal heart tone		

F

FIV	feline immunodeficiency virus		flutamide and leuprolide acetate depot
FIVC	forced inspiratory vital capacity		full lower denture
		FL Dtr	full lower denture
FIX	factor IX (nine)	FLE	frontal lobe epilepsy
FJB	facet joint block	FLe	fluorouracil and levamisole
FJN	familial juvenile nephrophthisis	flexsig	flexible sigmoidoscopy
FJP	familial juvenile polyposis	FLF	funny looking facies (see note under FLK)
FJROM	full joint range of motion		
FJS	finger joint size	FLGA	full-term, large for gestational age
FK506	tacrolimus (Prograf)		
FKA	formally known as	FLIC	Functional Living Index–Cancer
FKBP	FK-506 binding protein (tacrolimus)	FLIE	Functional Living Index—Emesis
FKD	Kinetic Family Drawing		
FKE	full knee extension	FLK	funny looking kid (should never be used: unusual facial features, is a better expression)
FL	fatty liver		
	femur length		
	fetal length		
	fluid	FLM	fetal lung maturity
	fluorescein	fl. oz.	fluid ounce
	flutamide and leuprolide acetate	FLP	fasting lipid profile
		FL REST	fluid restriction
	focal length	FLS	flashing lights and/or scotoma
	full liquids		
fL	femtoliter (10^{-15} liter)	FLT	fluorothymidine
F/L	father-in-law	FLU	fluconazole (Diflucan)
FLA	free-living amebic (ameba)		fludarabine (Fludara)
			flunisolide (Aero Bid)
	low-friction arthroplasty		fluoxetine (Prozac)
FLAIR	fluid attenuated inversion recovery		fluticasone propionate (Flonase)
			influenza
FLAP	fluorouracil, leucovorin, doxorubicin (Adriamycin), and cisplatin (Platinol AQ)	FLU A	influenza A virus
		FLUO	Fluothane
		fluoro	fluoroscopy
		FLUT	flutamide (Eulexin)
	5-lipoxygenase activating protein	FLV	Friend leukemia virus
		FLW	fasting laboratory work
FLASH	fast low-angle shot		
FLAVO	flavopiridol	FLZ	flurazepam (Dalmane)
FLB	funny looking beat	FM	face mask
FLBS	funny looking baby syndrome (see note under FLK)		fat mass
			fetal movements
			fine motor
FLC	follicular large cell lymphoma		floor manager
			fluorescent microscopy
FLD	fatty liver disease		foster mother
	fluid		

F & M	firm and midline (uterus)	FMX	full mouth x-ray
F-MACHOP	fluorouracil, methotrexate, cytarabine (ara-C), cyclophosphamide, doxorubicin (hydroxydaunorubicin), vincristine (Oncovin), and prednisone	FMZ	flumazenil (Romazicon)
		FN	facial nerve
			false negative
			febrile neutropenia
			finger-to-nose
			flight nurse
FMC	fetal movement count	F/N	fluids and nutrition
FMD	family medical doctor	F to N	finger to nose
	fibromuscular dysplasia	FNA	fine-needle aspiration
	foot and mouth disease	FNa	filtered sodium
FME	full mouth extraction	FNAB	fine-needle aspiration biopsy
FMF	familial Mediterranean fever	FNAC	fine-needle aspiratory cytology
	fetal movement felt	FNB	femoral nerve block
	forced midexpiratory flow	FNCJ	fine needle catheter jejunostomy
FMG	fine mesh gauze	FNF	femoral-neck fracture
	foreign medical graduate		finger nose finger
FMH	family medical history	FNH	focal nodular hyperplasia
	fibromuscular hyperplasia	FNHL	follicular non-Hodgkin's lymphoma
FmHx	family history		
FML®	fluorometholone	FNP	Family Nurse Practitioner
FMN	first malignant neoplasm	FNR	false negative rate
	flavin mononucleotide	FNS	food and nutrition services
FMOL	femtomole		functional neuromuscular stimulation
FMP	fasting metabolic panel		
	first menstrual period	F/NS	fever and night sweats
FMPA	full mouth periapicals	FNT	finger to nose test
FMR	fetal movement record	FNTC	fine needle transhepatic cholangiography
	focused medical review		
	functional magnetic resonance (imaging)	FO	foot orthosis
			foramen ovale
FMRD	full mouth restorative dentistry		foreign object
			fronto-occipital
fMRI	functional magnetic resonance imaging	FOB	father of baby
			fecal occult blood
FMS	fibromyalgia syndrome		feet out of bed
	fluorouracil, mitomycin, and streptozocin		fiberoptic bronchoscope
			foot of bed
	full mouth series	FOBT	fecal occult blood test
FMT	functional muscle test	FOC	father of child
FMTC	familial medullary thyroid carcinoma		fluid of choice
			fronto-occipital circumference
FMU	first morning urine		
FMV	fluorouracil, semustine (methyl-CCNU), and vincristine	FOD	fixing right eye
			free of disease
		FOEB	feet over edge of bed

F

FOG	Fluothane, oxygen and gas (nitrous oxide)	FPAL	full term, premature, abortion, living
	full-on gain	FPB	femoral-popliteal bypass
FOH	family ocular history		flexor pollicis brevis
FOI	flight of ideas	FPC	familial polyposis coli
FOIA	Freedom of Information Act		family practice center
		FPD	feto-pelvic disproportion
FOID	fear of impending doom		fixed partial denture
		FPDL	flashlamp-pumped pulsed dye laser
FOM	floor of mouth		
FOMi	fluorouracil, Oncovin, (vincristine), and mitomycin	FPE	first-pass effect
		FPG	fasting plasma glucose
		FPHx	family psychiatric history
FONSI	finding of no significant impact	FPIA	fluorescence-polarization immunoassay
FOOB	fell out of bed	FPL	flexor pollicis longus (tendon)
FOOSH	fell on outstretched hand		
FOP	fibrodysplasia ossificans progressiva		final printed labeling
		FPM	full passive movements
FOPS	fiberoptic proctosigmoid-oscopy	FPNA	first-pass nuclear angiocardiography
FORMIL	foreign military	FPOR	follicle puncture for oocyte retrieval
FOS	fiberoptic sigmoidoscopy		
	fixing left eye	FPU	family participation unit
	fosphenytoin (Cerebyx)	FPZ	fluphenazine
	future order screen	FPZ-D	fluphenazine decanoate
FOSC	freestanding outpatient surgery center	FQ	fluoroquinolones
		FR	fair
FOT	form of thought		father
	frontal outflow tract		Father (priest)
FOV	field of view		Federal Register
FOVI	field of vision intact		flow rate
FOW	fenestration of oval window		fluid restriction
			fluid retention
FP	fall precautions		fractional reabsorption
	false positive		frequent relapses
	familial porencephaly		Friends
	family planning		frothy
	family practice		full range
	family practitioner	F & R	force and rhythm (pulse)
	fibrous proliferation	FRA	fluorescent rabies antibody
	flat plate		
	fluorescence polarization	FRAC	fracture
	fluticasone propionate	FRACTS	fractional urines
	food poisoning	FRAG	fragment
	frozen plasma	FRAG-X	Fragile X Syndrome
F/P	fluid/plasma (ratio)	FRAP	Family risk assessment program
F-P	femoral popliteal		
fpA	fibrinopeptide A	FRC	frozen red cells

	functional residual capacity	FSALT	Fletcher suite after loading tandem
FRCPC	Fellow of the Royal College of Physicians of Canada	FSB	fetal scalp blood full spine board
		FSBG	fingerstick blood glucose
FRCPE	Fellow of the Royal College of Physicians of Edinburgh	FSBM	full strength breast milk
		FSBS	fingerstick blood sugar
		FSC	Fatigue Symptom Checklist
FRCSC	Fellow of the Royal College of Surgeons of Canada		flexible sigmoidoscopy
			fracture, simple, and comminuted
FRCSE	Fellow of the Royal College of Surgeons of Edinburgh		fracture, simple and complete
FRCSI	Fellow of the Royal College of Surgeons of Ireland	FSCC	fracture, simple, complete, and comminuted
		FSD	focal-skin distance
FRE	flow-related enhancement		fracture, simple and depressed
FRF	filtration replacement fluid	FSE	fast spin-echo
			fetal scalp electrode
FRJM	full range of joint movement	FSF	fibrin stabilizing factor
FRNT	focus-reduction neutralization test	FSG	fasting serum glucose
			focal and segmental glomerulosclerosis
FROA	full range of affect	FSGA	full-term, small for gestational age
FROM	full range of motion		
FROMAJE	functioning, reasoning, orientation, memory, arithmetic, judgment, and emotion (mental status evaluation)	FSGN	focal segmental glomerulonephritis
		FSGS	focal segmental glomerulosclerosis
		FSH	facioscapulohumeral follicle-stimulating hormone
FRP	follicle regulatory protein	FSHMD	facioscapulohumeral muscular dystrophy
	functional refractory period	FSIQ	Full-Scale Intelligence Quotient (part of Wechsler test)
FS	fetoscope		
	fibromyalgia syndrome	FSL	fasting serum level
	fingerstick	FSM	functional status measures
	flexible sigmoidoscopy		
	foreskin	F-SM/C	fungus, smear and culture
	fractional shortenings	FSME	Frühsommer-meningoencephalitis
	frozen section		
	full strength	FSO	for screws only (prosthetic cups)
	functional status		
F & S	full and soft		
FSA	Family Services Association	FSOP	French Society of Pediatric Oncology
FSALO	Fletcher suite after loading ovoids		

F

117

FSP	fibrin split products	F TIP	finger tip
FSR	fractionated stereotactic radiosurgery	FTIUP	full-term intrauterine pregnancy
	fusiform skin revision	FTKA	failed to keep appointment
FSS	fetal scalp sampling	FTLB	full-term living birth
	French steel sound (dilated to #24FSS)	FTLFC	full-term living female child
	frequency-selective saturation	FTLMC	full-term living male child
	full scale score	FTM	fluid thioglycollate medium
FSW	feet of sea water (pressure)	FTN	finger-to-nose
			full-term nursery
	field service worker	FTNB	full-term newborn
FT	family therapy	FTND	Fagerstrom Test for Nicotine Dependence
	feeding tube		
	filling time		full-term normal delivery
	finger tip	FTNSD	full-term, normal, spontaneous delivery
	flexor tendon		
	fluidotherapy	FTO	full-time occlusion (eye patch)
	follow through		
	foot (ft)	FTP	failure to progress
	free testosterone		full-term pregnancy
	full term	FTR	father
F_3T	trifluridine		failed to report
FT_3	free triiodothyronine		failed to respond
FT_4	free thyroxine		for the record
FT_4I	free thyroxine index	FTRAM	free transverse rectus abdominis myocutaneous (flap)
FTA	fluorescent titer antibody		
	fluorescent treponemal antibody		
		FTSD	full-term spontaneous delivery
FTB	fingertip blood		
FTBD	full-term born dead	FTSG	full-thickness skin graft
FTBI	fractionated total body irradiation	FTT	failure to thrive
			fetal tissue transplant
FTC	frames to come	Ftube	feeding tube
	full to confrontation	FTUPLD	full-term uncomplicated pregnancy, labor, and delivery
FTD	failure to descend		
	frontotemporal dementia		
	full-term delivery	FTV	functional trial visit
FTE	failure to engraft	FTW	failure to wean
FTEs	full-time equivalents	FU	fraction unbound
FTF	finger-to-finger		fluorouracil
	free thyroxine fraction	F & U	flanks and upper quadrants
FTFTN	finger-to-finger-to-nose		
FTG	full thickness graft	F/U	follow-up
FTI	farnesyl (protein) transferase inhibitor		fundus at umbilicus
		F↑U	fingers above umbilicus
	force-time integral	F↓U	fingers below umbilicus
	free thyroxine index	5-FU	fluorouracil

FUB	function uterine bleeding	Fx	fractional urine
FUCO	fractional uptake of carbon monoxide		fracture
		Fx-BB	fracture both bones
FUD	fear, uncertainty, and doubt	Fx-dis	fracture-dislocation
		F XI	Factor XI (eleven)
	full upper denture	FXN	function
FUDR®	floxuridine	FXR	fracture
FU Dtr	full upper denture	FYC	facultative yeast carrier
FUFA	fluorouracil and leucovorin (folinic acid)	FYI	for your information
		FZ	flutamide and goserelin acetate (Zoladex®)
FU/FL	full upper denture, full lower denture	FZRC	frozen red (blood) cells
FULG	fulguration		
5FU/LV	fluorouracil and leucovorin		
FUN	follow-up note		
FUNG-C	fungus culture		
FUNG-S	fungus smear		
FUO	fever of undetermined origin		
FUOV	follow-up office visit		
FU/LP	full upper denture, partial lower denture		
FUP	follow-up		
FUS	fusion		
FUV	follow-up visit		
FV	femoral vein		
FVC	false vocal cord(s)		
	forced vital capacity		
FVFR	filled voiding flow rate		
FVH	focal vascular headache		
F VIII	factor VIII (eight)		
FVL	femoral vein ligation		
	flow volume loop		
FVR	feline viral rhinotracheitis		
	forearm vascular resistance		
FW	fetal weight		
F/W	followed with		
F waves	fibrillatory waves		
	flutter waves		
FWB	full weight bearing		
	functional well-being		
FWD	fairly well developed		
FWHM	full width at half maximum		
FWS	fetal warfarin syndrome		
FWW	front wheel walker		

F

G

G	gallop
	gastrostomy
	gauge
	gavage feeding
	gingiva
	good
	grade
	gram (g)
	gravida
	guaiac
	guanine
G +	gram-positive
	guaiac positive
G −	gram-negative
	guaiac negative
↑g	increasing
↓g	decreasing
G1–4	grade 1–4
G-11	hexachlorophene
GA	Gamblers Anonymous
	gastric analysis
	general anesthesia
	general appearance
	gestational age
	ginger ale
	glycyrrhetinic acid
	granuloma annulare
	glucose/acetone
Ga	gallium
67Ga	gallium citrate Ga 67
GABA	gamma-aminobutyric acid
GABHS	group A beta hemolytic streptococci
GAD	generalized anxiety disorder
	glutamic acid decarboxylase
GAF	geographic adjustment factors
	Global Assessment of Functioning (scale)
GAG	glycosaminoglycan

GAL	galanthamine hydrobromide
	gallon
G'ale	ginger ale
GALI-PUT	galactose-1-phosphate uridye transferase enzyme
GALT	gut-associated lymphoid tissue
GAMT	guanidinoacetate methyltransferase
GAO	General Accounting Office
GAP	GTPase activating protein
GAR	gonnococcal antibody reaction
GARFT	glycinamide ribonucleotide formyl transferase
GAS	general adaption syndrome
	ginseng-abuse syndrome
	Glasgow Assessment Schedule
	Global Assessment Scale
	group A streptococci
Gas Anal F&T	gastric analysis, free and total
Ga scan	gallium scan
Gastroc	gastrocnemius
GAT	geriatric assessment team
	group adjustment therapy
GATB	General Aptitude Test Battery
GAU	geriatric assessment unit
Gaw	airway conductance
GB	gallbladder
	Ginkgo biloba
	Guillain-Barré (syndrome)
G & B	good and bad
GBA	gingivobuccoaxial
	ganglionic-blocking agent
GBBS	group B beta hemolytic streptococcus
GBE	*Ginkgo biloba* extract
GBG	gonadal-steroid binding globulin

GBH	gamma benzene hexachloride (lindane)	GCS	Glasgow Coma Scale
GBIA	Guthrie bacterial inhibition assay	G-CSF	filgrastrim (granulocyte colony-stimulating factor)
GBM	glioblastoma multiforme glomerular basement membrane	GCST	Gibson-Cooke sweat test
		GCT	general care and treatment
GBMI	guilty but mentally ill		germ cell tumor
GBP	gabapentin (Neurontin)		giant cell tumor
	gastric bypass		granulosa cell tumor
	gated blood pool (imaging)	GCU	gonococcal urethritis
		GCV	ganciclovir (Cytovene)
GBPS	gated blood pool scan		great cardiac vein
GBR	good blood return	GCVF	great cardiac vein flow
GBS	gallbladder series	GD	generalized delays
	gastric bypass surgery		gestational diabetes
	group B streptococci		good
	Guillain-Barré syndrome		gravely disabled
GBW	generalized body weakness		Graves' disease
		Gd	gadolinium
GBX	gall bladder extraction (cholecystectomy)	G & D	growth and development
		GDA	gastroduodenal artery
GC	gas chromatography	GDB	Guide Dogs for the Blind
	geriatric chair (Gerichair®)	Gd-BOPTA	gadolinium benzyloxypropionic tetra acetate
	gingival curettage		
	gonococci (gonorrhea)	GDC	Guglielmi detachable coil
	good condition	Gd-DTPA	gadopentetate (Magnevist)
	graham crackers	Gd-DTPA-BMA	gadodiamide
G−C	gram-negative cocci		
G+C	gram-positive cocci	GD FA	grandfather
GCA	giant cell arteritis	GDH	glutamic dehydrogenase
GCBP	gated cardiac blood pool	Gd-HPD03A	gadoteridol
GCC	guanylyl cyclase C		
GCE	general conditioning exercise	g/dl	grams per deciliter
		GDM	gestational diabetes mellitus
GCDFP	gross cystic disease fluid protein	GDM A-1	gestational diabetes mellitus, insulin controlled, Type I
GCI	General Cognitive Index		
GCIIS	glucose control insulin infusion system	GDM A-2	gestational diabetes mellitus, diet controlled, Type II
GCM	good central maintained		
GCMD	generalized cardiovascular metabolic disease	GDNF	glial-derived neurotrophic factor
		GDP	gel diffusion precipitin
GC-MS	gas chromatography-mass spectroscopy	GD MO	grandmother
		GDS	Global Deterioration Scale
GCP	good clinical practices		
GCR	gastrocolonic response glucocerebrosidase		

G

GE	gainfully employed	GFR	glomerular filtration rate
	gastric emptying		grunting, flaring, and retractions
	gastroenteritis		
	gastroesophageal		
GEA	gastroepiploic artery	GFS	glaucoma filtering surgery
GEC	galactose elimination capacity	GG	gamma globulin
GED	General Educational Development (Test)		guaifenesin (glyceryl guaiacolate)
GEE	Global Evaluation of Efficacy	G=G	grips equal and good
	glycine ethyl ester	GGE	Gastrografin enema
	graft-enteric erosion		generalized glandular enlargement
GEF	graft-enteric fistula	GGS	glands, goiter, and stiffness
GEJ	gastroesophageal junction		
GEM	gemcitabine (Gemzar)		group G streptococci
	gemfibrozil (Lopid)	GGT	gamma-glutamyl-transferase
GEMU	geriatric evaluation and management unit	GGTP	gamma-glutamyl-transpeptidase
GEN	genital	GH	general health
GEN/ ENDO	general anesthesia with endotracheal intubation		genetic hemochromatosis
GENT	gentamicin		gingival hyperplasia
GENTA/P	gentamicin-peak		glenohumeral
GENTA/T	gentamicin-trough		good health
GEP	gastroenteropancreatic		growth hormone
GEQ	generic equiavalent	GH₃	Gerovital
GER	gastroesophageal reflux	GHAA	Group Health Association of America
GERD	gastroesophageal reflux disease	GHB	gamma hydroxybutyrate
GES	gastric emptying scan	GHb	glycosylated hemoglobin
GET	gastric emptying time	GHD	growth hormone deficiency
	graded exercise test		
GET 1/2	gastric emptying half-time	GHDA	growth hormone deficiency (syndrome) in adults
GETA	general endotracheal anesthesia		
GEU	geriatric evaluation unit	GHJ	glenohumeral joint
GF	gastric fistula	G-H jt	glenohumeral joint
	gluten free	GHP(S)	gated heart pool (scan)
	grandfather	GHQ	General Health Questionnaire
GFAP	glial fibrillary acid protein		
GF-BAO	gastric fluid, basal acid output	GHRF	growth hormone releasing factor
GFCL	Goldmann fundus contact lens	GI	gastrointestinal
			granuloma inguinale
GFD	gluten-free diet	GIB	gastric ileal bypass
GFJ	grapefruit juice		gastrointestinal bleeding
GFM	good fetal movement	GIC	general immunocompe-
GFP	green-fluorescing protein		tence

GID	gastrointestinal distress		Good Laboratory Practice
	gender identity disorder		(Principles of)
GIDA	Gastrointestinal		group-living program
	Diagnostic Area	GLP-1	glucagon-like peptide-1
GIFD #3	colonoscope	GLR	gravity lumbar reduction
GIFT	gamete intrafallopian	GLU	glucose
	(tube) transfer	GLU 5	five hour glucose
GIH	gastrointestinal		tolerance test
	hemorrhage	GLUC	glucose
GIK	glucose-insulin-potassium	GLYCOS	glycosylated hemoglobin
GIL	gastrointestinal (tract)	Hb	
	lymphoma	GM	gastric mucosa
GING	gingiva		general medicine
	gingivectomy		geometric mean
G1K	greater than one thousand		gram (g)
GIOP	glucocorticoid (steroid)-		grand mal
	induced osteoporosis		grandmother
GIP	gastric inhibitory peptide	GM +	gram-positive
	giant cell interstitial	GM −	gram-negative
	pneumonia	gm %	grams per 100 milliliters
GIS	gas in stomach	GMC	general medical clinic
	gastrointestinal series	GMCD	grand mal convulsive
GIT	gastrointestinal tract		disorder
GITS	gastrointestinal	GM-CSF	sargramostim (granulo-
	therapeutic system		cyte-macrophage
	gut-derived infectious		colony-stimulating
	toxic shock		factor; Leukine)
GITSG	Gastrointestinal Tumor	GME	gaseous microemboli
	Study Group	GMF	general medical floor
GITT	glucose insulin tolerance	GMH	germinal matrix
	test		hemorrhage
GIWU	gastrointestinal work-up	GMP	general medical panel
giv	given		Good Manufacturing
GJ	gastrojejunostomy		Practices
GJT	gastrojejunostomy tube		guanosine monophosphate
G1K	greater than one thousand	GMS	galvanic muscle
GL	gastric lavage		stimulation
	glaucoma		general medical services
	greatest length		general medicine and
GLA	gamolenic acid		surgery
	gingivolinguoaxial		Gomori methenamine
	glucose-lowering agents		silver (stain)
GLC	gas-liquid chromatog-	GM&S	general medicine and
	raphy		surgery
GLIO	glioblastoma	GMSPS	Glasgow Meningococcal
GLN	glomerulonephritis		Septicemia Prognostic
GLOC	gravity induced loss of		Score
	consciousness	GMTs	geometric mean antibody
GLP	Gambro Liendia Plate		titers

G

123

GN	glomerulonephritis	transaminase (aspartate
	graduate nurse	aminotransferase)
	gram-negative	goals of treatment
GNB	ganglioneuroblastoma	GP	gabapentin
	gram-negative bacilli		general practitioner
	gram-negative bacteremia		globus pallidus
GNBM	gram-negative bacillary		glucose polymers
	meningitis		glycoprotein
GNC	gram-negative cocci		gram-positive
GND	gram-negative diplococci		grandparent
GNID	gram-negative		gutta percha
	intracellular diplococci	G/P	gravida/para
GNP	Geriatric Nurse	G_4P_{3104}	four pregnancies (gravid),
	Practitioner		3 went to term, one
GNR	gram-negative rods		premature, no abortion
GnRH	gonadotropin-releasing		(or miscarriage), and 4
	hormone		living children
GNS	gram-negative sepsis		(p = para)
GnSAF	gonadotropin surge	GPA	global program on AIDS
	attenuating factor	G#P#A#	gravida (number of
GNT	Graduate Nurse		pregnancies) para
	Technician		(number of live births)
GO	Graves' ophthalmopathy		abortion (number of
	Greek Orthodox		abortions)
GOAT	Galveston Orientation and	GPB	gram-positive bacilli
	Amnesia Test	GPC	giant papillary
GOBI	growth monitoring, oral		conjunctivitis
	rehydration, breast		glycerophosphorylcholine
	feeding, and		G-protein coupled
	immunization		gram-positive cocci
GOCS	Global Obsessive-	GPCL	gas permeable contact
	Compulsive Scale		lens
GOD	glucose oxidase	GPCR	G protein-coupled
GOG	Gynecologic Oncology		receptors
	Group	GPC/TP	glycerylphosphorylcholine
GOK	God only knows		to total phosphate
GOMER	get out of my emergency	G6PD	glucose-6-phosphate
	room		dehydrogenase
GON	gonococcal ophthalmia	GPGL	gamma probe guided
	neonatorum		lymphoscintigraphy
	greater occipital neuritis	GPI	general paralysis of the
GONA	glaucomatous optic nerve		insane
	atrophy		glucose-6-phosphate
GOO	gastric outlet obstruction		isomerase
GOR	gastro-oesophageal reflux	GPi	globus pallidus
	general operating room	G-PLT	giant platelets
GOS	Glasgow Outcome Scale	GPMAL	gravida, para, multiple
GOT	glucose oxidase test		births, abortions, and
	glutamic-oxaloacetic		live births

GPN	graduate practical nurse		gluteal sets
GPO	group purchasing organization		Gram stain grip strength
GPS	Goodpasture's syndrome	G/S	5% dextrose (glucose) and 0.9% sodium chloride (saline) injection
GPT	glutamic pyruvic transaminase		
GPX	glutathione peroxidase		
GR	gastric resection	GSAP	greatest single allergen present
gr	grain (approximately 60 mg) (this is a dangerous abbreviation)	GSCU	geriatric skilled care unit
		GSD	glucogen storage disease
G−R	gram-negative rods	GSD-1	glycogen storage disease, type 1
G+R	gram-positive rods		
GRA	granisetron (Kytril)	GSE	genital self-examination gluten sensitive enteropathy grip strong and equal
GRAS	generally recognized as safe		
GRASE	Generally Recognized as Safe and Effective		
GRASS	gradient recalled acquisition in a steady state	GSH	glutathione
		GSI	genuine stress incontinence
Grav.	gravid (pregnant)	GSM	grey-scale median
GRD	gastroesophageal reflux disease	GSMD	gestational sack and maternal date
GRD DTR	granddaughter	GSP	general survey panel
GRD SON	grandson	GSPN	greater superficial petrosal neurectomy
GRE	graded resistive exercise gradient-recalled echo gradient refocused echo		
		GSR	galvanic skin resistance (response) gastrosalivary reflex
GR-FR	grandfather		
GR-MO	grandmother	GSS	Gerstmann-Straüssler-Scheinker (syndrome)
GRN	granules green		
		GST	glutathione S-transferase gold sodium thiomalate
GRO	growth-related oncogene		
GRP	group	GSTM	gold sodium thiomalate
$Gr_1P_0AB_1$	one pregnancy, no births, and one abortion	GSUI	genuine stress urinary incontinence
GRP HM	group home	GSW	gunshot wound
GRT	gastric residence time glandular replacement therapy Graduate Respiratory Therapist grasp and release test	GSWA	gunshot wound to abdomen
		GT	gait gait training gastrotomy tube glucose tolerance great toe group therapy
GRTT	Graduate Respiratory Therapist Technician		
		GTA	glutaraldehyde
GS	gallstone generalized seizure general surgery	GTB	gastrointestinal tract bleeding

125

GTC	generalized tonic-clonic (seizure)	GVN	gentamicin, vancomycin, and nystatin
GTCS	generalized tonic-clonic seizure	GVS	gastric vertical stapling
GTD	gestational trophoblastic disease	G/W	dextrose (glucose) in water
GTE	general therapeutic exercise	G&W	glycerin and water (enema)
GTF	gastrostomy tube feedings	GWA	gunshot wound of the abdomen
	glucose tolerance factor	GWBI	General Well-Being Index
GTH	gonadotropic hormone	GWD	Guinea worm disease
GTN	gestational trophoblastic neoplasms	GWS	Gulf war syndrome
	glomerulo-tubulo-nephritis	GWT	gunshot wound of the throat
	glyceryl trinitrate (name for nitroglycerin in the United Kingdom)	GWX	guide wire exchange
		GXP	graded exercise program
		GXT	graded exercise test
GTP	glutamyl transpeptidase	Gy	gray (radiation unit)
	guanosine triphosphate	GYN	gynecology
GTR	granulocyte turnover rate	GZTS	Guilford-Zimmerman Temperament Survey
	gross total resection		
	guided tissue regeneration		
GTS	Gilles de la Tourette syndrome		
GTT	drops		
	glucose tolerance test		
GTT agar	gelatin-tellurite-taurocholate agar		
GTT3H	glucose tolerance test 3 hours (oral)		
GTTS	drops		
G-tube	gastrostomy tube		
GU	genitourinary		
	gonococcal urethritis		
GUAR	guarantor		
GUD	genital ulcer disease		
GUI	genitourinary infection		
GUS	genitourinary sphincter		
	genitourinary system		
GUSTO	Global Utilization of Streptokinase and TPA for Occluded Arteries		
GV	gentian violet		
GVF	Goldmann visual fields		
	good visual fields		
GVG	vigabatrin (gamma-vinyl GABA)		
GVHD	graft-versus-host disease		
GVL	graft-versus leukemia		

H

H	*Haemophilis*
	head
	heart
	height
	Helicobacter
	heroin
	Hispanic
	hour
	husband
	hydrogen
	hyperopia
	hypermetropia
	hyperphoria
	hypodermic
	objective angle
H′	hip
Ⓗ	hypodermic injection
H²	hiatal hernia
H₂	hydrogen
3H	high, hot, and a helluva lot
HA	headache
	hearing aid
	heart attack
	hemadsorption
	hemolytic anemia
	Hispanic American
	hospital admission
	hyaluronan
	hyaluronic acid
	hyperalimentation
	hypermetropic astigmatism
	hypothalmic amenorrhea
H/A	head-to-abdomen (ratio)
	holding area
HA-1A®	nebacumab
HAA	hepatitis-associated antigen
HAAB	hepatitis A antibody
HAART	highly active antiretroviral treatment
HABF	hepatic artery blood flow

HAc	acetic acid
HACCP	Hazard Analysis Critical Control Point
HACE	hepatic artery chemoembolization
	high-altitude cerebral edema
HACEK group	*Haemophilus parainfluenzae, H. aphrophilus,* and *H. paraphrophilus, Actinobacillus actinomycetemcomitans, Cardiobacterium hominis, Eikenella corrodens,* and *Kingella kingae*
HACS	hyperactive child syndrome
HAD	human adjuvant disease
	hypertonic acetate dextran
HADS	Hospital Anxiety and Depression Scale
HAE	hearing aid evaluation
	hepatic artery embolization
	herb-related adverse event
	hereditary angioedema
HAEC	Hirschprung's associated enterocolitis
HAF	hyperalimentation fluid
HAFM	hospital-acquired *Plasmodium falciparum* malaria
HAGG	hyperimmune antivariola gamma globulin
HAH	high-altitude headache
HAI	hemagglutination inhibition assay
	hepatic arterial infusion
HAIC	hepatic arterial infusional chemotherapy
HAK	hyperalimentation kit
HAL	hyperalimentation
HALO	halothane
	hours after light onset
HALRI	hospital-acquired lower respiratory infections
HAM	HTLV-1-associated myelopathy

H

127

	human albumin microspheres	HASHD	hypertensive arteriosclerotic heart disease
HAMA	human anti-murine (anti-mouse) antibody	HAT	head, arms, and trunk
HAM-A	Hamilton Anxiety (scale)		heterophile antibody titer
HAM D	Hamilton Depression (scale)		histone acetyltransferase
HAMS	hamstrings		hospital arrival time
HAN	heroin associated nephropathy		human African trypanosomiasis (sleeping sickness)
HANE	hereditary angioneurotic edema	HAV	hallux abducto valgus
HAO	hearing aid orientation		hepatitis A virus
HAP	hearing aid problem	HAZWO-PER	Hazardous Waste Operations and Emergency Response
	heredopathia atactica polyneuritiformis	HB	heart-beating (donor)
	hospital-acquired pneumonia		heart block
HAPC	hospital-acquired penetration contact		heel to buttock
			hemoglobin (Hb)
HAPD	home-automated peritoneal dialysis		hepatitis B
HAPE	high altitude pulmonary edema		high calorie
			hold breakfast
			housebound
HAPS	hepatic arterial perfusion scintigraphy	1^0HB	first degree heart block
		$HB1°$	first degree heart block
HAPTO	haptoglobin	$HB2°$	second degree heart block
HAQ	Headache Assessment Questionnaire	$HB3°$	third degree heart block
		HBAB	hepatitis B antibody
	Health Assessment Questionnaire	$Hb A_{1c}$	glycosylated hemoglobin
		HBAC	hyperdynamic beta-adrenergic circulatory
HAR	high altitude retinopathy		
	hyperacute rejection		
HARH	high altitude retinal hemorrhage	HbAS	sickle cell trait
		HBBW	hold breakfast for blood work
HARP	hypoprebetalipoproteinemia, acanthocytosis, retinitis pigmentosa, and pallidale degeneration (syndrome)	HBC	hereditary breast cancer
		HBcAb	hepatitis B core antibody (antigen)
		HBc AB	hepatitis B core antibody
HARS	Hamilton Anxiety Rating Scale	HBc Ag	hepatitis B core antigen
		HB core	hepatitis B core antigen
HAS	Hamilton Anxiety (Rating) Scale	HbCV	*Haemophilus* b conjugate vaccine
	home assessment service	HBD	has been drinking
	hyperalimentation solution		hydroxybutyrate dehydrogenase
HASCVD	hypertensive arteriosclerotic cardiovascular disease	HBDH	hydroxybutyrate dehydrogenase

HBE	hepatitis B epsilon		honey-bee venom
HBED	hydroxybenzylethylene-diamine diacetic acid	HBVP	high biological value protein
HbF	fetal hemoglobin	HBW	high birth weight
HBF	hepatic blood flow	H/BW	heart-to-body weight (ratio)
HBGA	had it before, got it again	HC	hairy cell
HBGM	home blood glucose monitoring		handicapped
			head circumference
HBH	Health Belief Model		heart catheterization
HBHC	hospital based home care		heel cords
HBI	Harvey-Bradshaw Index		Hickman catheter
	hemibody irradiation		home care
HBID	hereditary benign intraepithelial dyskeratosis		hot compress
			housecall
			Huntington's chorea
HBIG	hepatitis B immune globulin		hydrocephalus
			hydrocortisone
Hb Kansas	mutant hemoglobin with a low affinity for oxygen	4-HC	4-hydroperoxycyclo-phosphamide
HBLV	B-lymphotropic virus human	H & C	hot and cold
		HCA	health care aide
HBM	human bone marrow		heterocyclic antidepres-sant
HBNK	heparin-binding neurotrophic factor		hypothermic circulatory arrest
HBO	hyperbaric oxygen (HBO$_2$ preferred)	H-CAP	altretamine (hexamethyl-melamine), cyclophosphamide, doxorubicin (Adriamycin), and cisplatin (Platinol AQ)
HBO$_2$	Hyperbaric oxygen		
HbO$_2$	hemoglobin, oxygenated		
	hyperbaric oxygen (HBO$_2$ preferred)		
HBOC	hemoglobin-based oxygen carrier		
		HCB	hexachlorobenzene
HBO$_2$T	hyperbaric oxygen treatment	HCC	hepatocellular carcinoma
		HCD	herniate cervical disk
HBP	high blood pressure		
HBPM	home blood pressure monitoring		hydrocolloid dressing
		HCFA	Health Care Financing Administration
HBS	Health Behavior Scale		
HbS	sickle cell hemoglobin	HCFC	hydrochlorofluorocarbon
HBsAg	hepatitis B surface antigen	hCG	human chorionic gonadotropin
HbSC	sickle cell hemoglobin C	HCH	hexachlorocyclohexane
HBSS	Hank's balanced salt solution		hygroscopic condenser humidifier
HbSS	sickle cell anemia	HCI	home care instructions
HBT	hydrogen breath test	HCL	hairy cell leukemia
HBV	hepatitis B vaccine	HCl	hydrochloric acid
	hepatitis B virus		hydrochloride

H

HCLF	high carbohydrate, low fiber (diet)	HCVD	hypertensive cardiovascular disease
HCLs	hard contact lenses	HCWs	health-care workers
HCLV	hairy cell leukemia variant	HCY	homocysteine
		HCYS	homocysteine
HCM	health care maintenance	HD	haloperidol decanoate
	heterogeneous cation-exchange membrane		Hansen's disease
			hearing distance
	hypercalcemia of malignancy		heart disease
			Heller-Dor (procedure)
	hypertropic cardiomyopathy		heloma durum
			hemodialysis
HCMV	human cytomegalovirus		herniated disk
HCO₃	bicarbonate		high dose
HCP	handicapped		hip disarticulation
	healthcare provider		Hodgkin's disease
	hearing conservation programs		hospital day
			hospital discharge
	hereditary coporphyria		house dust
	hexachlorophene		Huntington's disease
	home chemotherapy program	HDA	high-dose arm
		HD-AC	high-dose cytarabine
HCPCS	Health Care Common Procedure Coding System	HD-ara-C	high-dose cytarabine (ara-C)
HCQ	hydroxychloroquine	HDBQ	Hilton Drinking Behavior Questionnaire
HCR	health care review	HDC	habilitative day care
HCS	human chorionic somatomammotropin		high-dose chemotherapy
		HDCC	high-dose combination chemotherapy
17-HCS	17-hydroxycorticosteroids		
HCSE	horse chestnut seed extract	HD-CPA	high-dose cyclophosphamide
HCT	head computerized (axial) tomography	HDCPT	high-dose cyclophosphamide therapy
	hematocrit	HDC-SCR	high-dose chemotherapy with stem-cell rescue
	histamine challenge test		
	human chorionic thyrotropin	HDCT	high-dose chemotherapy
	hydrochlorothiazide (this is a dangerous abbreviation)	HDCV	rabies virus vaccine, human diploid (human diploid cell vaccine)
		HDF	hemodiafiltration
		HDH	high-density humidity
	hydrocortisone	HDI	high-definition imagine
HCTU	home cervical traction unit	HDL	high-density lipoprotein
		HDL-C	high-density lipoprotein cholesterol
HCTZ	hydrochlorothiazide (this is a dangerous abbreviation)		
		HDLW	hearing distance for watch to be heard in left ear
HCV	hepatitis C virus		

HDM	home-delivered meals	H&E	hematoxylin and eosin
	house dust mite		hemorrhage and exudate
HDMEC	human dermal		heredity and environment
	microvascular	HEA	health
	endothelial cells	HEAR	hospital emergency
HD-MTX	high-dose methotrexate		ambulance radio
HD-MTX-	high-dose methotrexate	HEAT	human erythrocyte
CF	and leucovorin		agglutination test
	(citrovorum factor)	HEB	hydrophilic emollient base
HD-MTX	high-dose methotrexate	HEC	Health Education Center
/LV	and leucovorin	HeCOG	Hellenic Cooperative
HDN	hemolytic disease of the		Oncology Group
	newborn	HEDIS	Health Employer Data
	heparin dosing nomogram		and Information Set
	high-density nebulizer	HEENT	head, eyes, ears, nose,
HDNS	Hodgkin's disease,		and throat
	nodular sclerosis	HEK	human embryonic kidney
HDP	high-density polyethylene	HEL	human embryonic lung
	hydroxymethyline	HeLa	Helen Lake (tumor cells)
	diphosphonate	HELLP	hemolysis, elevated liver
HDPAA	heparin-dependent	Syn-	enzymes, and low
	platelet-associated	drome	platelet count
	antibody	HEMA	hydroxyethylmethacrylate
HDPC	hand piece	HEMI	hemiplegia
HDR	heparin dose response	HEMOSID	hemosiderin
	husband to delivery	HEMPAS	hereditary erythrocytic
	room		multinuclearity with
HDRA	histoculture drug response		positive acidified serum
	assay		test
HDRB	high-dose rate	HEMS	helicopter emergency
	brachytherapy		medical services
HDRS	Hamilton Depression	HEN	hemorrhages, exudates,
	Rating Scale		and nicking
HDRW	hearing distance for watch		home enteral nutrition
	to be heard in right ear	He-Ne	helium-neon
HDS	Hamilton Depression	HEP	hemoglobin
	(Rating) Scale		electrophoresis
	herniated disk syndrome		heparin
HDSCR	health deviation self-care		hepatic
	requisite		hepatoerythropoietic
HDT	habilitative day treatment		porphyria
HDU	hemodialysis unit		hepatoma
HDV	hepatitis D virus		histamine equivalent
HDW	hearing distance (with)		prick
	watch		home exercise program
HDYF	how do you feel	HEPA	hamster egg penetration
HE	hard exudate		assay
	health educator		high-efficiency particulate
	hepatic encephalopathy		air (filter)

H

hep cap	heparin cap	HFJV	high-frequency jet ventilation
HERP	human exposure (dose)/rodent potency (dose)	H flu	*Haemophilus influenzae*
		HFO	high-frequency oscillation
HES	hetastarch (hydroxyethyl starch)	HFOV	high-frequency oscillatory ventilation
	hypereosinophilic syndrome	HFPPV	high-frequency positive pressure ventilation
HEs	hypertensive emergencies	HFRS	hemorrhagic fever with renal syndrome
HETF	home enteral tube feeding		
HEV	hepatitis E virus	HFS	hand-foot syndrome
	hepato-encephalomyelitis virus	HFSH	human follicle-stimulating hormone
	high endothelial venule	HFST	hearing-for-speech test
Hex	altretamine (hexamethylmelamine)	HFUPR	hourly fetal urine production rate
Hexa-CAF	altretamine (hexamethylmelamine), cyclophosphamide, methotrexate (amethopterin), and fluorouracil	HFV	high-frequency ventilation
		HFX RT	hyperfractionated radiation therapy
		HG	handgrasp
			handgrip
			hemoglobin
HF	Hageman factor	Hg	mercury
	hard feces	HGA	high grade astrocytomas
	hay fever	Hgb	hemoglobin
	head of fetus	Hgb ELECT	hemoglobin electrophoresis
	heart failure		
	high-frequency	Hgb F	fetal hemoglobin
	Hispanic female	Hgb S	sickle cell hemoglobin
	hot flashes	HGE	human granulocytic ehrlichiosis
	house formula		
HFA	health facility administrator	HGES	handgrasp equal and strong
	hydrofluoroalkane-134a	HGF	hepatocyte growth factor
HFAS	hereditary flat adenoma syndrome	HGG	human gamma globulin
		HGH	human growth hormone
HFB	high-frequency band	HGI	Human Genome Initiative
HFC	hydrofluorocarbon	HGM	home glucose monitoring
HFCC	high frequency chest compression	HGN	hypogastric nerve
		HGO	hepatic glucose output
HFD	high-fiber diet		hip guidance orthosis
	high-forceps delivery	HGPRT	hypoxanthine-guanine phosphoribosyl-transferase
	high-frequency discharges		
hFH	heterozygous familial hypercholesterolemia		
		HGSIL	high-grade squamous intraepithelial lesion
HFHL	high-frequence hearing loss		
		HGV	hepatitis G virus
HFI	hereditary fructose intolerance	HH	hard of hearing
			head hood

132

	hiatal hernia	HIA	hemagglutination inhibition antibody
	home health		
	homonymous hemiopia	HIAA	hydroxyindoleacetic acid
	household	5-HIAA	5-hydroxyindoleacetic acid
	hypogonadotropic hypogonadism	HIAP	human intracisternal A-type particle
	hypoeninemic hypoaldosteronism	HIB	*Haemophilus influenzae* type b (vaccine)
H/H	hemoglobin/hematocrit		
H&H	hematocrit and hemoglobin	HIB-C	*Haemophilus-influenzae* B vaccine conjugate
HHA	health hazard appraisal		
	hereditary hemolytic anemia	HIC	Human Investigation Committee
	home health agency	hi-cal	high caloric
	home health aid	HID	headache, insomnia, and depression
HHC	home health care		
HHD	Doctor of Holistic Health		herniated intervertebral disk
	home hemodialysis		
	hypertensive heart disease	HIDA	hepato-iminodiacetic acid (lidofenin)
HHFM	high-humidity face mask		
HHM	high-humidity mask	HiDAC	high-dose cytarabine (ara-C)
	humoral hypercalcemia of malignancy	HIDS	hyperimmunoglobulinemia D syndrome
HHN	hand held nebulizer		
HHNC	hyperosmolar hyperglycemic nonketotic coma	HIE	hyperimmunoglobuline-mia E
			hypoxic-ischemic encephalopathy
HHNK	hyperglycemic hyperosmolar nonketotic (coma)	HIF	*Haemophilus influenzae*
			higher integrative functions
HHS	Health and Human Service (US Department of)	HIHA	high impulsiveness, high anxiety
HHT	hereditary hemorrhagic telangiectasis	HIHARS	hyperventilation-induced high-amplitude rhythmic slowing
HHTC	high-humidity trach collar		
HHTM	high-humidity trach mask	HII	hepatic-iron index
HHTS	high-humidity tracheostomy shield	HIIC	heated intraoperative intraperitoneal chemotherapy
HHV-8	human herpesvirus 8		
HI	*Haemophilus influenzae*	HIL	hypoxic-ischemic lesion
	head injury	HILA	high impulsiveness, low anxiety
	health insurance		
	hearing impaired	HILP	hyperthermic isolated limb perfusion
	hemagglutination inhibition		
	homicidal ideation	HIM	health information management
	hospital insurance	HINI	hypoxic-ischemic neuronal injury
	human insulin		

HIO	health insuring organization			heel-to-knee
				hexokinase
HIP	health insurance plan	HKAFO	hip-knee-ankle-foot orthosis
HIPAA	Health Insurance Portability and Accountability Act of 1996	HKAO	hip-knee-ankle orthosis
		HKMN	Hickman (catheter)
		HKO	hip-knee orthosis
HIPC	hormone-independent prostate cancer	HKS	heel-knee-shin (test)
		HKT	heterotopic kidney transplant
hi-pro	high protein		
HIR	head injury routine	HL	hairline
HIS	Hanover Intensive Score		half-life
	Health Intention Scale		hallux limitus
	high intermittent suction		haloperidol
	histidine		harelip
	Home Incapacity Scale		hearing level
	hospital information system		hearing loss
			heavy lifting
HISMS	How I See Myself Scale		hemilaryngectomy
HISTO	histoplasmin skin test		heparin lock
	histoplasmosis		hepatic lipase
HIT	heparin induced thrombocytopenia		Hickman line
		H&L	heart and lung
	histamine inhalation test	HLA	human leukocyte antigen
			human lymphocyte antigen
	home infusion therapy		
HITTS	heparin-induced thrombotic thrombocytopenia syndrome	HLA negative	heart, lungs, and abdomen negative
		HLB	head, limbs, and body
		HLD	haloperidol decanoate
HIU	head injury unit		herniated lumbar disk
HIV	human immunodeficiency virus	HLDP	hypoglossia-limb deficiency phenotype
HIV-1	human immunodeficiency virus type 1	HLGR	high-level gentamicin resistance
HIV-2	human immunodeficiency virus type 2	HLH	hemophagocytic lymphohistiocytosis
HIVAT	home intravenous antibiotic therapy		human luteinizing hormone
HIVD	herniated intervertebral disk	HLHS	hypoplastic left heart syndrome
HIV-D	human immunodeficiency virus-related dementia	HLK	heart, liver, and kidneys
		HLP	hyperlipoproteinemia
hi-vit	high vitamin	hLS	human lung surfactant
HIVMP	high-dose intravenous methylprednisolone	HLT	heart-lung transplantation (transplant)
HJB	Howell-Jolly bodies	HLV	herpes-like virus
HJR	hepato jugular reflux		hypoplastic left ventricle
HK	hand-to-knee	HM	hand motion

134

	head movement	HMPAO	hexylmethylpropylene amineoxine
	heart murmur		
	heavily muscled	HMR	histocytic medullary reticulosis
	heloma molle		
	Hispanic male		Hoechst Marion Roussel
	Holter monitor		
	human milk	¹H-MRS	proton magnetic resonance spectroscopy
	human semisynthetic insulin	HMS	hyperactive malarial splenomegaly
	humidity mask		
HMA	hemorrhages and microaneurysms		hypodermic morphine sulfate (this is a dangerous abbreviation)
HMB	homatropine methylbromide	HMS®	medrysone
HMBA	hexamethylene bisacetamide	hMSCs	human mesenchymal stem cells
HMC-CoA	hydroxymethylglutaryl-coenzyme A	HMSN I	hereditary motor and sensory neuropathy type I
HMD	hyaline membrane disease		
HMDP	hydroxymethyline diphosphonate	HMSR	high medical-social risk
		HMSS	hyperactive malarial splenomegaly syndrome
HME	heat and moisture exchanger		
	heat, massage, and exercise	HMWK	high molecular weight kininogen
	home medical equipment	HMX	heat massage exercise
	human monocytic ehrlichiosis	HN	head and neck
			head nurse
			high nitrogen
HMETSC	heavy metal screen		home nursing
HMF	human milk fortifier	H&N	head and neck
HMG	human menopausal gonadotropin	HN2	mechlorethamine HCl
		HNC	head and neck cancer
HMG CoA	hepatic hydroxymethyl glutaryl coenzyme A		human neutrophil collagenase
HMI	healed myocardial infarction		hyperosmolar nonketotic coma
	history of medical illness	HNCa	head and neck cancer
HMIS	hospital medical information system	HNCCG	Head and Neck Cancer Cooperative Group
HMK	homemaking	HNE	human neutrophil elastase
HM & LP	hand motion and light perception	HNI	hospitalization not indicated
HMM	altretamine (hexamethyl-melamine)	HNKDC	hyperosomolar nonketotic diabetic coma
HMO	Health Maintenance Organization	HNKDS	hyperosmolar nonketotic diabetic state
HMP	health maintenance plan		
	hexose monophosphate	HNLN	hospitalization no longer necessary
	hot moist packs		

HNN	hybrid neural network	HOTV	letter symbols used in pediatric visual acuity testing
HNP	herniated nucleus pulposus		
HNPCC	heredity nonpolyposis colorectal cancer	HOVT	letter symbols used in pediatric visual acuity testing
HNRNA	heterogeneous nuclear ribonucleic acid	HP	hard palate
HNS	0.45% sodium chloride injection (half normal saline)		Harvard pump
			Helicobacter pylori
			hemipelvectomy
			hemiplegia
	head and neck surgery		high-protein (supplement)
	head, neck, and shaft		hot packs
HNSCC	squamous cell carcinoma of the head and neck		house physician
HNSN	home, no services needed		hydrogen peroxide
HNV	has not voided		hydrophilic petrolatum
HNWG	has not worn glasses	Hp	*Helicobacter pylori*
HO	hand orthosis	H&P	history and physical
	Hemotology-Oncology	HPA	hybridization protection assay
	heterotropic ossification		
	hip orthosis		hypothalamic-pituitary-adrenal (axis)
	house officer		
H/O	history of	HPAE-PAD	high pH anion exchange chromatography coupled with pulsed amperometric detection
H₂O	water		
H₂O₂	hydrogen peroxide		
HOA	hip osteoarthritis		
HOB	head of bed	HPAT	home parenteral antibiotic therapy
HOB UPSOB	head of bed up for shortness of breath		
HOC	Health Officer Certificate	HPB	Health Protection Branch (the Canadian equivalent of the U.S. Food and Drug Administration)
HOCM	high-osmolality contrast media		
	hypertrophic obstructive cardiomyopathy		
HOG	halothane, oxygen, and gas (nitrous oxide)	HPC	hereditary prostate cancer
HOH	hard of hearing		history of present condition (complaint)
HOI	hospital onset of infection		
HOM	high-osmolar contrast media	HPCE	high-performance capillary electrophore-sis
HONK	hyperosmolar nonketotic (coma)		
		HPD	high-protein diet
HOP	hourly output		home peritoneal dialysis
HOPI	history of present illness	HpD	hematoporphyrin derivative
HORF	high-output renal failure		
HORS	Hemiballism/Hemichorea Outcome Rating Score	HP&D	hemoprofile and differential
HOSP	hospital hospitalization	HPE	hemorrhage, papilledema, exudate

	history and physical examination	HPV	human papilloma virus
			human parvovirus
HPET	*Helicobacter pylori* eradication therapy	*H pylori*	*Helicobacter pylori*
		HPZ	high pressure zone
HPF	high-power field	HQC	hydroquinone cream
HPFH	hereditary persistence of fetal hemoglobin	HQL	health-related quality of life
HPG	human pituitary gonadotropin	HR	hallux rigidus
			Harrington rod
HPI	history of present illness		hazard ratio
HPL	human placenta lactogen		heart rate
	hyperplexia		hemorrhagic retinopathy
HPLC	high-pressure (performance) liquid chromatography		hospital record
			hour
		Hr 0	zero hour (when treatment starts)
HPM	hemiplegic migraine		
HPN	home parenteral nutrition	Hr -2	minus two hours (two hours prior to treatment)
HPNI	hemodialysis prognostic nutrition index		
HPNS	high pressure nervous syndrome	H & R	hysterectomy and radiation
HPO	hydrophilic ointment	HRA	high right atrium
	hypertrophic pulmonary osteoarthropathy		histamine releasing activity
HPOA	hypertrophic pulmonary osteoarthropathy	H2RA	H2-receptor antagonist
		HRC	Human Rights Committee
2HPP	2-hour postprandial (blood sugar)	HRCT	high-resolution computed tomography
2HPPBS	2-hour postprandial blood sugar	HRD	human retroviral disease
		HRE	high-resolution electrocardiography
HPPM	hyperplastic persistent pupillary membrane	HRF	Harris return flow
			health-related facility
HPS	hantavirus pulmonary syndrome		histamine releasing factor
	hepatopulmonary syndrome	HRIF	histamine inhibitory releasing factor
	hypertrophic pyloric stenosis	HRL	head rotated left
		HRLA	human reovirus-like agent
HPT	heparin protamine titration	HRLM	high-resolution light microscopy
	histamine provocation test	hRLX-2	synthetic human relaxin
	hyperparathyroidism	HRMPC	hormone-refractory metastatic prostate cancer
HPTD	highly permeable transparent dressing		
hPTH	human parathyroid hormone I$_{34}$ (teriparatide)	HRNB	Halstead-Reitan Neuropsychological Battery
HPTM	home prothrombin time monitoring	HRP	high-risk pregnancy
			horseradish peroxidase

HRP-2	histidine-rich protein-2		autonomic neuropathy
HRPC	hormone-refractory		(types I–IV)
	prostate cancer	HSB	husband
HRQL	health-related quality of	HSBG	heel stick blood gas
	life	HSC	hematopoietic stem cell
HRQOL	health-related quality of	HSCL	Hopkins Symptom Check
	life		List
HRR	head rotated right	HSD	hypoactive sexual desire
HRRC	Human Research Review		(disorder)
	Committee	HSE	herpes simplex
HRS	Haw River syndrome		encephalitis
	hepatorenal syndrome		human skin equivalent
HRSD	Hamilton Rating Scale for		hypertonic saline-
	Depression		epinephrine
HRST	heat, reddening, swelling,	HSES	hemorrhagic shock and
	or tenderness		encephalopathy
HRT	heart rate	HSG	herpes simplex genitalis
	heparin response test		hysterosalpingogram
	high-risk transfer	H-SIL	high-grade squamous
	hormone replacement		intraepithelial lesions
	therapy	HSK	herpes simplex keratitis
HRV	heart rate variability	HSL	herpes simplex labialis
HS	bedtime		hormone sensitive
	half strength		lipase
	hamstrings	HSM	hepatosplenomegaly
	hamstring sets		holosystolic murmur
	Hartman's solution	HSN	Hansen-Street nail
	(lactated Ringer's)		heart sounds normal
	heart size	HSP	heat shock protein
	heart sounds		Henoch-Schönlein
	heavy smoker		purpura
	heel spur		hereditary spastic
	heel stick		paraplegia
	hereditary spherocytosis		hysterosalpingography
	herpes simplex	HSPE	high-strength pancreatic
	hidradenitis suppurativa		enzymes
	high school	HSQ	Health Status
	hippocampal sclerosis		Questionnaire
	Hurlers syndrome	HSR	heated serum reagin
H→S	heel to shin	HSS	half-strength saline
H&S	hearing and speech		(0.45% Sodium
	hemorrhage and shock		Chloride)
	hysterectomy and	HSSE	high soap suds enema
	sterilization	HS-tk	herpes simplex thymidine
HSA	Health Systems Agency		kinase
	human serum albumin	HSV	herpes simplex virus
	hypersomnia-sleep		highly selective vagotomy
	apnea	HSV-1	herpes simplex virus
HSAN	hereditary sensory and		type 1

HSV-2	herpes simplex virus type 2		Hematest® stools
		HTSCA	human tumor stem cell assay
HSVE	herpes simplex virus encephalitis	H-TSH	human thyroid-stimulating hormone
HT	hammertoe		
	hearing test	HTT	hand thrust test
	heart	HTV	herpes-type virus
	heart transplant	HTVD	hypertensive vascular disease
	height		
	high temperature	HTX	hemothorax
	hormonotherapy	HU	head unit
	Hubbard tank		hydroxyurea
	hypermetropia		hypertensive urgencies
	hyperopia	Hu	Hounsfield units
	hypertension	HUCB	human umbilical cord blood
	hyperthermia		
	hyperthyroid	HUH	Humana Hospital
H/T	heel and toe (walking)	HUI	Health Utilities Index
H&T	hospitalization and treatment	HUIFM	human leukocyte interferon meloy
H(T)	intermittent hypertropia	HUK	human urinary kallikrein
5-HT	serotonin (5-hydroxytryptamine)	HUM	heat, ultrasound, and massage
ht. aer.	heated aerosol	HUM 70/30	human insulin, regular 30 units/mL with human insulin isophane suspension 70 units/mL (Humulin® 70/30 insulin)
HTAT	human tetanus antitoxin		
HTB	hot tub bath		
HTC	heated tracheostomy collar		
	hypertensive crisis		
HTF	house tube feeding	HUMARA	human androgen receptor assay
HTGL	hepatic triglyceride lipase		
HTK	heel to knee	HUM L	human insulin zinc suspension (Humulin® L Insulin)
HTL	hearing threshold level		
	human T-cell leukemia		
	human thymic leukemia	HUM N	human insulin isophane suspension (Humulin® N Insulin)
HTLV III	human T-cell lymphotrophic virus type III		
		HUM R	human insulin, regular (Humulin® R Insulin)
HTM	*Haemophilus* test medium		
	high threshold mechanoceptors	HUR	hydroxyurea
		HUS	head ultrasound
HTN	hypertension		hemolytic uremic syndrome
HTO	high tibia osteotomy		
HTP	House-Tree-Person-test		husband
5-HTP	serotonin (5-hydroxytryptophan)	husb	husband
		HUT	head-upright tilt (test)
HTR	hard tissue replacement		hyperplasia of usual type
HTS	head traumatic syndrome		
	heel-to-shin		

H

HUVEC	human umbilical vein endothelial cells	Hy	hypermetropia
		HYDRO	hydronephrosis
HV	hallux valgus		hydrotherapy
	Hantavirus	HYG	hygiene
	has voided	HYPER	above
	Hemovac®		higher than
	hepatic vein	Hyper Al	hyperalimentation
	herpesvirus	Hyper K	hyperkalemia
	home visit	HYPER T	hypertrophic tonsils and
H&V	hemigastrecomy and	& A	adenoids
	vagotomy	HYPO	below
HVA	homovanillic acid		hypodermic injection
HVD	hypertensive vascular		lower than
	disease	Hypo K	hypokalemia
HVDO	hypovitaminosis D	hypopit	hypopituitarism
	osteopathy	HYs	healthy years of life
HVE	high voltage	Hyst	hysterectomy
	electrophoresis	Hz	Hertz
HVES	high voltage electrical	HZ	herpes zoster
	stimulation	HZO	herpes zoster
HVF	Humphrey visual field		ophthalmicus
HVGS	high volt galvanic	HZV	herpes zoster virus
	stimulation		
HVL	half value layer		
	hippocampal volume loss		
HVOO	hepatic venous outflow obstruction		
HVPC	high voltage pulsed current		
HVPG	hepatic venous pressure gradient		
HYPT	hyperventilation provocation test		
HVS	hyperventilation syndrome		
HW	heparin well		
	homework		
	housewife		
HWB	hot water bottle		
HWFE	housewife		
HWG	has worn glasses		
HWH	halfway house		
HWP	hot wet pack		
HWPG	has worn prescription glasses		
Hx	history		
	hospitalization		
HXM	altretamine (hexamethylmelamine)		
Hx & Px	history and physical (examination)		

I

I	impression		intermittent androgen deprivation
	incisal		intractable atopic dermatitis
	independent	IADHS	inappropriate antidiuretic hormone syndrome
	initial		
	inspiration	IADL	Instrumental Activities of Daily Living
	intact (bag of waters)		
	intermediate	IA DSA	intra-arterial digital subtraction arteriography
	iris		
	one		
I_2	iodine	IAGT	indirect antiglobulin test
I^{131}	radioactive iodine	IAHA	immune adherence hemagglutination
I-3+7	idarubicin and cytarabine		
IA	incidental appendectomy	IAHD	idiopathic acquired hemolytic disease
	incurred accidentally		
	intra-amniotic	IAI	intra-abdominal infection
	intra-arterial		intra-amniotic infection
I & A	irrigation and aspiration	IALD	instrumental activities of daily living
IAA	ileoanal anastomosis		
	insulin autoantibodies	IAM	internal auditory meatus
	interrupted aortic arch	IAN	intern's admission note
IAB	incomplete abortion	IAO	immediately after onset
	induced abortion	IAP	independent adjudicating panel
	intermittent androgen blockade		
			intermittent acute porphyria
IABC	intra-aortic balloon counterpulsation		intracarotid amobarbital procedure
IABCP	intra-aortic balloon counterpulsation	IARC	International Agency for Research on Cancer
IABP	intra-aortic balloon pump	IART	intra-atrial reentrant tachycardia
	intra-arterial blood pressure	IAS	idiopathic ankylosing spondylitis
IAC	internal auditory canal		intermittent androgen suppression
	intra-arterial chemotherapy		internal anal sphincter
	isolated adrenal cell	IASD	interatrial septal defect
IAC-CPR	interposed abdominal compressions—cardio-pulmonary resuscitation	IAT	immunoaugmentive therapy
			indirect antiglobulin test
			intracarotid amobarbital test
IACG	intermittent angle-closure glaucoma		intraoperative autologous transfusion
IACP	intra-aortic counterpulsa-tion	IAV	intermittent assist ventilation
IAD	implantable atrial defibrillator	IB	ileal bypass

	insulin receptor binding test		incipient cataract (grade 1+ to 4+)
	isolation bed		incomplete
IB1A	interferon beta-1a (Avonex)		indirect calorimetry
			indirect Coombs (test)
IBAM	idiopathic bile acid malabsorption		individual counseling
			informed consent
IBBB	intra-blood-brain barrier		inspiratory capacity
IBBBB	incomplete bilateral bundle branch block		intensive care
			intercostal
IBC	invasive bladder cancer		intercourse
	iron binding capacity		intermediate care
IBD	infectious bursal disease		intermittent catheterization
	inflammatory bowel disease		interstitial changes
IBDQ	Inflammatory Bowel Disease Questionnaire		interstitial cystitis
			intracerebral
IBG	iliac bone graft		intracranial
IBI	intermittent bladder irrigation		intraincisional
			irritable colon
ibid	at the same place	I/C	imipenem-cilastatin (Primaxin®)
IBILI	indirect bilirubin		
IBM	ideal body mass	ICA	ileocolic anastomosis
	inclusion body myositis		intermediate care area
IBMI	initial body mass index		internal carotid artery
			intracranial abscess
IBMTR	International Bone Marrow Transplant Registry		intracranial aneurysm
			islet-cell antibody
IBNR	incurred but not reported	ICAM	intracellular adhesion molecule
IBOW	intact bag of waters	ICAM-1	intercellular adhesion molecule-1
IBPS	Insall-Burstein posterior stabilizer	ICAO	internal carotid artery occlusion
IBR	immediate breast reconstruction	ICAS	intermediate coronary artery syndrome
	infectious bovine rhinotracheitis	ICAT	infant cardiac arrest tray
IBRS	Inpatient Behavior Rating Scale	ICB	intracranial bleeding
		ICBG	iliac crest bone graft
IBS	irritable bowel syndrome	ICBT	intercostobronchial trunk
IBT	ink blot test (Rorschach test)	ICC	immunocytochemistry
			Indian childhood cirrhosis
IBTR	intra-breast tumor recurrence		intraclass correlation coefficient
IBU	ibuprofen		islet cell carcinoma
IBW	ideal body weight	ICCE	intracapsular cataract extraction
IC	between meals		
	immune complex	ICCU	intensive coronary care unit
	immunocompromised		

	intermediate coronary care unit	ICLE	intracapsular lens extraction
ICD	implantable cardioverter defibrillator	ICM	intercostal margin
	indigocarmine dye		intercostal muscle
	informed consent document	ICN	infection control nurse
			intensive care nursery
	instantaneous cardiac death	ICN2	neonatal intensive care unit level II
	isocitrate dehydrogenase	ICP	inductively coupled plasma
	irritant contact dermatitis		intracranial pressure
ICDA	International Classification of Disease, Adapted	ICPP	intubated continuous positive pressure
ICDB	incomplete database	ICR	intercostal retractions
ICDC	implantable cardioverter defibrillator catheter		intrastromal corneal ring
		ICRF-159	razoxane
ICD 9 CM	International Classification of Diseases, 9th Revision, Clinical Modification	ICS	ileocecal sphincter
			inhaled corticosteroid(s)
			intercostal space
		ICSH	interstitial cell-stimulating hormone
ICDO	International Classification of Diseases for Oncology	ICSI	intracytoplasmic sperm injection
ICE	ice, compression, and elevation	ICSR	intercostal space retractions
		ICT	icterus
	ifosfamide, carboplatin, and etoposide		indirect Coombs' test
	individual career exploration		inflammation of connective tissue
	interleukin-1 alpha converting enzyme		intensive conventional therapy
	interleukin-1 beta converting enzyme		intermittent cervical traction
+ ice	add ice		intracranial tumor
ICES	ice, compression, elevation, and support		intracutaneous test
			islet cell transplant
ICF	intermediate care facility	ICTX	intermittent cervical traction
	intracellular fluid	ICU	intensive care unit
ICG	indocyanine green		intermediate care unit
ICGA	indocyanine green angiography	ICV	intracerebroventricular
		ICVH	ischemic cerebrovascular headache
ICH	immunocompromised host	ICW	in connection with
	intracerebral hemorrhage		intercellular water
	intracranial hemorrhage	ID	identification
ICIT	intensified conventional insulin therapy		identify
			idiotype
ICL	intracorneal lens		ifosfamide, mesna

I

	uroprotection, and doxorubicin	IDR	idarubicin
	immunodiffusion		idiosyncratic drug reaction
	induction delivery		intradermal reaction
	infectious disease (physician or department)	IDS	infectious disease service integrated delivery system
	initial diagnosis	IDT	intradermal test
	initial dose	IDTP	immunodiffusion tube precipitin
	intradermal	IDU	idoxuridine
id	the same		infectious disease unit
I & D	incision and drainage		injecting drug user
IDA	idarubicin	IDV	indinavir (Crixivan)
	iron deficiency anemia		intermittent demand ventilation
IDAM	infant of drug abusing mother	IDVC	indwelling venous catheter
IDB	incomplete database		
IDC	idiopathic dilated cardiomyopathy	IE	ifosfamide, and etoposide with mesna
	invasive ductal cancer		immunoelectrophoresis induced emesis
IDCF	immunodiffusion complement fixation		infective endocarditis inner ear
IDD	insulin-dependent diabetes iodine-deficiency disorders		international unit (European abbreviation)
IDDM	insulin-dependent diabetes mellitus	I & E	ingress and egress (tubes) internal and external
IDDS	implantable drug delivery system	*i.e.*	that is
IDE	Investigational Device Exemption	IEC	independent ethics committee inpatient exercise center
IDFC	immature dead female child	IEF	isoelectric focusing
IDH	isocitric dehydrogenase	IEL	intestinal-intraepithelial lymphocyte
IDI	Interpersonal Dependency Inventory	IEM	immune electron microscopy
	intrathecal drug infusion		inborn errors of metabolism
IDK	internal derangement of knee	iEMG	integrated electromyography
IDL	intermediate-density lipoprotein	IEP	immunoelectrophoresis
IDM	infant of a diabetic mother		Individualized Education Plan
IDMC	immature dead male child	IEPA	immunoelectrophoresis analysis
IDP	initiate discharge planning inosine diphosphate	I:E ratio	inspiratory to expiratory time ratio
IDPN	intradialytic parenteral nutrition		

144

IET	infantile estropia	IgM	immunoglobulin M
IF	idiopathic flushing	IGP	interstitial glycoprotein
	ifosfamide	IGR	intrauterine growth
	immunofluorescence		retardation
	injury factor	IGT	impaired glucose
	interferon		tolerance
	interfrontal	IGTN	ingrown toenail
	intermaxillary fixation	IH	indirect hemagglutination
	internal fixation		infectious hepatitis
	intrinsic factor		inguinal hernia
	involved field	IHA	immune hemolytic anemia
	(radiotherapy)		indirect
IFA	immunofluorescent assay		hemagglutination
	indirect fluorescent		infusion hepatic
	antibody		arteriography
IFAT	immunofluorescence	IHC	idiopathic hypercalciuria
	antibody test		immobilization
	(technique)		hypercalcemia
IFE	immunofixation		immunohistochemistry
	electrophoresis		inner hair cell (in
	in-flight emergency		cochlea)
IFL	indolent follicular	IHD	intraheptic duct (ule)
	lymphoma		ischemic heart disease
IFM	internal fetal monitoring	IHDN	integrated health delivery
IFN	interferon		network
IFNB	interferon beta-1 b	IHH	idiopathic hypogona-
	(Betaseron®)		dotrophic hypogo-
IFO	ifosfamide (Ifex)		nadism
IFOS	ifosfamide (Ifex)	IHO	idiopathic hypertrophic
IFP	inflammatory fibroid		osteoarthropathy
	polyps	IHP	idiopathic hypoparathy-
IFSE	internal fetal scalp		roidism
	electrode		inferior hypogastric
IgA	immunoglobulin A		plexus
IGCS	inpatient geriatric	IHPH	intrahepatic portal
	consultation services		hypertension
IgD	immunoglobulin D	IHR	inguinal hernia repair
IGDE	idiopathic gait disorders		intrinsic heart rate
	of the elderly	IHS	Indian Health Service
IGDM	infant of gestational		integrated healthcare
	diabetic mother		system
IgE	immunoglobulin E		Iodiopathic Headache
IGF-I	insulin-like growth		Score
	factor I	IHs	iris hamartomas
IgG	immunoglobulin G	IHSA	iodinated human serum
IGIM	immune globulin		albumin
	intramuscular	IHSS	idiopathic hypertrophic
IGIV	immune globulin		subaortic stenosis
	intravenous	IHT	insulin hypoglycemia test
		IHU	inpatient hospice unit

I

IHW	inner heel wedge		interstitial lung disease
II	internal iliac (artery)		ischemic leg disease
IIA	internal iliac artery	ILE	infantile lobar emphysema
IICP	increased intracranial pressure	ILF	indicated low forceps
		ILFC	immature living female child
IICU	infant intensive care unit		
IIEF	International Index of Erectile Function	ILI	influenza-like illness
		ILM	internal limiting membrane
IIF	indirect immunofluorescence		
		ILMC	immature living male child
IIH	idiopathic infantile hypercalcemia		
		ILMI	inferolateral myocardial infarct
IIH	iodine-induced hyperthyroidism		
		ILP	interstitial laser photocoagulation
IIHT	iodide-induced hyperthyroidism		
			isolated limb perfusion
IIP	idiopathic interstitial pneumonitis	ILQTS	idiopathic long QT (interval) syndrome
IIPF	idiopathic interstitial pulmonary fibrosis	ILVEN	inflammatory linear verrucal epidermal nevus
IJ	ileojejunal		
	internal jugular	IM	ice massage
I&J	insight and judgment		infectious mononucleosis
IJC	internal jugular catheter		intermetatarsal
IJD	inflammatory joint disease		internal medicine
IJO	idiopathic juvenile osteoporosis		intramedullary
			intramuscular
IJP	internal jugular pressure	IMA	inferior mesenteric artery
IJR	idiojunctional rhythm		
IJT	idiojunctional tachycardia		internal mammary artery
IJV	internal jugular vein	IMAC	ifosfamide, mesna uroprotection, doxorubicin (Adriamycin), and cisplatin
IK	immobilized knee		
	interstitial keratitis		
IL	immature lungs		
	interleukin (1, 2, etc.)		
	intralesional		immobilized metal affinity chromatography
	Intralipid®		
ILA	insulin-like activity	IMAE	internal maxillary artery embolization
ILB	incidental Lewy body		
ILBBB	incomplete left bundle branch block	IMAG	internal mammary artery graft
ILBW	infant, low birth weight	IMARD	immunomodulating antirheumatic drugs
ILC	interstitial laser coagulation		
		IMB	intermenstrual bleeding
	invasive lobular cancer	IMBP	immobilized mismatch binding protein
ILD	indentation load deflection		
		IMC	intermittent catheterization
	intermediate density lipoproteins		
			intramedullary catheter

IMCU	intermediate care unit		intima to media (wall) thickness
IME	independent medical examination (evaluation)	IMU	intermediate medicine unit
IMF	idiopathic myelofibrosis	IMV	inferior mesenteric vein
	ifosfamide, mesna uroprotection, methotrexate, and fluorouracil		intermittent mandatory ventilation
	immobilization mandibular fracture		intermittent mechanical ventilation
	inframammary fold	IMVP-16	ifosfamide, mesna uroprotection,
	intermaxillary fixation		methotrexate, and
IMG	internal medicine group		etoposide
IMGU	insulin-mediated glucose uptake	IN	insulin intranasal
IMH	idiopathic myocardial hypertrophy	In	inches indium
IMH test	indirect microhemaggluti-nation test	INAD	in no apparent distress Investigational New Animal Drug
IMI	imipramine	INB	intercostal nerve blockade
	impending myocardial infarction	INC	incisal incision
	inferior myocardial infarction		incomplete incontinent
	intramuscular injection		increase
131I-MIBG	iodine131-metaiodobenzyl-guanidine (iobenguane 131I)		inside-the-needle catheter
		INCC	Institut National du Cancer du Canada
IMIG	intramuscular immunoglobulin	Inc Spir	incentive spirometer
IMLC	incomplete mitral leaflet closure	IND	induced Investigational New Drug (application)
IMM	immunizations		
IMN	internal mammary (lymph) node	INDA	Investigational New Drug Application
IMP	impacted important	INDIGO	interstitial laser ablation of the prostate
	impression improved	INDM	infant of nondiabetic mother
	inosine monophoshate	INDO	indomethacin
IMPX	impaction	111In-DTPA	indium pentetate
IMR	infant mortality rate		
IMRA	immunoradiometric assay	INE	infantile necrotizing
IMS	immunosuppressants		encephalomyelopathy
	incurred in military service	INEX	inexperienced
		INF	infant
IMT	inspiratory muscle training		infarction infected

I

	infection		intraoperative
	inferior	I&O	intake and output
	information	IOA	intact on admission
	infused	IOC	intern on call
	infusion		intraoperative
	intravenous nutritional		cholangiogram
	fluid	IOCG	intraoperative
INFC	infected		cholangiogram
	infection	IOD	interorbital distance
ING	inguinal	IODM	infant of diabetic
✔ ing	checking		mother
INH	isoniazid	IOF	intraocular fluid
INI	intranuclear inclusion	IOFB	intraocular foreign body
inj	injection	IOFNA	intraoperative fine needle
	injury		aspiration
INK	injury not known	IOH	idiopathic orthostatic
INN	International		hypotension
	Nonproprietary Name	IOI	intraosseous infusion
INO	internuclear ophthal-	IOL	intraocular lens
	moplegia	IOLI	intraocular lens
INOP	internodal ophthal-		implantation
	moplegia	IOM	Institute of Medicine
inpt	inpatient	ION	ischemic optic neuropathy
INQ	inferior nasal quadrant	IONIS	indirect optic nerve injury
INR	international normalized		syndrome
	ratio (for anticoagulant	IONTO	iontophoresis
	monitoring)	IOOA	inferior oblique
INS	idiopathic nephrotic		overaction
	syndrome	IOP	intraocular pressure
	insurance	IOR	ideas of reference
INST	instrumental delivery		immature oocyte retrieval
INT	intermittent needle		inferior oblique recession
	therapy	IO-RB	intraocular retinoblastoma
	internal	IORT	intraoperative radiation
Int mon	internal monitor		therapy
INTERP	interpretation	IOS	intraoperative sonography
Int Med	internal medicine	IOT	intraocular tension
intol	intolerance	IOUS	intraocular ultrasound
int-rot	internal rotation	IOV	initial office visit
int trx	intermittent traction	IP	ice pack
intub	intubation		incubation period
inver	inversion		individualized plan
INVOS	in vivo optical		in plaster
	spectroscopy		interphalangeal
IO	inferior oblique		interstitial pneumonia
	initial opening		intestinal permeability
	intestinal obstruction		intraperitoneal
	intraocular pressure	I/P	iris/pupil
	intra-Ommaya	IP3	inositol triphosphate

IPA	independent practice association		hyperthermic chemotherapy
	interpleural analgesia	IPI	International Prognostic Index
	invasive pulmonary aspergillosis	IPJ	interphalangeal joint
	isopropyl alcohol	IPK	intractable plantar keratosis
IPAA	ileo-pouch anal anastamosis	IPM	intrauterine pressure monitor
IPAP	inspiratory positive airway pressure	IPMI	inferoposterior myocardial infarct
IPB	infrapopliteal bypass	IPN	infantile periarteritis nodosa
IPC	indirect pulp cavity		intern's progress note
	intermittent pneumatic compression (boots)		interstitial pneumonia
	intraperitoneal chemotherapy	IPOF	immediate postoperative fitting
IPCD	idiopathic paroxysmal cerebral dysrhythmia	IPOP	immediate postoperative prosthesis
	infantile polycystic disease	IPP	inflatable penile prosthesis
IPCK	infantile polycystic kidney (disease)		intrapleual pressure
			isolated pelvic perfusion
IPCT	intraperitoneal chemotherapy	IPPA	inspection, palpation, percussion, and
IPD	idiopathic Parkinson's disease		auscultation
	immediate pigment darkening	IPPB	intermittent positive pressure breathing
	inflammatory pelvic disease	IPPF	immediate postoperative prosthetic fitting
	intermittent peritoneal dialysis	IPPI	interruption of pregnancy for psychiatric indication
	interpupillary distance	IPPV	intermittent positive pressure ventilation
IPF	idiopathic pulmonary fibrosis	IPS	infundibular pulmonic stenosis
	interstitial pulmonary fibrosis		initial prognostic score
IPFD	intrapartum fetal distress		intermittent photic stimulation
IPG	impedance plethysmography	IPSCs	islet-producing stem cells
	individually polymerized grass	IPSF	immediate postsurgical fitting
IPH	idiopathic pulmonary hemosiderosis	IPSID	immunoproliferative small intestinal disease
	interphalangeal	IPSP	inhibitory postsynaptic potential
	intraparenchymal hemorrhage	I PSY	intermediate psychiatry
IPHP	intraperitoneal	IPT	intermittent pelvic traction

iPTH	parathyroid hormone by radioimmunoassay	IRED	infrared emission detection
IPTX	intermittent pelvic traction	IRF	internal rotation in flexion
IPV	inactivated poliovirus vaccine	IRH	intraretinal hemorrhage
IPVC	interpolated premature ventricular contraction	IRI	immunoreactive insulin
IPW	interphalangeal width	IRIV	immunopotentiating reconstituted influenza virosomes
IQ	intelligence quotient		
IQR	interquartile range	IRMA	immediate response mobile analysis (blood analysis system)
IR	immediate-release (tablets)		
	inferior rectus		immunoradiometric assay
	infrared		intraretinal microvascular abnormalities
	insulin resistance		
	internal reduction	IRMS	isotope-ratio mass spectrometry
	internal resistance		
	internal rotation	IROS	ipsilateral routing of signals
I&R	insertion and removal		
IRA-EEA	ileorectal anastomoses with end-to-end anastomosis	IRR	infrared radiation
			intrarenal reflux
			irregular rate and rhythm
IRAP	interleukin-1 receptor antagonist protein	IRRC	Institutional Research Review Committee
IRB	Institutional Review Board	irreg	irregular
IRBBB	incomplete right bundle branch block	IRR HYDRO	irreversible hydrocolloid
IRBC	immature red blood cell	IRS	Information and Referral Society
	irradiated red blood cells		
IRBP	interphotoreceptor retinoid-binding protein	IRSB	intravenous regional sympathetic block
		IRT	immunoreactive trypsin
IRC	indirect radionuclide cystography	IRV	inspiratory reserve volume
	infrared coagulation		inverse ratio ventilation
	Institutional Review Committee (Board)	IS	incentive spirometer
			induced sputum
IRCU	intensive respiratory care unit		*in situ*
			intercostal space
IRD	immune renal disease(s)		inventory of systems
IRDM	insulin-resistant diabetes mellitus		ipecac syrup
		I-S	Ionescu-Shiley (prosthetic heart valve)
IRDS	idiopathic respiratory distress syndrome	I/S	instruct/supervise
		ISA	ileosigmoid anastomosis
	infant respiratory distress syndrome		Incest Survivors Anonymous
IRE	internal rotation in extension		intrinsic sympathomimetic activity

ISADH	inappropriate secretion of antidiuretic hormone	ISOK	isokinetic
		ISOM	isometric
ISB	incentive spirometry breathing	ISOs	isoenzymes
		ISP	inferior spermatic plexus
ISBP	interscalen brachial plexus		interspace
ISC	indwelling subclavian catheter	ISQ	as before; continue on (*in status quo*)
	infant servo-control	ISR	integrated secretory response
	infant skin control		
	intermittent straight catheterization	ISS	idiopathic short stature
			Individual Self-Rating Scale
	isolette servo-control		Injury Severity Score
I/SCN	urinary iodine/thiocyanate ratio		irritable stomach syndrome
ISCOM	immunostimulating complex		Integrated Summary of Safety
ISCs	irreversible sickle cells	IS10S	10% invert sugar in 0.9% sodium chloride (saline) injection
ISCU	infant special care unit		
ISD	inhibited sexual desire		
	initial sleep distur- bance	ISSP	Infant Support Services Program
	intrinsic (urethral) sphincter deficiency	IST	injection sclerotherapy
	isosorbide dinitrate		insulin sensitivity test
ISDN	isosorbide dinitrate		insulin shock therapy
ISE	ion-sensitive electrode	ISU	intermediate surgical unit
ISEL	*in situ* end labeling	ISW	interstitial water
ISF	interstitial fluid	IS10W	10% invert sugar injection (in water)
ISG	immune serum globulin (immune globulin)	ISWI	incisional surgical wound infection
ISH	isolated systolic hypertension	IT	incentive therapy
			individual therapy
ISHLT	International Society for Heart and Lung Transplantation		inferior-temporal
			Inhalation Therapist
ISHT	isolated systolic hypertension		inhalation therapy
			inspiratory time
ISI	International Sensitivity Index		intensive therapy
			intermittent traction
ISK	isokinetic		intertrochanteric
ISMA	infantile spinal muscular atrophy		intertuberous
			intrathecal (dangerous)
ISMN	isosorbide mononitrate		intratracheal (dangerous, could be interupted as intrathecal)
ISMO®	isosorbide mononitrate		
ISO	isodose	ITA	individual treatment assessment
	isolette		
	isoproterenol		inferior temporal artery
ISOE	isoetharine		itasetron
ISOF	isoflurane (Florane)		

ITAG	internal thoracic artery graft	ITVAD	indwelling transcutaneous vascular access device
ITAL	intrathoracic artificial lung	ITX	immunotoxin(s)
ITB	iliotibial band	IU	international unit (this is a dangerous abbreviation as it is read as intravenous)
	intrathecal baclofen		
ITC	Incontinence Treatment Center		
	in the canal (hearing aid)	IUC	intrauterine catheter
		IUCD	intrauterine contraceptive device
ITCP	idiopathic thrombocytopenic purpura	IUD	intrauterine death
			intrauterine device
ITCU	intensive thoracic cardiovascular unit	IUDR	idoxuridine
		IUFB	intrauterine foreign body
ITE	insufficient therapeutic effect	IUFD	intrauterine fetal death
			intrauterine fetal distress
	in-the-ear (hearing aid)	IUFT	intrauterine fetal transfusion
ITF	inpatient treatment facility		
ITFF	intertrochanteric femoral fracture	IUGR	intrauterine growth retardation (restriction)
ITGV	intrathoracic gas volume	IUI	intrauterine insemination
ITMTX	intrathecal methotrexate	IUP	intrauterine pregnancy
ITN	irinotecan (Camptosar)	IUPC	intrauterine pressure catheter
ITOC	intratracheal oxygen catheter	IUPD	intrauterine pregnancy delivered
ITOP	intentional termination of pregnancy	IUP,TBCS	intrauterine pregnancy, term birth, cesarean section
ITOU	intensive therapy observation unit		
ITP	idiopathic thrombocytopenic purpura	IUP,TBLC	intrauterine pregnancy, term birth, living child
		IUR	intrauterine retardation
	interim treatment plan	IUT	intrauterine transfusion
ITPA	Illinois Test of Psycholinguistic Ability	IUTD	immunizations up to date
		IV	four
ITQ	inferior temporal quadrant		interview
			intravenous (i.v.)
ITR	isotretinoin (Accutane)		intravertebral
ITRA	itraconazole (Sporanox)		invasive
ITSCU	infant-toddler special care unit		symbol for class 4 controlled substances
ITT	identical twins (raised) together	IVA	Intervir-A
		IVAD	implantable venous access device
	insulin tolerance test		
	intention-to-treat (analysis)		implantable vascular access device
ITU	infant-toddler unit	IVBAT	intravascular bronchoalveolar tumor
	intensive therapy unit		
	intensive treatment unit	IVC	inferior vena cava

	inspiratory vital capacity	IVO	intraoral vertical osteotomy
	intravenous chemotherapy	IVOX	intravascular oxygenator (oxygenation)
	intravenous cholangio-gram	IVP	intravenous push (this is a dangerous meaning as it is read as intravenous pyelogram)
	intraventricular catheter		
IVCD	intraventricular conduction defect (delay)		
IVCP	inferior vena cava pressure		intravenous pyelogram
		IVPB	intravenous piggyback
IVCV	inferior venacavography	IVPF	isovolume pressure flow
IVD	intervertebral disk	IVPU	intravenous push
	intravenous drip	IVR	idioventricular rhythm
IVDA	intravenous drug abuse		interactive voice-response (system)
IVDSA	intravenous digital subtraction angiography		intravenous retrograde
IVDU	intravenous drug user		intravenous rider (this is a dangerous abbreviation as it has been read as IVP-IV push)
IVET	*in vivo* expression technology		
IVF	intervertebral foramina		
	intravenous fluid(s)		isovolumic relaxation (time)
	in vitro fertilization		
IVFA	intravenous fluorescein angiography	IVRAP	intravenous retrograde access port
IVFE	intravenous fat emulsion	IVRG	intravenous retrograde
IVF-ET	*in vitro* fertilization-embryo transfer	IV-RNV	intravenous radionuclide venography
IVFT	intravenous fetal transfusion	IVRO	intraoral vertical ramus osteotomy
IVGG	intravenous gamma globulin	IVRT	isovolumic relation time
		IVS	intraventricular septum
IVGTT	intravenous glucose tolerance test		irritable voiding syndrome
IVH	intravenous hyperalimen-tation	IVSD	intraventricular septal defect
	intraventricular hemorrhage	IVSE	interventricular septal excursion
IVIG	intravenous immunoglob-ulin	IVSO	intraoral vertical segmental osteotomy
IVJC	intervertebral joint complex	IVSS	intravenous Soluset®
		IVT	intravenous transfusion
IVL	intravenous lock	IVTTT	intravenous tolbutamide tolerance test
IVLBW	infant of very low birth weight	IVU	intravenous urography (urogram)
IVMP	intravenously administered methylprednisolone	IVUC	intravenous ultrasound catheter
IVNC	isolated ventricular noncompaction	IVUS	intravascular ultrasound
		IW	inspiratory wheeze

I

IWI	inferior wall infarction
IWL	insensible water loss
IWMI	inferior wall myocardial infarct
IWML	idiopathic white matter lesion
IWT	ice-water test
	impacted wisdom teeth

J

J	Jaeger measure of near vision with 20/20 about equal to J1
	jejunostomy
	Jewish
	joint
	joule
	juice
JA	joint aspiration
Jack	jacknife position
JAFAR	Juvenile Arthritis Functional Assessment Report
JAMA	*Journal of the American Medical Association*
JAMG	juvenile autoimmune myasthenia gravis
JAN	Japanese Accepted Name
JAR	junior assistant resident
JARAN	junior assistant resident admission note
JBE	Japanese B encephalitis
JBS	Johanson Blizzard syndrome
JC	junior clinicians (medical students)
JCA	juvenile chronic arthritis
JCAHO	Joint Commission on Accreditation of Healthcare Organizations
JCOG	Japanese Clinical Oncology Group
JD	jaundice
JDG	jugulodigastric
JDM	juvenile diabetes mellitus
JDMS	juvenile dermatomyositis
JE	Japanese encephalitis
JEB	junctional escape beat
JEJ	jejunum
JER	junctional escape rhythm
JET	jejunal extension tube

	junctional ectopic tachycardia	JR	junctional rhythm
JEV	Japanese encephalitis virus	JRA	juvenile rheumatoid arthritis
JF	joint fluid	JRAN	junior resident admission note
JFS	Jewish Family Service	Jr BF	junior baby food
JGCT	juvenile granulosa cell tumor	JRC	joint replacement center
		JSF	Japanese spotted fever
JHR	Jarisch-Herxheimer reaction	JT	jejunostomy tube
JI	jejunoileal		joint
JIB	jejunoileal bypass		junctional tachycardia
JIS	juvenile idiopathic scoliosis	JTF	jejunostomy tube feeding
		JTP	joint projection
JJ	jaw jerk	JTPS	juvenile tropical pancreatitis syndrome
J & J	Johnson & Johnson Health Care Systems, Inc.	J-Tube	jejunostomy tube
		JUV	juvenile
JLP	juvenile laryngeal papillomatosis	JV	jugular vein
		JVC	jugular venous catheter
JM-9	iproplatin	JVD	jugular venous distention
JME	juvenile myoclonic epilepsy	JVP	jugular venous pressure
			jugular venous pulsation
JMS	junior medical student		jugular venous pulse
JNB	jaundice of newborn	JVPT	jugular venous pulse tracing
JNCL	juvenile-onset neuronal ceroid lipofuscinosis	JW	Jehovah's Witness
JND	just noticeable difference	Jx	joint
JNT	joint	JXG	juvenile xanthogranuloma
JNVD	jugular neck vein distention		
JODM	juvenile onset diabetes mellitus		
JOMAC	judgment, orientation, memory, abstraction, and calculation		
JOMACI	judgment, orientation, memory, abstraction, and calculation intact		
JP	Jackson-Pratt (drain) Jobst pump joint protection		
JPB	junctional premature beats		
JP BS	Jackson-Pratt to bulb suction		
JPC	junctional premature contraction		
JPS	joint position sense		

J

K

K	cornea
	kelvin
	ketamine (Super K)
	Kosher
	potassium
	thousand
	vitamin K
K'	knee
K⁺	potassium
K_1	phytonadione
K_2	menatetrenone
K_3	menadione
K_4	menadiol sodium diphosphate
17K	17-ketosteroids
KA	kainic acid
	keratoacanthoma
	ketoacidosis
Ka	first order absorption constant in hr.⁻¹
KAB	knowledge, attitude, and behavior
K-ABC	Kaufman Assessment Battery for Children
KABINS	knowledge, attitude, behavior, and improvement in nutritional status
KAFO	knee-ankle-foot orthosis
KAO	knee-ankle orthosis
KAS	Katz Adjustment Scale
KASH	knowledge, abilities, skills, and habits
kat	katal
K-A units	King-Armstrong units
KB	ketone bodies
	knee bearing
KBD	Kashin-Beck disease
KC	keratoconjunctivitis
	keratoconus
	knees to chest
	Korean conflict
kcal	kilocalorie

KCCT	kaolin cephalin clotting time
kCi	kilocurie
KCl	potassium chloride
KCS	keratoconjunctivitis sicca
KCZ	ketoconazole (Nizoral)
KD	Kawasaki's disease
	Keto Diastix®
	ketogenic diet
	kidney donors
	knee disarticulation
	knowledge deficit
Kd	kilodalton
KDA	known drug allergies
KDC®	brand name of infant warmer
KDU	Kidney Dialysis Unit
KE	first order elimination rate constant in hr.⁻¹
KED	Kendrick extrication device
k_{el}	elimination rate constant
KET	ketoconazole (Nizoral)
	ketones
KETO	ketoconazole (Nizoral)
17 Keto	17 ketosteroids
keV	kilo-electron volts
KEVD	Krupin eye valve with disk
KF	kidney function
KFA	kinetic fibrinogen assay
KFAB	kidney-fixing antibodies
KFAO	knee-foot-ankle orthosis
KFD	Kyasanur Forrest disease
KFR	Kayser-Fleischer ring
KFS	Klippel-Feil syndrome
kg	kilogram
K-G	Kimray-Greenfield (filter)
KGF	keratinocyte growth factor
KGC	Keflin, gentamicin, and carbenicillin
KHF	Korean hemorrhagic fever
K24H	potassium, urine 24 hour
kHz	kilohertz
KI	karyopyknotic index
	knee immobilizer

	potassium iodide	KSE	knee sling exercises
KID	keratitis, ichthyosis, and deafness (syndrome)	KSHV	Kaposi's sarcoma-associated herpesvirus
	kidney	KS/OI	Kaposi's sarcoma and opportunistic infections
kilo	kilogram	KSR	potassium chloride sustained release (tablets)
	thousand		
KISS	saturated solution of potassium iodide	KSW	knife stab wound
KIT	Kahn Intelligence Test	KT	kidney transplant
KIU	kallikrein inhibitor units		kinesiotherapy
KJ	kilojoule		known to
	knee jerk	KTC	knee to chest
KJR	knee jerk reflex	KTP	potassium-titanyl-phosphate (laser)
KK	knee kick		
	knock-knee	KTU	kidney transplant unit
KL-BET	Kleihauer-Betke		known to us
Kleb	*Klebsiella*	KUB	kidney(s), ureter(s), and bladder
KLH	keyhole limpet hemocyanin		kidney ultrasound biopsy
K-Lor®	potassium chloride tablets		
KLS	kidneys, liver, and spleen	KUS	kidney(s), ureter(s), and spleen
KM	kanamycin		
KMG	kangaroo-mother care	KV	kilovolt
KMnO₄	potassium permanganate	KVO	keep vein open
KMV	killed measles vaccine	KVP	kilovolt peak
KN	knee	KW	Keith-Wagener (ophthalmoscopic finding, graded I-IV)
KNO	keep needle open		
KO	keep open		
	knee orthosis		Kimmelstiel-Wilson
	knocked out	KWB	Keith, Wagener, Barker
KOH	potassium hydroxide	KWIC	keywork in context
KOR	keep open rate	K-wire	Kirschner wire
KP	hot pack		
	keratoprecipitate		
	kinetic perimetry		
KPE	Kelman phacoemulsification		
KPM	kilopounds per minute		
KPS	Karnofsky performance status (scores)		
Kr	krypton		
K-rod	Küntscher rod		
KS	Kawasaki syndrome		
	Kaposi's sarcoma		
	kidney stone		
	Klinefelter's syndrome		
17-KS	17-ketosteroids		
KSA	knowledge, skills, and abilities		

K

L

			long arm cast
		LAc	Licensed Acupuncturist
		LACC	locally advanced cervical carcinoma
		LACT-ART	lactate arterial
L	fifty	LAD	left anterior descending
	left		left axis deviation
	lente insulin		leukocyte adhesion deficiency
	levorotatory		
	lingual	LADA	left anterior descending (coronary) artery
	liter		
	liver	LADCA	left anterior descending coronary artery
	lumbar		
	lung	LADD	left anterior descending diagonal
l	levorotatory		
L'	lumbar	LAD-MIN	left axis deviation minimal
Ⓛ	left		
$L_1...L_5$	lumbar nerve 1 through 5	LADPG	laparoscopically assisted distal partial gastrectomy
	lumbar vertebra 1 through 5		
LA	language age	LAE	left atrial enlargement
	latex agglutination		long above elbow
	Latin American	LAEC	locally advanced esophageal cancer
	left arm		
	left atrial	LAF	laminar air flow
	left atrium		Latin-American female
	light adaptation		low animal fat
	linguoaxial		lymphocyte-activating factor
	linoleic acid		
	local anesthesia	LAFB	left anterior fascicular block
	long acting		
	lupus anticoagulant	LAFF	lateral arm free flap
L + A	light and accommodation	LAFM	locally acquired *Plasmodium falciparum* malaria
	living and active		
LAA	left atrium and its appendage		
		LAFR	laminar airflow room
LAAM	levomethadyl acetate (L-alpha acetylmeth-adol)	LAG	lymphangiogram
		LAH	left anterior hemiblock
			left atrial hypertrophy
LAB	laboratory	LAHB	left anterior hemiblock
	left abdomen	LAIT	latex agglutination inhibition test
LABBB	left anterior bundle branch block		
		LAK	lymphokine-activated killer
LABC	locally advanced breast cancer	LAL	left axillary line
			limulus amebocyte lysate
LAC	laceration	LALLS	low-angle laser light scattering
	left atrial catheter		
	locally advanced cancer		

LAM	laminectomy	LASER	light amplification by
	laminogram		stimulated emission of
	Latin-American male		radiation
lam✓	laminectomy check	LASIK	laser *in situ*
LAMB	mucocutaneous lentigines,		keratomileusis
	atrial myxoma, and	L-ASP	asparaginase
	blue nevus (syndrome)	LAST	left anterior small
L-AMB	liposomal amphotericin B		thoracotomy
LAMMA	laser microprobe mass	LAT	lateral
	analysis		latex agglutination test
LANC	long arm navicular cast		left anterior thigh
LAN	lymphadenopathy	LATCH	literature attached to chart
LAO	left anterior oblique	lat.men.	lateral meniscectomy
LAP	laparoscopy	LATS	long-acting thyroid
	laparotomy		stimulator
	left atrial pressure	LAUP	laser-assisted uvula-
	leucine amino peptidase		palatoplasty
	leukocyte alkaline	LAV	lymphadenopathy
	phosphatase		associated virus
LAPA	locally advanced	LAVA	laser-assisted vasal
	pancreatic		anastomosis
	adenocarcinoma	LAVH	laparoscopically assisted
LAP-	laparoscopic		vaginal hysterectomy
APPY	appendectomy	LAW	left atrial wall
LAP	laparoscopic	LAWER	life-terminating acts
CHOLE	cholecystectomy		without the explicit
LAPMS	long arm posterior		request
	molded splint	LAX	laxative
LAPW	left atrial posterior wall	LB	large bowel
LAQ	long arc quad		lateral bend
LAR	left arm, reclining		left breast
	long-acting release		left buttock
	low anterior resection		live births
LARM	left arm		low back
LARSI	lumbar anterior-root		lung biopsy
	stimulator implants		lymphoid body
LAS	laxative abuse syndrome		pound
	left arm, sitting	L&B	left and below
	leucine acetylsalicylate	LB3	colonoscope
	long arm splint	LBA	laser balloon angioplasty
	low-amplitude signal	LBB	left breast biopsy
	lymphadenopathy		long back board
	syndrome	LBBB	left bundle branch block
	lymphangioscintigraphy	LBBx	left breast biopsy
	lysine acetylsalicylate	LBCD	left border of cardiac
LASA	Linear Analogue		dullness
	Self-Assessment	L/B/Cr	electrolytes, blood urea
	(scales)		nitrogen, and serum
	lipid-associated sialic acid		creatinine

L

LBD	large bile duct	LCAH	life care at home
	left border dullness	LCAL	large-cell anaplastic lymphoma
	Lewy body dementia		
	low back disability	LCAT	lecithin cholesterol acyltransferase
LBE	long below elbow		
LBG	Landry-Guillain-Barré (syndrome)	LCB	left costal border
		LCCA	left common carotid artery
LBH	length, breadth, and height		
			leukocytoclastic angiitis
LBM	last bowel movement	LCCS	low cervical cesarean section
	lean body mass		
	loose bowel movement	LCD	coal tar solution (*liquor carbonis detergens*)
LBMI	last body mass index		
LBNA	lysis bladder neck adhesions		localized collagen dystrophy
			low calcium diet
LBNP	lower body negative pressure	LCDC	Laboratory Centre for Disease Control (Canada)
LBO	large bowel obstruction		
LBP	low back pain	LCDCP	low-contact dynamic compression plate
	low blood pressure		
LBQC	large base quad cane	LCDE	laparoscopic common duct exploration
LBS	low back syndrome		
	pounds	LCE	laparoscopic cholecystectomy
LBT	low back tenderness		
	low back trouble		left carotid endarterec- tomy
LBV	left brachial vein		
	low biological value	LCF	left circumflex
LBW	lean body weight	LCFA	long-chain fatty acid
	low birth weight (less than 2,500 g)	LCFM	left circumflex marginal
		LCGU	local cerebral glucose utilization
LBWI	low birth weight infant		
		LCH	Langerhans' cell histiocytosis
LC	Laënnec's cirrhosis		
	laparoscopic cholecystectomy		local city hospital
		LCIS	lobular cancer *in situ*
	left circumflex	LCL	lateral collateral ligament
	leisure counseling		
	level of consciousness	LCLC	large cell lung carcinoma
	living children	LCM	left costal margin
	low calorie		lower costal margin
	lung cancer		lymphocytic choriomeningitis
3LC	triple lumen catheter		
LCA	Leber's congenital amaurosis	LCMI	left ventricular mass index
	left circumflex artery	LCN	lidocaine
	left coronary artery	LCO	low cardiac output
	light contact assist	LCP	long, closed, posterior (cervix)
LCAD	long-chain acyl-coenzyme A dehydrogenase		

LCPD	Legg-Calvé-Perthes disease	L/D	labor and delivery
			light to dark (ratio)
LCPUFAs	long-chain polyunsaturated fatty acids	LD-1	lactic dehydrogenase 1
		LD-5	lactic dehydrogenase 5
		LD_{50}	median lethal dose
LCR	late cortical response	LDA	low density areas
	late cutaneous reaction		low-dose arm
	ligase chain reaction	LDB	Legionnaires disease bacterium
LCS	low constant suction		
	low continuous suction	LDCOC	low-dose combination oral contraceptive
LCSG	left cardiac sympathetic ganglionectomy	LDD	laser disk decompression
	lost child support group		Lee and Desu's D (test)
LCSS	Lung Cancer Symptom Score		light-dark discrimination
		LDDS	local dentist
LCSW	Licensed Clinical Social Worker	LDEA	left deviation of electrical axis
	low continuous wall suction	LDF	laser Doppler flowmetry
LCT	long chain triglyceride	LDH	lactic dehydrogenase
	low cervical transverse	LDIH	left direct inguinal hernia
	lymphocytotoxicity	LDIR	low dose of ionizing radiation
LCTCS	low cervical transverse cesarean section	LDL	low-density lipoprotein
		LDLC	low-density lipoprotein cholesterol
LCTD	low-calcium test diet		
LCV	leucovorin	LDMRT	low-dose mediastinal radiation therapy
	leukocytoclastic vasculitis	LDNF	lung-derived neurotrophic factor
	low cervical vertical		
LCX	left circumflex coronary artery	l-dopa	levodopa
		LD-PCR	limiting dilution polymerase chain reaction
LD	lactic dehydrogenase (formerly LDH)		
	last dose	LDR	labor, delivery, and recovery
	latissimus dorsi		length-to-diameter ratio
	learning disability	LDR/P	labor, delivery, recovery, and postpartum
	learning disorder		
	left deltoid	LDT	left dorsotransverse
	Legionnaire's disease	LD-T	lactic dehydrogenase total
	lethal dose	LDUB	long double upright brace
	levodopa	LDUH	low-dose unfractionated heparin
	Licensed Dietician		
	liver disease	LDV	laser Doppler velocimetry
	living donor	LE	left ear
	loading dose		left eye
	long dwell		lens extraction
	low density		live embryo
	low dosage		lower extremities
	Lyme disease		
L&D	labor and deliver		

161

	lupus erythematosus	LESI	lumbar epidural steroid injection
LEA	lower extremity amputation	LESP	lower esophageal sphincter pressure
	lumbar epidural anesthesia	LET	left esotropia
LEAD	lower extremity arterial disease		leukocyte esterase test
LEAP	Lower Extremity Amputation Prevention (program)		lidocaine, epinephrine and tetracaine gel
			linear energy transfer
LEB	lumbar epidural block	LEU	leucine
LEC	lens epithelial cell	LEV	levamisole
LECBD	laparoscopic exploration of the common bile duct		levator muscle
		LEVA	levamisole (Ergamisol)
LED	liposomal encapsulated doxorubicin	LF	laparoscopic fundoplications
	lowest effective dose		Lassa fever
	lupus erythematosus disseminatus		left foot
			living female
LEEP	loop electrosurgical excision procedure		low fat
			low forceps
LEF	lower extremity fracture		low frequency
LEH	liposome-encapsulated hemoglobin	LFA	left femoral artery
			left forearm
LEHPZ	lower esophageal high pressure zone		left fronto-anterior
			leukocyte function-associated antigen
LEJ	ligation of the esophagogastric junction		low friction arthroplasty
			lymphocyte function-associated antigen
LEM	lateral eye movements	LFA-1	leukocyte function-associated antigen-1
	light electron microscope	LFB	low frequency band
LEP	leptospirosis	LFC	living female child
	lower esophageal pressure		low fat and cholesterol
LEP 2	leptospirosis 2	LFCS	low flap cesarean section
LE prep	lupus erythematosus preparation	LFD	lactose-free diet
L-ERX	leukoerythroblastic reaction		low fat diet
			low fiber diet
LES	local excitatory state		low forceps delivery
	lower esophageal sphincter		lunate fossa depression
	lumbar epidural steroids	LFGNR	lactose fermenting gram-negative rod
	lupus erythematosus systemic	LFL	left frontolateral
		LFM	lateral force microscopy
LESEP	lower extremity somatosensory evoked potential	LFP	left frontoposterior
		LFS	leukemia-free survival
			Li-Fraumeni syndrome
			liver function series
LESG	Late Effects Study Group	LFT	latex flocculation test

	left fronto-transverse	LHON	Leber's hereditary optic
	liver function tests		neuropathy
	low flap transverse	LHP	left hemiparesis
LFU	limit flocculation	LHR	leukocyte histamine
	unit		release
	lost to follow-up	LHRH	luteinizing hormone-
LG	large		releasing hormone
	laryngectomy	LHRH-A	luteinizing hormone-
	left gluteal		releasing hormone
	linguogingival		analogue
	lymphography	LHRT	leukocyte histamine
LGA	large for gestational age		release test
	left gastric artery	LHS	left hand side
LGI	lower gastrointestinal		long-handled sponge
	(series)	LHSH	long-handled shoe horn
LGIOS	low-grade intraosseous-	LHT	left hypertropia
	type osteosarcoma	LI	lactose intolerance
LGL	large granular lymphocyte		lamellar ichthyosis
	low-grade lymphoma(s)		large intestine
	Lown-Ganong-Levine		laser iridotomy
	(syndrome)		learning impaired
LGLS	Lown-Ganong-Levine		linguoincisal
	syndrome		liver involvement
LGM	left gluteus medius	Li	lithium
	(maximus)	LIA	laser interference acuity
LGN	lateral geniculate leaflet		left iliac artery
	lobular glomerulonephritis	LIB	left in bottle
LG-NHL	low-grade non-Hodgkin's	LIC	left iliac crest
	lymphoma		left internal carotid
LGS	Lennox-Gastaut syndrome		leisure interest class
	low Gomco suction	LICA	left internal carotid artery
LGSIL	low grade squamous	LICD	lower intestinal Crohn's
	intraepithelial lesion		disease
LGV	lymphogranuloma	LICM	left intercostal margin
	venerum	Li_2CO_3	lithium carbonate
LH	learning handicap	LICS	left intercostal space
	left hand	Lido	lidocaine
	left hemisphere	LIF	left iliac fossa
	left hyperphoria		left index finger
	luteinizing hormone		leukemia-inhibiting factor
LHA	left hepatic artery		liver (migration)
LHC	left heart catheterization		inhibitory factor
LHF	left heart failure	LIFE	laser-induced fluorescence
LHG	left hand grip		emission
LHH	left homonymous		lung imaging fluorescence
	hemianopsia		endoscopy
LHI	Labor Health Institute	LIG	ligament
LHL	left hemisphere lesions		lymphocyte immune
	left hepatic lobe		globulin

L

163

LIGHTS	phototherapy lights	LITHO	lithotripsy
LIH	laparoscopic inguinal herniorrhaphy	LITT	laser-induced thermotherapy
	left inguinal hernia	LIV	left innominate vein
LIHA	low impulsiveness, high anxiety	L-IVP	limited intravenous pyelogram
LIJ	left internal jugular	LIVB	live birth
LILA	low impulsiveness, low anxiety	LIVC	left inferior vena cava
		LIVPRO	liver profile
LIM	limited toxicology screening	LIWS	low intermittent wall suction
LIMA	left internal mammary artery (graft)	LJL	lateral joint line
		LJM	limited joint mobility
LINDI	lithium-induced nephrogenic diabetes insipidus	LK	lamellar keratoplasty
			left kidney
		LKA	Lazare-Klerman-Armour (Personality Inventory)
LING	lingual		
LIO	laser indirect ophthalmoscope	LKM-3	liver-kidney microsomal antibodies type 3
	left inferior oblique (muscle)	LKS	Landau-Kleffner syndrome
LIOU	laparoscopic intraoperative ultrasound		liver, kidneys, spleen
		LKSB	liver, kidneys, spleen, and bladder
LIP	lithium-induced polydipsia	LKSNP	liver, kidneys, and spleen not palpable
	lymphocytic interstitial pneumonia	L — M K — O — S — T	liver, kidneys, and spleen negative, no masses, or tenderness
LIPV	left inferior pulmonary vein		
		LL	large lymphocyte
LIQ	liquid		left lateral
	liquor		left leg
	lower inner quadrant		left lower
LIR	left iliac region		left lung
	left inferior rectus		lid lag
LIS	left intercostal space		long leg (brace or cast)
	locked-in syndrome		lower lid
	low intermittent suction		lower lip
			lower lobe
	lung injury score		lumbar laminectomy
LISS	low ionic strength saline		lumbar length
			lymphocytic leukemia
LISW	Licensed Independent Social Worker		lymphoblastic lymphoma
		L&L	lids and lashes
LIT	literature	LL2	limb lead two
	liver injury test	LLA	lids, lashes, and adnexa
LITA	left internal thoracic artery		limulus lysate assay
		LLAT	left lateral
LITH	lithotomy	LLB	last living breath

	left lateral bending	LMC	living male child
	left lateral border	LMCA	left main coronary artery
	long leg brace		left middle cerebral artery
LLC	laparoscopic laser cholecystectomy	LMCAT	left middle cerebral artery thrombosis
	long leg cast	LMCL	left midclavicular line
LLBCD	left lower border of cardiac dullness	LMD	local medical doctor low molecular weight
LLD	left lateral decubitus		dextran
	left length discrepancy	LME	left mediolateral
LLE	left lower extremity		episiotomy
	little league elbow	LMEE	left middle ear
LLETZ	large-loop excision of the transformation zone	LMF	exploration left middle finger
LLFG	long leg fiberglas (cast)		melphalan (L-PAM),
LLG	left lateral gaze		methotrexate, and
LL-GXT	low-level graded exercise test	L/min	fluorouracil liters per minute
LLL	left lower lid	LML	left medial lateral
	left lower lobe (lung)		left middle lobe
LLLE	lower lid left eye	LMLE	left mediolateral
LLLNR	left lower lobe, no rales		episiotomy
LLO	Legionella-like organism	LMM	lentigo maligna melanoma
LLOD	lower lid, right eye	LMN	lower motor neuron
	lower limit of detection	LMNL	lower motor neuron lesion
LLOS	lower lid, left eye	LMP	last menstrual period
LLP	long leg plaster		left mentoposterior
LLQ	left lower quadrant (abdomen)	LMR	low malignant potential left medial rectus
LLR	left lateral rectus	LMRM	left modified radical
LLRE	lower lid, right eye		mastectomy
LLS	lazy leukocyte syndrome	LMS	lateral medullary
LLSB	left lower sternal border		syndrome
LLT	left lateral thigh	LMT	left main trunk
	lowest level term		left mentotransverse
LLWC	long leg walking cast	LMW	low molecular weight
LLX	left lower extremity	LMWD	low molecular weight
LM	left main		dextran
	light microscopy	LMWH	low molecular weight
	linguomesial		heparins
	living male	LN	latent nystagmus
	lung metastases		left nostril (nare)
L/M	liters per minute		lymph nodes
LMA	laryngeal mask airway	LN_2	liquid nitrogen
	left mentoanterior	LNA	alpha-linolenic acid
	liver membrane autoantibody	LNB	lymph node biopsy
		LNCs	lymph node cells
LMB	Laurence-Moon-Biedl syndrome	LND	light-near dissociation lonidamine

L

	lymph node dissection	LOHF	late-onset hepatic failure
LNE	lymph node enlargement	L-OHP	oxaliplatin
	lymph node excision	LOIH	left oblique inguinal
LNF	laparoscopic Nissen		hernia
	fundoplication	LOI	level of injury
LNG	levonorgestrel		Leyton Obsessional
LNM	lymph node metastases		Inventory
LNMC	lymph node mononuclear	LOINC	Logical Observation
	cells		Identifier Names and
LNMP	last normal menstrual		Codes
	period	LOL	laughing out loud
LNNB	Luria-Nebraska		left occipitolateral
	Neuropsychological		little old lady
	Battery	LOM	left otitis media
LNS	lymph node sampling		limitation of motion
LNT	late neurological toxicity		little old man
LO	lateral oblique (x-ray		loss of motion
	view)		low-osmolar (contrast)
	linguo-occlusal		media
	lumbar orthosis	LOMSA	left otitis media,
5-LO	5-lipoxygenase		suppurative, acute
LOA	late-onset agammaglobu-	LOMSC	left otitis media,
	linemia		suppurative, chronic
	leave of absence	LoNa	low sodium
	left occiput anterior	LOO	length of operation
	looseness of associations	LOP	laparoscopic orchiopexy
	lysis of adhesions		leave on pass
LOAD	late-onset Alzheimer's		left occiput posterior
	disease		level of pain
LOAEL	lowest observed adverse	LOQ	limit(s) of quantitation
	effect level		lower outer quadrant
LOB	loss of balance	LOR	loss of resistance
LOC	laxative of choice	LORS-I	Level of Rehabilitation
	level of care		Scale-I
	level of comfort	LOS	length of stay
	level of concern		loss of sight
	level of consciousness	LOT	left occiput transverse
	local		Licensed Occupational
	loss of consciousness		Therapist
LOCM	low-osmolality contrast	LOV	loss of vision
	media	LOVA	loss of visual acuity
LOD	limit of detection	LOZ	lozenge
	line of duty	LP	light perception
LOF	leaking of fluids		linguopulpal
	leave on floor		lipoprotein
LOFD	low outlet forceps		low protein
	delivery		lumbar puncture
LOG	Logmar chart	L/P	lactate-pyruvate
LOH	loss of heterozygosity		ratio

LP5	Life-Pak 5	LPO	left posterior oblique
LPA	left pulmonary artery		light perception only
Lp(a)	lipoprotein (a)	LPPC	leukocyte-poor packed
LPA%	left pulmonary artery		cells
	oxygen saturation	LPPH	late postpartum
L-PAM	melphalan		hemorrhage
LPC	laser photocoagulation	LPS	last Pap smear
	Licensed Professional		lipopolysaccharide
	Counselor	LP	lumboperitoneal shunt
LPCC	Licensed Professional	SHUNT	
	Certified Counselor	LP$\bar{s}$P	light perception without
LPC-L	lymphoplasmacytoid		projection
	lymphoma	LPT	Licensed Physical
LP$\bar{c}$P	light perception with		Therapist
	projection	LPTN	Licensed Psychiatric
LPD	leiomyomatosis		Technical Nurse
	peritonealis disseminata	LPV	left portal vein
	low potassium dextran		left pulmonary vein
	low protein diet	LQTS	long QT interval
	luteal phase defect		syndrome
	luteal phase deficiency	LR	labor room
	lymphoproliferative		lactated Ringer's
	disease		(injection)
LPDA	left posterior descending		lateral rectus
	artery		left-right
LPEP	left pre-ejection period		light reflex
LPF	liver plasma flow	L&R	left and right
	low-power field	L→R	left to right
	lymphocytosis-promoting	LR1A	labor room 1A
	factor	LRA	left radial artery
LPFB	left posterior fascicular		left renal artery
	block	LRC	lower rib cage
LPH	left posterior hemiblock	LRCP	Licentiate of the Royal
LPHB	left posterior hemiblock		College of Physicians
LPI	laser peripheral	LRCS	Licentiate of the Royal
	iridectomy		College of Surgeons
	leukotriene pathway	LRD	limb reduction
	inhibitor		defects
LPICA	left posterior internal		living-related donor
	carotid artery		living renal donor
LPIH	left-posterior-inferior	LRDT	living-related donor
	hemiblock		transplant
LPL	left posterolateral	LRE	localization-related
	lipoprotein lipase		epilepsy
LPLND	laparoscopic pelvic lymph	LREH	low renin essential
	node dissection		hypertension
LPM	latent primary malignancy	LRF	left rectus femoris
	liters per minute	L&R gtt	Levophed and Regitine
LPN	Licensed Practical Nurse		drip (infusion)

L

LRHT	living-related hepatic transplantation		lymphosarcoma
		LSB	left scapular border
LRI	lower respiratory infection		left sternal border
			local standby
LRLT	living-related liver transplantation		lumbar spinal block
			lumbar sympathetic block
LRM	left radical mastectomy		
	local regional metastases	LS BPS	laparoscopic bilateral partial salpingectomy
LRMP	last regular menstrual period		
		LSC	last sexual contact
LRND	left radical neck dissection		late systolic click
			left subclavian (artery) (vein)
LRO	long range objective		
Lrot	left rotation		lichen simplex chronicus
LRP	lung-resistance protein		
LRQ	lower right quadrant	LSCA	left scapuloanterior
LROU	lateral rectus, both eyes	LSCP	left scapuloposterior
LRR	light reflection rheography	LSCS	lower segment cesarean section
LRRT	locoregional radiotherapy	LSD	least significant difference
LRS	lactated Ringer's solution		low salt diet
LRT	living renal transplant		lysergide
	local radiation therapy	LSE	local side effects
	lower respiratory tract	LSed	level of sedation
LRTD	living relative transplant donor	LSF	low saturated fat
		LSFA	low saturated fatty acid (diet)
LRTI	ligament reconstruction with tendon interposition		
		L-SIL	low-grade squamous intraepithelial lesions
	lower respiratory tract infection		
		LSK	liver, spleen, and kidneys
LRV	left renal vein	LSKM	liver-spleen-kidney-megalgia
	log reduction value		
LRZ	lorazepam	LSL	left sacrolateral
LS	left side		left short leg (brace)
	legally separated	LSLF	low sodium, low fat (diet)
	Leigh's syndrome	LSM	laser scanning microscope
	liver scan		late systolic murmur
	liver-spleen		least squares mean
	low salt		limited sampling model
	lumbosacral		liver, spleen masses
L/S	lecithin-sphingomyelin ratio	LSMT	life-sustaining medical treatment
L&S	ligation and stripping	LSO	left salpingo-oophorectomy
	liver and spleen		left superior oblique
L5-S1	lumbar fifth vertebra to sacral first vertebra		lumbosacral orthosis
		LSP	left sacrum posterior
LSA	left sacrum anterior		liver-specific (membrane) lipoprotein
	lipid-bound sialic acid		

L–Spar	Elspar (asparaginase)	LTC₄	leukotriene C_4
L-SPINE	lumbar spine	LTC-101	long-term care form-101
LSQ	Life Situation Questionnaire	LTCCS	low transverse cervical cesarean section
LSR	left superior rectus	LTCF	long-term care facility
L/S ratio	lecithin/sphingomyelin ratio	LTC-IC	long-term culture-initiating cells
LSS	limb sparing surgery	LTCS	low transverse cesarean section
	liver-spleen scan	LTD	largest tumor dimension
	lumbar spinal stenosis		leg transfer device
LSSS	Liverpool Seizure Severity Scale	LTD₄	leukotriene D_4
LST	left sacrum transverse	LTE	less than effective
LSTC	laparoscopic tubal coagulation	LTE₄	leukotriene E_4
		LTFU	long-term follow-up
LSTL	laparoscopic tubal ligation	LTG	lamotrigine
L's & T's	lines and tubes		long-term goal
LSU	life support unit	LTGA	low tension glaucoma
LSV	left subclavian vein		left transposition of great artery
LSVC	left superior vena cava		
LSW	left-side weakness	LTH	luteotropic hormone
	Licensed Social Worker	LTK	laser thermal keratoplasty
LT	laboratory technician	LTL	laparoscopic tubal ligation
	left		
	left thigh	LTM	long-term memory
	left triceps		long-term monitoring
	leukotrienes	LTOT	long-term oxygen therapy
	Levin tube	LTP	laser trabeculoplasty
	light		long-term plan
	light touch		long-term potentiation
	low transverse	LTR	long terminal repeats
	lumbar traction		lower trunk rotation
	lung transplantation	LTRA	leukotriene receptor antagonist
	lunotriquetral		
	lymphotoxin	LTS	laparoscopic tubal sterilization
L&T	lettuce and tomato		long-term survivors
LT4	levothyroxine	LTT	lactose tolerance test
LTA	laryngotracheal applicator		lymphocyte transformation test
	laryngeal tracheal anesthesia		
		LTUI	low transverse uterine incision
	local tracheal anesthesia		
LTAS	left transatrial septal	LTV	long term variability
LTB	laparoscopic tubal banding		Luche tumor virus
		LTV+	long-term variability–average to moderate
	laryngotracheobronchitis		
LTB₄	leukotriene B_4		
LTC	left to count	LTV 0	long-term variability–absent
	long-term care		
	long thick closed		

169

L

LTVC	long-term venous catheter	LVAS	left ventricular assist system
LTZ	letrozole (Femara)		
LU	left upper	LVAT	left ventricular activation time
	left ureteral		
	living unit	LVBP	left ventricle bypass pump
	Lutheran	LVD	left ventricular dimension
L & U	lower and upper		left ventricular dysfunction
LUA	left upper arm		
LUD	left uterine displacement	LVDP	left ventricular diastolic pressure
LUE	left upper extremity		
Lues I	primary syphilis	LVDT	linear variable differential transformer
Lues II	secondary syphilis		
Lues III	tertiary syphilis	LVDV	left ventricular diastolic volume
LUL	left upper lid		
	left upper lobe (lung)	LVE	left ventricular enlargement
LUNA	laparoscopic uterosacral nerve ablation		
		LVEDP	left ventricular end diastolic pressure
LUOB	left upper outer buttock		
LUOQ	left upper outer quadrant	LVEDV	left ventricular end-diastolic volume
LUQ	left upper quadrant		
LURD	living unrelated donor	LVEF	left ventricular ejection fraction
LUS	laparoscopic ultrasonography		
		LVEP	left ventricular end pressure
	lower uterine segment		
LUSB	left upper scapular border	LVESVI	left ventricular end systolic volume index
	left upper sternal border		
LUST	lower uterine segment transverse	LVET	left ventricular ejection time
LUT	lower urinary tract	LVF	left ventricular failure
LUTS	lower urinary tract symptoms		left visual field
		LVFP	left ventricular filling pressure
LUTT	lower urinary tract tumor		
LUX	left upper extremity	LVFU	leucovorin and fluorouracil
LV	leave		
	left ventricle	LVG	left ventrogluteal
	leucovorin	LVH	left ventricular hypertrophy
	live virus		
LVA	left ventricular aneurysm	LVID	left ventricular internal diameter
LVC	laser vision correction		
	low viscosity cement	LVIDd	left ventricle internal dimension diastole
	low vision clinic		
LVAD	left ventricular assist device	LVIDs	left ventricle internal dimension systole
LV Angio	left ventricular angiogram	LVL	large volume leukapheresis
L-VAM	leuprolide acetate, vinblastine, doxorubicin (Adriamycin), and mitomycin		left vastus lateralis
		LVM	left ventricular mass
		LVMI	left ventricular mass index

LVMM	left ventricular muscle mass	LWCT	left without completing treatment
LVN	Licensed Visiting Nurse	LWOP	leave without pay
	Licensed Vocational Nurse	LWOT	left without treatment
		LWP	large whirlpool
LVO	left ventricular overactivity	LX	larynx local irradiation lower extremity
LVOP	left ventricular outflow tract	LXC	laxative of choice
		LXT	left exotropia
LVP	large volume parenteral left ventricular pressure	LYCD	live yeast cell derivative
		LYEL	lost years of expected life
LVPW	left ventricular posterior wall	LYG	lymphomatoid granulomatosis
LVR	leucovorin	LYM	lymphocytes
LVRS	lung volume reduction surgery	lymphs	lymphocytes
		LYS	large yellow soft (stools) lysine
LVRT	liver volume replaced by tumor	lytes	electrolytes (Na, K, Cl, etc.)
LVS	left ventricular strain	LZ	landing zone
LVS EMI	left ventricular subendocardial myocardial ischemia	LZP	lorazepam
LVSP	left ventricular systolic pressure		
LVSW	left ventricular stroke work		
LVSWI	left ventricular stroke work index		
LVV	left ventricular volume live varicella vaccine		
LVW	left ventricular wall		
LVWI	left ventricular work index		
LVWMA	left ventricular wall motion abnormality		
LVWMI	left ventricular wall motion index		
LVWT	left ventricular wall thickness		
LW	lacerating wound living will		
L & W	Lee and White (coagulation) living and well		
LWAQ	Living with Asthma Questionnaire		
LWCT	Lee-White clotting time		
LWBS	left without being seen		
LWC	leave without consent		

L

M

M	male
	manual
	marital
	married
	masked (audiology)
	mass
	medial
	memory
	mesial
	meta
	meter (m)
	mild
	million
	minimum
	molar
	Monday
	monocytes
	mother
	mouth
	murmur
	muscle
	Mycobacterium
	Mycoplasma
	myopia
	myopic
	thousand
Ⓜ	murmur
M_1	first mitral sound
M1	left mastoid
M1 to M7	categories of acute nonlymphoblastic leukemia
M_2	second mitral sound
m^2	square meters (body surface)
M2	right mastoid
M-2	vincristine, carmustine, cyclophosphamide, melphalan, and prednisone
M_3	third mitral sound
M-3	medical student 3rd year
3M	mitomycin, mitoxantrone, and methotrexate
M-3+7	mitoxantrone and cytarabine
M-4	medical student 4th year
MA	machine
	Master of Arts
	mean arterial (blood pressure)
	medical assistance
	medical authorization
	megestrol acetate
	menstrual age
	mental age
	Mexican American
	microaneurysms
	Miller-Abbott (tube)
	milliamps
	monoclonal antibodies
	motorcycle accident
M/A	mood and/or affect
MA-1	Bennett volume ventilator
MAA	macroaggregates of albumin
	Marketing Authorization Application (European Union)
MAB	maximum androgen blockade
Mab	monoclonal antibody
MABP	mean arterial blood pressure
MAC	macrocytic erythrocytes
	macrophage
	macula
	maximal allowable concentration
	medial arterial calcification
	membrane attack complex
	methotrexate, dactinomycin (Actinomycin D), and cyclophosphamide
	mid-arm circumference
	minimum alveolar concentration
	monitored anesthesia care

172

	multi-access catheter	MAFO	molded ankle/foot orthosis
	Mycobacterium avium	MAFP	maternal alpha-fetoprotein
	complex	MAG	medication administration
MACC	methotrexate,		guideline (record)
	doxorubicin,	mag cit	magnesium citrate
	(Adriamycin)	MAGP	meatal advancement
	cyclophosphamide, and		glandulophaleoplasty
	lomustine (Cee Nu)	mag sulf	magnesium sulfate
MACCC	Master Arts, Certified	MAHA	macroangiopathic
	Clinical Competence		hemolytic anemia
MACE	Malon antegrade	MAI	maximal aggregation
	continence enema		index
MACOP-B	methotrexate,		minor acute illness
	doxorubicin,		*Mycobacterium*
	(Adriamycin)		*avium-intracellulare*
	cyclophosphamide,	MAID	mesna, doxorubicin
	vincristine (Oncovin),		(Adriamycin),
	prednisone,		ifosfamide, and
	and bleomycin with		dacarbazine
	leucovorin rescue	MAL	malignant
MACRO	macrocytes		midaxillary line
MACS	magnetic activated cell	MALDI	matrix assisted laser
	sorting		desorption ionization
MACs	malignancy-associated	MALG	Minnesota antilympho-
	changes		blast globulin
MACTAR	McMaster-Toronto	malig	malignant
	Arthritis Patient	MALT	mucosa-associated
	Reference (Disability		lymphoid tissue
	Questionnaire)	MALToma	lymphoma of mucosa-
MAD	mind altering drugs		associated lymphoid
	moderate atopic dermatitis		tissue
MADD	Mothers Against Drunk	MAM	mammogram
	Driving		Mexican-American male
MADRS	Montgomery-Åsburg		monitored administration
	Depression Rating		of medication
	Scale	MAMC	mid-arm muscle
MAE	medical air evacuation		circumference
	moves all extremities	Mammo	mammography
MAES	moves all extremities	m-AMSA	amsacrine
	slowly	MAN	malignancy associated
MAEEW	moves all extremities		neutropenia
	equally well	Mand	mandibular
MAEW	moves all extremities	MANE	Morrow Assessment of
	well		Nausea and Emesis
MAF	metabolic activity factor	MANOVA	multivariate analysis of
	Mexican-American female		variance
MAFAs	movement-associated fetal	MAO	maximum acid output
	(heart rate)	MAO-A	monoamine oxidase type
	accelerations		A

M

MAO-B	monoamine oxidase type B		stimulated emission of radiation
MAOI	monoamine oxidase inhibitor	MASH POT	mashed potatoes
MAOP	Mid-Atlantic Oncology Program	MAST	mastectomy
			medical antishock trousers
MAP	magnesium, ammonium, and phosphate (Struvite stones)		Michigan Alcoholism Screening Test
			military antishock trousers
	mean airway pressure	MAT	manual arts therapy
	mean arterial pressure		maternal
	Medical Assistance Program		maternity
			mature
	megaloblastic anemia of pregnancy		medication administration team
	mitogen-activated protein		Miller-Abbott tube
	mitomycin, doxorubicin (Adriamycin), and cisplatin (Platinol)		multifocal atrial tachycardia
		MAU	microalbuminuria
	morning after pill (oral contraceptives)	MAVR	mitral and aortic valve replacement
	muscle-action potential	max	maxillary
MAPI	Millon Adolescent Personality Inventory		maximal
		MAX A	maximum assistance (assist)
MAPS	Make a Picture Story	MAXCONT	maximum contrast method
MAR	marital		
	medication administration record	MAxL	mid-axillary line
		MAYO	mayonnaise
	mineral apposition rates	MB	buccal margin
MARE	manual active-resistive exercise		mandible
			Mallory body
MARSA	methicillin-aminoglycoside-resistant *Staphylococcus aureus*		Medical Board
			medulloblastoma
			mesiobuccal
MAS	macrophage activation syndrome		methylene blue
		M/B	mother/baby
	meconium aspiration syndrome	MBA	Master of Business Administration
	Memory Assessment Scale	M-BACOD	methotrexate (high-dose), bleomycin, doxorubicin (Adriamycin), cyclophosphamide, vincristine (Oncovin), and dexamethasone with leucovorin rescue
	minimum-access surgery		
	mobile arm support		
MASA	mutant allele-specific amplification		
MASDA^SM	Multiple-Allele-Specific Diagnostic Assay	MBC	male breast cancer
MASER	microwave amplification (application) by		maximum bladder capacity

	maximum breathing capacity		mitoxantrone and cytarabine
	metastatic breast cancer		mitral commissurotomy
	methotrexate, bleomycin, and cisplatin		mixed cellularity
	minimal bactericidal concentration		molluscum contagiosum
MB-CK	a creatinine kinase isoenzyme		monocomponent highly purified pork insulin
MBD	metabolic bone disease		*Moraxella catarrhalis*
	methylene blue dye		mouth care
MBEST	modulus blipped echo-planar single-pulse technique	m + c	myocarditis morphine and cocaine
		MCA	Medicines Control Agency (United Kingdom)
MBD	minimal brain damage minimal brain dysfunction		megestrol, cyclophospha- mide, and doxorubicin (Adriamycin)
MBE	may be elevated medium below elbow		metacarpal amputation
MBF	meat base formula myocardial blood flow		micrometastases clonogenic assay
MBFC	medial brachial fascial compartment		middle cerebral aneurysm middle cerebral artery
MBHI	Millon Behavioral Health Inventory		monoclonal antibodies motorcycle accident
MBI	methylene blue installation		multichannel analyzer multiple congenital anomalies
MBL	mannose-binding lectin menstrual blood loss	2-MCA	2-methyl citric acid
MBM	mother's breast milk	MCAD	medium-chain acyl-CoA dehydrogenase
MBNW	multiple-breath nitrogen washout	MCAF	monocyte chemoattractant and activity factor
MBO	mesiobuccal occlusion	MCAO	middle cerebral artery occlusion
MBP	malignant brachial plexopathy	MCAT	Medical College Admission Test
	mannan-binding protein mannose-binding protein	MCB	Medicines Control Board (United Kingdom's equivalent to the United States Food and Drug Administration)
	medullary bone pain mesiobuccopulpal myelin basic protein		
MBq	megabecquerels		mid-cycle bleeding
MBS	modified barium swallow		middle chamber bubbling
MBT	maternal blood type	McB pt	McBurney's point
MC	male child	MCC	microcrystalline cellulose
	medium-chain (triglycerides)		midstream clean-catch
	metacarpal	MCCU	mobile coronary care unit
	metatarso - cuneiform	MCD	malformation of cortical development
	mini-laparotomy cholecystectomy		

M

	mean cell diameter	MCP	mean carotid pressure
	minimal-change disease		metacarpophalangeal joint
	multicystic dysplasia		metoclopramide (Reglan)
MCDT	mast cell degranulation test		monocyte chemotactic protein
MCF	multicentric foci	MCR	Medicare
MCFA	medium chain fatty acid		metabolic clearance rate
mcg	microgram (μg)		myocardial revascularization
MCG	magnetocardiogram magnetocardiography	MC=R	moderately constricted and equally reactive
MCGN	minimal-change glomerular nephritis	MCRC	metastatic colorectal cancer
MCH	mean corpuscular hemoglobin	MCS	microculture and sensitivity
	microfibrillar collagen hemostat		moderate constant suction
	muscle contraction headache		multiple chemical sensitivity
MCHC	mean corpuscular hemoglobin concentration		myocardial contractile state
mCi	millicurie	MCSA	minimal cross-sectional area
MCID	minimum clinically important difference(s)	M-CSF	macrophage colony-stimulating factor
MCL	mantle cell lymphoma	MC-SR	moderately constricted and slightly reactive
	maximum comfort level		
	medial collateral ligament	MCT	manual cervical traction
	midclavicular line		mean circulation time
	midcostal line		medium chain triglyceride
	modified chest lead		medullary carcinoma of the thyroid
	most comfortable level		
mcL	microliter (1/1,000 of an mL)		microwave coagulation therapy
MCLL	most comfortable listening level	MCTC	metrizamide computed tomography cisternogram
MCLNS	mucocutaneous lymph node syndrome	MCTD	mixed connective tissue disease
MCMI	Millon Clinical Multiaxial Inventory	MCU	micturating cystourethrogram
mcmol	micromoles	MCV	mean corpuscular volume
MCN	minimal change nephropathy	MCVRI	minimal coronary vascular resistance index
MCNS	minimal change nephrotic syndrome		
MCO	managed care organization	MD	macula degeneration
			maintenance dialysis
	mupirocin calcium ointment (Bactroban Nasal)		maintenance dose
			major depression
			mammary dysplasia

	manic depression	MDM	mid-diastolic murmur
	medical doctor		minor determinant mix
	mediodorsal		(of penicillin)
	mental deficiency	MDMA	methylenedioxy-
	mesiodistal		methamphetamine
	movement disorder		(ecstasy)
	multiple dose	MDNT	midnight
	muscular dystrophy	MDO	mentally disordered
	myocardial damage		offender
MD-50®	diatrizoate sodium	MDP	methylene diphosphonate
	injection 50%	MDPH	Michigan Department of
MDA	malondialdehyde		Public Health
	manual dilation of the	MDPI	maximum daily
	anus		permissible intake
	methylenedioxyamphet-	MDR	Medical Device Reporting
	amine		(regulation)
	micrometastases detection		minimum daily
	assay		requirement
	motor discriminative		multi-drug resistance
	acuity	MD=R	moderately dilated and
MDAC	multiple-dose activated		equally reactive
	charcoal	MDR-1	multidrug resistance gene
MDACC	MD Anderson Cancer	MDRE	multiple-drug-resistant
	Center		enterococci
MDA LDL	malondialdehydeconju- gated low-density	MDREF	multidrug resistant enteric fever
	lipoprotein	MDRTB	multidrug-resistant
MDC	medial dorsal cutaneous		tuberculosis
	(nerve)	MDS	maternal deprivation
MDCM	mildly dilated congestive		syndrome
	cardiomyopathy		Minimum Data Set
MDD	major depressive disorder		myelodysplastic
	manic depressive disorder		syndromes
MDE	major depressive episode	MD-SR	moderately dilated and
MDF	myocardial depressant		slightly reactive
	factor	MDSU	medical day stay unit
MDGF	macrophage-derived	MDT	maggot debridement
	growth factor		therapy
MDI	manic depressive illness		motion detection
	metered dose inhaler		threshold
	methylenedioxyindenes		multidisciplinary team
	multiple daily injection		multidrug therapy
	multiple dosage insulin	MDTM	multidisciplinary team
MDIA	Mental Development		meeting
	Index, Adjusted	MDTP	multidisciplinary
MDII	multiple daily insulin		treatment plan
	injection	MDU	maintenance dialysis unit
MDIS	metered-dose inhaler-	MDUO	myocardial disease of
	spacer (device)		unknown origin

M

MDV	Marek's disease virus	MED-LARS	Medical Literature Analysis and Retrieval System
	multiple dose vial		
MDY	month, date, and year		
ME	macula edema	MEDS	medications
	manic episode	MEE	maintenance energy expenditure
	medical events		
	medical evidence		measured energy expenditure
	medical examiner		
	mestranol		middle ear effusion
	Methodist	MEF	maximum expired flow rate
	middle ear		
	myalgic encephalomyelitis		middle ear fluid
M/E	myeloid-erythroid (ratio)	MEFR	mid expiratory flow rate
M&E	Mecholyl and Eserine	MEFV	maximum expiratory flow-volume
	mucositis and enteritis		
MEA-I	multiple endocrine adenomatosis type I	MEG	magnetoencephalogram
			magnetoencephalography
MEB	Medical Evaluation Board	Meg-CSF	megakaryocytic colony-stimulating factor
	methylene blue		
MEC	meconium	MEGX	monoethylglycinexylidide
	middle ear canal(s)	MEI	medical economic index
MeCCNU	semustine	MEIA	microparticle enzyme immunoassay
MECG	maternal electrocardiogram		
		MEKC	micellar electrokinetic (capillary) chromatography
MeCP	semustine (methyl CCNU) cyclophosphamide, and prednisone		
		MEL	melatonin
		MELAS	myopathy, encephalopathy, lactic acidosis, and stroke-like episodes (syndrome)
MED	medial		
	median erythrocyte diameter		
	medical	MEL B	melarsoprol (Arsobal)
	medication	MEM	memory
	medicine		monocular estimate method (near retinoscopy)
	medium		
	medulloblastoma		
	minimal erythema dose	MEN	meningeal
	minimum effective dose		meninges
MEDAC	multiple endocrine deficiency Addison's disease (autoimmune) candidiasis		meningitis
		MEN (II)	multiple endocrine neoplasia (type II)
		MENS	microcurrent electrical neuromuscular stimulation
MEDCO	Medcosonolator		
MEDDRA	Medical Dictionary for Drug Regulatory Affairs		mini-electrical nerve stimulator
MEDEX	medication administration record	MEO	malignant external otitis

MeOH	methyl alcohol		*Malassezia furfur*
MEOS	microsomal ethanol oxidizing system		masculinity/femininity
			meat free
MEP	maximal expiratory pressure		mesial facial
	meperidine		methotrexate and fluorouracil
	multimodality evoked potential		midcavity forceps
			mid forceps
mEq	milliequivalent		mother and father
mEq/24 H	milliequivalents per 24 hours		mycosis fungoides
			myelofibrosis
mEq/L	milliequivalents per liter		myocardial fibrosis
		M & F	male and female
MER	medical evidence of record		mother and father
		MFA	malaise, fatigue, and anorexia
	methanol-extracted residue (of phenol-treated BCG)	MFAT	multifocal atrial tachycardia
M/E ratio	myeloid/erythroid ratio	MFB	metallic foreign body
MERRF	myoclonic epilepsy and ragged red fibers		multiple-frequency bioimpedance
MES	mesial	MFC	medial femoral condyle
MESS	Mangled Extremity Severe Score	MFCU	Medicaid Fraud Control Unit
MET	medical emergency treatment	MFD	Memory for Designs
	metabolic		midforceps delivery
	metamyelocytes		milk-free diet
	metastasis		multiple fractions per day
	metronidazole	MFEM	maximal forced expiratory maneuver
META	metamyelocytes	MFFT	Matching Familiar Figures Test
METH	methicillin		
MetHb	methemoglobin	MFH	malignant fibrous histiocytoma
	methemoglobinemia		
methyl CCNU	semustine	MFI	mean fluorescent intensity
		MFPS	myofascial pain syndrome
methyl G	mitroguazone dihydrochloride	MFR	mid-forceps rotation
			myofascial release
methyl GAG	mitroguazone dihydrochloride	MFS	Miller-Fisher syndrome
			mitral first sound
METS	metabolic equivalents (multiples of resting oxygen uptake)		monofixation syndrome
		MFT	muscle function test
	metastases	MFVNS	middle fossa vestibular nerve section
METT	maximum exercise tolerance test	MFVPT	Motor Free Visual Perception Test
MEV	million electron volts	MFVR	minimal forearm vascular resistance
MEX	Mexican		
MF	Malassezia folliculitis	MG	Marcus Gunn

M

	Michaelis-Gutmann (bodies)	MGT	management
	milligram (mg)	*mgtt*	minidrop (60 drops = 1 mL)
	myasthenia gravis	MGUS	monoclonal gammopathy of undetermined significance
mg	milligram		
Mg	magnesium		
mG	milligauss	MGW	multiple gunshot wound
μg	microgram (1/1000 of a milligram)	MGW enema	magnesium sulfate, glycerin, and water enema
M&G	myringotomy and grommets		
mg%	milligrams per 100 milliliters	M-GXT	multi-stage graded exercise test
MGBG	mitoguazone	mGy	milligray (radiation unit)
MGCT	malignant glandular cell tumor	MH	malignant hyperthermia marital history
MGD	meibomian gland dysfunction		medical history menstrual history
MGDF	megakaryocyte growth and development factor		mental health moist heat
mg/dl	milligrams per 100 milliliters	MHA	Mental Health Assistant methotrexate,
MGF	macrophage growth factor mast cell growth factor maternal grandfather		hydrocortisone, and cytarabine (ara-C)
MGGM	maternal great grandmother		microangiopathic hemolytic anemia
MGHL	middle glenohumeral ligament	MHA-TP	microhemagglutination microhemagglutination- *Treponema pallidum*
mg/kg	milligram per kilogram		
mg/kg/d	milligram per kilogram per day	MHB	maximum hospital benefits
mg/kg/hr	milligram per kilogram per hour	MHb	methemoglobin
MGM	maternal grandmother milligram (mg is correct)	MHBSS	modified Hank's balanced salt solution
MGMA	Medical Group Management Association	MHC	major histocompatibility complex
MGN	membranous glomerulonephritis		mental health center (clinic) mental health counselor
MgO	magnesium oxide	M/hct	microhematocrit
MG/OL	molecular genetics/oncology laboratory	mHg	millimeters of mercury
		MHH	mental health hold
MGP	Marcus Gunn pupil	MHI	Mental Health Index (information)
MGR	murmurs, gallops, or rubs		
MGS	malignant glandular schwannoma	MHIP	mental health inpatient
		MH/MR	mental health and mental retardation
MgSO₄	magnesium sulfate (Epsom salt)	MHN	massive hepatic necrosis

MHO	medical house officer	MICR	methacholine inhalation challenge response
MHRI	Mental Health Research Institute	MICRO	microcytes
MHS	major histocompatibility system	MICU	medical intensive care unit
	malignant hyperthermia susceptible		mobile intensive care unit
	multihospital system	MID	mesioincisodistal
MHT	mental health team		minimal ineffective dose
	Mental Health Technician		multi-infarct dementia
MHTAP	microhemagglutination assay for antibody to *Treponema pallidum*	MIDCAB	minimally invasive direct coronary artery bypass
		MID EPIS	midline episiotomy
		Mid I	middle insomnia
MHW	medial heel wedge	MIE	maximim inspiratory effort
	mental health worker		meconium ileus equivalent (cystic fibrosis)
MHX	methohexital sodium		
MHxR	medical history review		medical improvement expected
MHz	megahertz		
MI	membrane intact	MIEI	medication-induced esophageal injury
	mental illness		
	mental institution	MIF	Merthiolate, iodine, and formalin
	mesial incisal		
	mitral insufficiency		migration inhibitory factor
	myocardial infarction	MIFR	mid-inspiratory flow rate
MIA	medically indigent adult	MIF 50%VC	mid-inspiratory flow at 50% of vital capacity
	missing in action		
MIBI	technetium 99m sestamibi (a myocardial perfusion agent, Cardiolite)	MIG	measles immune globulin
		MIH	migraine with interparoxysmal headache
MIBG	iobenguane sulfate I 123 (meta-iodobenzyl guanidine I 123)		myointimal hyperplasia
		MIL	military
MIBK	methylisobutylketone		mesial incisal lingual (surface)
MIC	maternal and infant care		
	methacholine inhalation challenge		mother-in-law
		MIMCU	medical intermediate care unit
	medical intensive care microscope		
		MIN	mammary intraepithelial neoplasia
	microcytic erythrocytes		
	minimum inhibitory concentration		melanocytic intraepidermal neoplasia
MICA	mentally ill chemical abuser		mineral
			minimum
MICE	mesna, ifosfamide, carboplatin, and etoposide		minor
			minute (min)
MICN	mobile intensive care nurse	MIN A	minimal assistance (assist)

M

181

MIME	mitoguazone, ifosfamide, methotrexate, and etoposide with mesna		multiple injection therapy (of insulin)
		MITO-C	mitomycin
MINE	mesna, ifosfamide, mitoxantrone (Novantrone), and etoposide	MIU	million international units
		mIU	milli-international unit (one-thousandth of an International unit)
	medical improvement not expected	MIVA	mivacurium (Mivacron)
		MIW	mental inquest warrant
MIO	minimum identifiable odor	mix mon	mixed monitor
		MJ	marijuana
	monocular indirect ophthalmoscopy		megajoule
		MJD	Machado Joseph Disease
MIP	macrophage inflammatory protein	MJL	medial joint line
		MJS	medial joint space
	maximum inspiratory pressure	MJT	Mead Johnson tube
		μkat	microkatal (micro-moles/sec)
	maximum-intensity projection	MKAB	may keep at bedside
	mean intrathoracic pressure	MKB	married, keeping baby
		MK-CSF	megakaryocyte colony-stimulating factor
	mean intravascular pressure	MKI	mitotic-karyorrhectic index
	medical improvement possible	MKM	microgram per kilogram per minute
	metacarpointerphalangeal	ML	malignant lymphoma
MIRD	medical internal radiation dose		middle lobe
MIRP	myocardial infarction rehabilitation program		midline
		mL	milliliter
		M/L	monocyte to lymphocyte (ratio)
MIRS	Medical Improvement Review Standard		mother-in-law
MIS	management information systems	MLA	medical laboratory assay
			mento-laeva anterior
	minimally invasive surgery	MLAC	minimum local analgesic concentration
	mitral insufficiency	MLAP	mean left atrial pressure
	moderate intermittent suction	MLBW	moderately low birth weight
MISC	miscarriage	MLC	metastatic liver cancer
	miscellaneous		minimal lethal concentration
M Isch	myocardial ischemia		mixed lymphocyte culture
MISO	misonidazole		multilevel care
MISS	Modified Injury Severity Score (scale)		multilumen catheter
MIT	meconium in trachea		myelomonocytic leukemia, chronic
	miracidia immobilization test	MLD	masking level difference

	metachromatic leukodystrophy		multiple myeloma
	microlumbar diskectomy		muscle movement
	microsurgical lumbar	mM.	myelomeningocele
	diskectomy	mm	millimole (mmol)
	minimal lethal dose		millimeter
MLE	midline (medial)	M&M	milk and molasses
	episiotomy		morbidity and mortality
MLF	median longitudinal	MMA	methylmalonic acid
	fasciculus		methylmethacrylate
MLN	manifest latent nystagmus	MMC	mitomycin (mitomycin C)
MLNS	minimal lesions nephrotic	MMD	malignant metastatic
	syndrome		disease
	mucocutaneous lymph		myotonic muscular
	node syndrome		dystrophy
	(Kawasaki syndrome)	MMECT	multiple monitor
MLO	mesiolinguo-occlusal		electroconvulsive
MLP	mento-laeva posterior		therapy
	mesiolinguopulpal	MMEFR	maximal mid-expiratory
	mid-level provider		flow rate
MLPN	Medical Licensed	MMF	mean maximum flow
	Practical Nurse		mycophenolate mofetil
MLR	middle latency response		(CellCept)
	mixed lymphocyte	MMFR	maximal mid-expiratory
	reaction		flow rate
	multiple logistic	MMG	mechanomyography
	regression	mmHg	millimeters of mercury
MLS	mediastinal B-cell	MMK	Marshall-Marchetti-Krantz
	lymphoma with		(cystourethropexy)
	sclerosis	MMM	mitoxantrone,
MLT	melatonin		methotrexate, and
	mento-laeva transversa		mitomycin
MLU	mean length of utterance		mucous membrane
MLV	monitored live voice		moist
MM	major medical (insurance)		myelofibrosis with
	malignant melanoma		myeloid metaplasia
	malignant mesothelioma	MMMT	metastatic mixed
	Marshall-Marchetti		müllerian tumor
	medial malleolus	MMOA	maxillary mandibular
	member months		odontectomy
	meningococcic meningitis	mmol	alveolectomy
	mercaptopurine and	μmol	millimole
	methotrexate	MMP	micromole
	methadone maintenance		matrix metallopro-
	millimeter (mm)		teinase
	mist mask		multiple medical
	morbidity and mortality	MMP-8	problems
	motor meal	MMPI	metalloproteinase-8
	mucous membrane		matrix metalloproteinase inhibitor

M

	Minnesota Multiphasic Personality Inventory	MNM	mononeuritis multiplex
MMPI-D	Minnesota Multiphasic Personality Inventory-Depression Scale	MNNB	Monas-Nitz Neuropsychological Battery
6-MMPR	6-methylmercaptopurine riboside	MNR	marrow neutrophil reserve
MMR	measles, mumps, and rubella	MNSc	Master of Nursing Science
	midline malignant reticulosis	MnSOD	manganese superoxide dismutase
MMS	Mini-Mental State (examination)	Mn SSEPS	median nerve somatosensory evoked potentials
	Mohs' micrographic surgery	MNTB	medial nucleus of the trapezoid body
MMSE	Mini-Mental State Examination	MNX	meniscectomy
MMT	malignant mesenchymal tumors	MNZ	metronidazole
	manual muscle test	MO	medial oblique (x-ray view)
	Mini Mental Test		mesio-occlusal
	mixed müllerian tumors		mineral oil
MMTP	Methadone Maintenance Treatment Program		month (mo)
			months old
MMTV	malignant mesothelioma of the tunica vaginalis		morbidly obese
	monomorphic ventricular tachycardia		mother
		Mo	molybdenum
	mouse mammary tumor virus	MOA	mechanism of action
			metronidazole, omeprazole, and amoxicillin
MMV	mandatory minute volume		
MMWR	*Morbidity and Mortality Weekly Report*	MoAb	monoclonal antibody
		MOB	medical office building
MN	midnight	MOB-PT	mitomycin, vincristine (Oncovin), bleomycin, and cisplatin (Platinol AQ)
	mononuclear		
Mn	manganese		
M&N	morning and night		
	Mydriacyl and Neo-Synephrine	MOC	medial olivocochlear
			Medical Officer on Call
MNC	monomicrobial necrotizing cellulitis		metronidazole, omeprazole, and clarithromycin
	mononuclear leukocytes		mother of child
MNCV	motor nerve conduction velocity	MOCI	Maudsley Obsessive-Compulsive Inventory
MND	modified neck dissection	MOD	maturity onset diabetes
	motor neuron disease		medical officer of the day
MNF	myelinated nerve fibers		mesio-occlusodistal
MNG	multinodular goiter		moderate
			mode of death
			moment of death

	multiorgan dysfunction		months
MOD A	moderate assistance (assist)	mOsm	milliosmol
		MOSF	multiple organ system failure
MODM	mature-onset diabetes mellitus		
		MOS sf-20	Medical Outcomes Study, short form 20
MODS	multiple organ dysfunction syndrome	MOS sf-36	Medical Outcomes Study, short form, 36 items
MODY	maturity onset diabetes of youth	mOsmol	milliosmole
MOE	movement of extremities	MOT	motility examination
MOF	mesial occlusal facial	MOTS	mucosal oral therapeutic system
	methotrexate, vincristine (Oncovin), and fluorouracil	MOTT	mycobacteria other than tubercle
	methoxyflurane	MOU	medical oncology unit
MOFS	multiple-organ failure syndrome		memorandum of understanding
MOH	Ministry of Health	MOUS	multiple occurrences of unexplained symptoms
MoICU	mobile intensive care unit		
MOJAC	mood orientation, judgement, affect, and content	MOV	minimum obstructive volume
			multiple oral vitamin
MOM	milk of magnesia	MOW	Meals on Wheels
	mother	MP	malignant pyoderma
	mucoid otitis media		melphalan and prednisone
MoM	multiples of the median		menstrual period
MOMP	major outer membrane protein		mercaptopurine
			metacarpal phalangeal joint
MON	maximum observation nursery		moist park
	monitor		monitor pattern
MONO	infectious mononucleosis		monophasic
	monocyte		motor potential
	monospot		mouthpiece
mono, di	monochorionic, diamniotic		myocardial perfusion
		M & P	Millipore and phase
mono, mono	monochorionic, monoamniotic	4 MP	methylpyrazole (fomepizole; Antizol)
MOP	medical outpatient	6-MP	mercaptopurine
8 MOP	methoxsalen	MPA	main pulmonary artery
MOPP	mechlorethamine, vincristine (Oncovin), procarbazine, and prednisone		medroxyprogesterone acetate
		MPa	megapascal
		MPAC	Memorial Pain Assessment Card
MOPV	monovalent oral poliovirus vaccine	MPAP	mean pulmonary artery pressure
MOR	morphine		
MOS	Medical Outcome Study	MPAQ	McGill Pain Assessment Questionnaire
	mirror optical system		

M

MPB	male pattern baldness		mesiopulpolingual
	mephobarbital	MPL®	monophosphoryl lipid A
MPBFV	mean pulmonary-blood-flow velocity	MPLC	medium pressure liquid chromatography
MPBNS	modified Peyronie bladder neck suspension	MPM	malignant pleural mesothelioma
MPC	meperidine, promethazine, and chlorpromazine		Mortality Prediction Model
	mucopurulent cervicitis	MPN	monthly progress note
MPCN	microscopically positive and culturally negative		most probable number multiple primary neoplasms
M-PCR	multiplex polymerase chain reaction	MPO	male pattern obesity myeloperoxidase
MPCU	medical progressive care unit	MPOA	medial preoptic area
MPD	maximum permissable dose	MPP	massive periretinal proliferation
	methylphenidate (Ritalin)		maximum pressure picture
	moisture permeable dressing	MPQ	McGill Pain Questionnaire
	multiple personality disorder	MPPT	methylprednisolone pulse therapy
	myofascial pain dysfunction (syndrome)	MPR	massive periretinal retraction
MPE	malignant pleural effusion	MPS	mean particle size
	mean prediction error		mononuclear phagocyte system
MPEC	multipolar electrocoagulation		mucopolysaccharidosis
MPEG	methoxypolyethylene glycol		multiphasic screening
MPF	methylparaben free	MPSS	massively parallel signature sequencing
m-PFL	methotrexate, cisplatin (Platinol), fluorouracil, and leucovorin		methylprednisolone sodium succinate
MPGN	membranoproliferative glomerulonephritis	MPT	multiple parameter telemetry
MPH	massive pulmonary hemorrhage	MPTRD	motor, pain, touch, and reflex deficit
	Master of Public Health	MPU	maternal pediatric unit
	methylphenidate	MPV	mean platelet volume
	miles per hour	MQ	memory quotient
MPI	Maudsley Personality Inventory	MR	Maddox rod
	myocardial perfusion imaging		magnetic resonance manifest refraction
MPJ	metacarpophalangeal joint		may repeat
MPK	milligram per kilogram		measles-rubella medial rectus
MPL	maximum permissable level		medical record mental retardation milliroentgen

	mitral regurgitation	MR FIT	Multiple Risk Factor
	moderate resistance		Intervention Trial
M&R	measure and record	MRG	murmurs, rubs, and
MR × 1	may repeat times one		gallops
	(once)	MRH	Maddox rod hyperphoria
MRA	magnetic resonance	MRHD	maximum recommended
	angiography		human dose
	main renal artery	MRHT	modified rhyme hearing
	medical record		test
	administrator	MRI	magnetic resonance
	medical research associate		imaging
	midright atrium	M & R	measure and record input
	multivariate regression	I & O	and output
	analysis	MRL	minimal response level
mrad	millirad		moderate rubra lochia
MRAN	medical resident admitting	MRLVD	maximum residue limits
	note		of veterinary drugs
MRAP	mean right atrial pressure	MRLT	mesalamine-related lung
MRAS	main renal artery stenosis		toxicity
MRC	Master of Rehabilitation	MRM	modified radical
	Counseling		mastectomy
MRCA	magnetic resonance	MRN	magnetic resonance
	coronary angiography		neurography
MRCC	metastatic renal cell		medical record number
	carcinoma		medical resident's note
MRCP	magnetic resonance	mRNA	messenger ribonucleic
	cholangiopancreatography		acid
	Member of the Royal	MROU	medial rectus, both eyes
	College of Physicians	MRP	multidrug resistance
	mental retardation,		associated protein
	cerebral palsy	MRPN	medical resident progress
MRCPs	movement-related cortical		note
	potentials	MRS	magnetic resonance
MRCS	Member of the Royal		spectroscopy
	College of Surgeons		methicillin-resistant
MRD	margin reflex distance		*Staphylococcus aureus*
	Medical Records	MRSA	methicillin-resistant
	Department		*Staphylococcus aureus*
	minimal residual disease	MRSE	methicillin-resistant
MRDD	maximum recommended		*Staphylococcus*
	daily dose		*epidermidis*
	Mental Retardation and	MRT	magnetic resonance
	Development		tomography
	Disabilities		modified rhyme test
MRDM	malnutrition-related	MRTA	magnetic resonance
	diabetes mellitus		tomographic
MRE	manual resistance exercise		angiography
MRFC	mouse rosette-forming	MRV®	mixed respiratory vaccine
	cells	MR × 1	may repeat once

M

MS	mass spectroscopy	MSCs	mesenchymal stem cells
	Master of Science	MSCU	medical special care unit
	medical student	MSCWP	musculoskeletal chest
	mental status		wall pain
	milk shake	MSD	microsurgical diskectomy
	minimal support		mid-sleep disturbance
	mitral sounds	MSDBP	mean sitting diastolic
	mitral stenosis		blood pressure
	moderately susceptible	MSDS	material safety data
	morning stiffness		sheet
	morphine sulfate	MSE	Mental Status
	motile sperm		Examination
	multiple sclerosis	Msec	milliseconds
	muscle spasm	MSEL	myasthenic syndrome of
	muscle strength		Eaton-Lambert
	musculoskeletal	MSER	mean systolic ejection
M & S	microculture and		rate
	sensitivity		Mental Status
3MS	Modified Mini-Mental		Examination Record
	Status (examination)	MSF	meconium-stained fluid
MS III	third-year medical student		megakaryocyte
MSA	Medical Savings		stimulating factor
	Accounts	MSG	methysergide
	membrane-stabilizing		monosodium glutamate
	activity	MSH	melanocyte-stimulating
	microsomal autoantibod-		hormone
	ies	MSHA	mannose-sensitive
	multiple system atrophy		hemagglutinin
MSAF	meconium-stained	MSI	magnetic source imaging
	amniotic fluid		multiple subcortical
MSAFP	maternal serum alpha-		infarction
	fetoprotein		musculoskeletal
MSAP	mean systemic arterial		impairment
	pressure	MSIR®	morphine sulfate
MSAS	Mandel Social		immediate release
	Adjustment Scale		tablets
MSAS-SF	Memorial Symptom	MSIS	Multiple Severity of
	Assessment		Illness System
	Scale – short form	MSK	medullary sponge kidney
MSB	mainstem bronchus	MSKCC	Memorial Sloan-Kettering
MSBOS	maximum surgical blood		Cancer Center
	order schedule	MSL	midsternal line
MSC	major symptom complex	MSLT	multiple sleep latency test
	midsystolic click	MSM	magnetic starch
	MS Contin®		microspheres
MSCA	McCarthy Scales of		men who have sex with
	Children's Abilities		men
MSCCC	Master Sciences, Certified		methsuximide
	Clinical Competence		mid-systolic murmur

MSN	Master of Science in Nursing	mSv	millisievert (radiation unit)
MSNA	muscle sympathetic nerve activity	MSW	Master of Social Work multiple stab wounds
MSO	managed services organization	MT	empty macular target
	mentally stable and oriented		maggot therapy maintenance therapy
	mental status, oriented		malaria therapy
	most significant other		malignant teratoma
MSO₄	morphine sulfate (this is a dangerous abbreviation)		Medical Technologist metatarsal
MSOF	multi-system organ failure		middle turbinate
MSPN	medical student progress notes		monitor technician muscles and tendons
MSPU	medical short procedure unit		muscle tone music therapy (Therapist)
			myringotomy tube(s)
MSQ	Mental Status Questionnaire	M/T	masses of tenderness myringotomy with tubes
	meters squared	M & T	*Monilia* and *Trichomonas*
MSR	muscle stretch reflexes		muscles and tendons
MSRPP	Multidimensional Scale for Rating Psychiatric Patients	MTA	myringotomy and tubes Medical Technical Assistant
MSS	Marital Satisfaction Scale		multi-targeted antifolate
	mean sac size	MTAD	tympanic membrane of
	minor surgery suite		the right ear
MSSA	methicillin-susceptible *Staphylococcus aureus*	MT/AK	music therapy/ audiokinetics
MSS-CR	mean sac size and crown-rump length	MTAS	tympanic membrane of the left ear
MSSP	Maternal Support Services Program	MTAU	tympanic membranes of both ears
MSSU	mid-stream specimen of urine	MTB	*Mycobacterium tuberculosis*
MST	mean survival time	MTBC	Music Therapist-Board
	median survival time		Certified
	mental stress test	MTBE	methyl tert-butyl ether
	multiple subpial transection	MTC	magnetization transfer contrast
MSTA®	mumps skin test antigen		medullary thyroid
MSTI	multiple soft tissue injuries		carcinoma metoclopramide
MSU	maple syrup urine		mitomycin
	midstream urine	MTD	maximum tolerated dose
MSUD	maple-syrup urine disease		metastatic trophoblastic
MSUs	midstream specimens of urine		disease minimum toxic dose

M

189

	Monroe tidal drainage	MU	million units
	Mycobacterium		Murphy unit
	tuberculosis direct (test)	mU	milliunits
MTDI	maximum tolerable daily intake	MUA	manipulation under anesthesia
MTDT	*Mycobacterium tuberculosis* direct test	MUAC	middle upper arm circumference
MTE	multiple trace elements	MUD	matched unrelated donor
MTET	modified treadmill exercise testing	MUDDLES	miosis, urination, diarrhea, diaphoresis,
MTF	medical treatment facility		lacrimation, excitation
MTG	middle temporal gyrus (gyri)		of central nervous system, and salivation
	mid-thigh girth		(effects of
MTHFR	methylene tetrahydrofolate reductase		cholinesterase inhibitors)
MTI	magnetization transfer imaging	MUDPILES	*m*ethanol, metformin; *u*remia; *d*iabetic ketoacidosis;
	malignant teratoma intermediate		*p*henformin, paraldehyde; *i*ron,
MTJ	mid-tarsal joint		*i*soniazid, ibuprofen;
MTLE	medial temporal-lobe epilepsy		*l*actic acidosis; *e*thanol, ethylene glycol; and
MTM	modified Thayer-Martin medium		*s*alicylates, sepsis (causes of metabolic
MTP	master treatment plan		acidosis)
	medical termination of pregnancy	MUE	medication use evaluation
	metatarsophalangeal	MUGA	multigated (radionuclide) angiogram
	microsomal triglyceride transfer protein		multiple gated acquisition (scan)
MTR _	mother	MUGX	multiple gated acquisition
MTR-O	no masses, tenderness, or rebound		exercise
MTRS	Licensed Master Therapeutic Recreation Specialist	MULE	microcomputer upper limb exerciser
		MuLV	murine leukemia virus
MTS	mesial temporal sclerosis	MUNSH	Memorial University of Newfoundland Scale of
MTST	maximal treadmill stress test		Happiness
MTT	mamillothalamic tract	MUO	metastasis of unknown origin
	mean transit time		
	methylthiotetrazole	MUPAT	multiple-site perineal applicator technique
MTU	malignant teratoma undifferentiated	MUSE®	Medicated Urethral System for Erection
	methylthiouracil		(alprostadil urethral
MTX	methotrexate		suppository)
MTZ	mitoxantrone	mus-lig	musculoligamentous

MUU	mouse uterine units	MVPP	mechlorethamine, vinblastine, procarbazine, and prednisone
MV	mechanical ventilation		
	millivolts		
	minute volume		
	mitoxantrone and etoposide	MVPS	mitral valve prolapse syndrome
	mitral valve	MVR	massive vitreous retraction
	mixed venous		micro-vitreoretinal (blade)
	multivesicular		mitral valve regurgitation
MVA	malignant vertricular arrhythmias		mitral valve replacement
		MVRI	mixed vaccine respiratory infections
	manual vacuum aspiration		
	mitral valve area	MVS	mitral valve stenosis
	motor vehicle accident		motor, vascular, and sensory
M-VAC	methotrexate, vinblastine doxorubicin (Adriamycin), and cisplatin	MVT	multiform ventricular tachycardia
			multivitamin
MVB	methotrexate and vinblastine	MVU	Montevideo units
		MVV	maximum ventilatory volume
	mixed venous blood		
MVC	maximal voluntary contraction		maximum voluntary ventilation
			mixed vespid venom
	motor vehicle collision	MWB	minimal weight bearing
MVc	mitral valve closure	MWD	microwave diathermy
MVD	microvascular decompression	M-W-F	Monday-Wednesday-Friday
	microvessel density	MWI	Medical Walk-In (Clinic)
	mitral valve disease	MWS	Mickety-Wilson syndrome
	multivessel disease	MWT	maintenance of wakefulness test
MVE	mitral valve (leaflet) excursion		Mallory-Weiss tear
	Murray Valley encephalitis		malpositioned wisdom teeth
MV Grad	mitral valve gradient	Mx	manifest refraction
MVI	multiple vitamin injection		mastectomy
MVI®	trade name for parenteral multivitamins		maxilla
			movement
MVI 12®	trade name for parenteral multivitamins		myringotomy
MVO	mixed venous oxygen saturation	My	myopia
		MYD	mydriatic
MVO₂	myocardial oxygen consumption	myelo	myelocytes
			myelogram
MVP	mean venous pressure	MyG	myasthenia gravis
	mitomycin, vinblastine, and cisplatin (Platinol AQ)	MYOP	myopia
		MYR	myringotomy
	mitral valve prolapse	MYS	medium yellow soft (stools)

M

MZ   monozygotic
MZL   marginal zone lymphocyte
MZT   monozygotic twins

N

N	nausea
	negative
	Negro
	Neisseria
	nerve
	neutrophil
	never
	newton
	nipple
	nitrogen
	no
	nodes
	nonalcoholic
	none
	normal
	not
	notified
	noun
	NPH insulin
	size of sample
N I thru	first through twelfth
N XII	cranial nerves
O.1 N	tenth-normal
N₂	nitrogen
5'-N	5'-nucleotidase
Na	sodium
Na⁺	sodium
NA	Narcotics Anonymous
	Native American
	Negro adult
	nicotinic acid
	nonalcoholic
	normal axis
	not admitted
	not applicable
	not available
	nurse aide
	nurse's aid
	Nurse Anesthetist
	nursing assistant
N & A	normal and active
NAA	neutron activation analysis

	no apparent abnormalities	NAG	narrow angle glaucoma
NAAC	no apparent anesthesia complications	NaHCO₃	sodium bicarbonate
		NAI	no action indicated
NAA/Cr	N-acetyl aspartate/creatine ratio		no acute inflammation
			nonaccidental injury
NAATPT	not available at the present time	NaI	sodium iodide
		NAION	nonarteritic ischemic optic neuropathy
NAB	not at bedside		
NABS	normoactive bowel sounds	NAIT	neonatal alloimmune thrombocytopenia
NABX	needle aspiration biopsy	NAL	nasal angiocentric lymphoma
NAC	acetylcysteine (N-acetylcysteine; Mucomyst)	NAM	Native American male
			normal adult male
	neoadjuvant chemotherapy	NANB	non-A, non-B (hepatitis) (hepatitis C)
	no acute changes	NANBH	non-A, non-B hepatitis (hepatitis C)
NACD	no anatomical cause of death	NANC	nonadrenergic, noncholinergic
NaClO	sodium hypochlorite		
NaCl	sodium chloride (salt)	NANDA	North American Nursing Diagnosis Association (taxonomy)
NaCMC	sodium carboxymethyl cellulose		
NACT	neoadjuvant chemotherapy	NAP	narrative, assessment, and plan
NAD	nicotinamide adenine dinucleotide		nosocomial acquired pneumonia
	no active disease	NAPA	N-acetyl procainamide
	no acute distress	NAPD	no active pulmonary disease
	no apparent distress		
	no appreciable disease	Na Pent	Pentothal Sodium
	normal axis deviation	NAR	no action required
	nothing abnormal detected		no adverse reaction
			nonambulatory restraint
NADA	New Animal Drug Application		not at risk
		NARC	narcotic(s)
NADPH	nicotinamide adenine dinucleotide phosphate	NAS	nasal
			neonatal abstinence syndrome
NADSIC	no apparent active disease seen in chest		no abnormality seen
			no added salt
NaE	exchangeable sodium	NASBA	nucleic-acid sequencing based amplification
NaF	sodium fluoride		
NAF	nafcillin	NAS-NRC	National Academy of Sciences – National Research Council
	Native American female		
	Negro adult female		
	normal adult female	NASTT	nonspecific abnormality of ST segment and T wave
	Notice of Adverse Findings (FDA post-audit letter)		

NAT	N-acetyltransferase	NBT	nitroblue tetrazolium
	no action taken		reduction (tests)
	no acute trauma		normal breast tissue
	nonaccidental trauma	NBTE	nonbacterial thrombotic
	nonspecific abnormality		endocarditis
	of T wave	NBTNF	newborn, term, normal
$Na^{99m}Tc0_4^-$	sodium pertechnetate		female
	Tc 99m	NBTNM	newborn, term, normal,
NAUC	normalized area under the		male
	curve	NBW	normal birth weight
NAW	nasal antral window		(2,500–3,999 g)
NAWM	normal-appearing white	NC	nasal cannula
	matter		Negro child
NB	nail bed		neurologic check
	needle biopsy		no change
	newborn		no charge
	nitrogen balance		no complaints
	note well		noncontributory
NBC	newborn center		normocephalic
	nonbed care		nose clamp
NBCCS	nevoid basal-cell		nose clips
	carcinoma syndrome		not classified
NBD	neurologic bladder		not completed
	dysfunction		not cultured
	no brain damage	NCA	neurocirculatory asthenia
NBF	not breast fed		no congenital
NBH	new bag (bottle) hung		abnormalities
NBHH	newborn helpful hints	N/CAN	nasal cannula
NBI	no bone injury	NCAP	nasal continuous airway
NBICU	newborn intensive care		pressure
	unit	NCAS	zinostatin
NBL/OM	neuroblastoma and		(neocarzinostatin)
	opsoclonus-myoclonus	NC/AT	normocephalic atraumatic
NBM	no bowel movement	NCB	natural childbirth
	normal bone marrow		no code blue
	normal bowel movement	NCC	no concentrated
	nothing by mouth		carbohydrates
NBN	newborn nursery		nursing care card
NBP	needle biopsy of prostate	NCCLS	National Committee for
	no bone pathology		Clinical Laboratory
NBQC	narrow base quad cane		Standards
NBR	no blood return	NCCN	National Comprehensive
NBS	newborn screen (serum		Cancer Network
	thyroxine and	NCCTG	North Central Cancer
	phenylketonuria)		Treatment Group
	Nijmegen breakage	NCCU	neurosurgical continuous
	syndrome		care unit
	no bacteria seen	NCD	no congenital deformities
	normal bowel sounds		normal childhood diseases

	not considered disabling		not clinically significant
NCDB	National Cancer Data Base		zinostatin (neocarzinostatin)
NCE	new chemical entity	NCSE	nonconvulsive status epilepticus
NCEP	National Cholesterol Education Program	NCT	neutron capture therapy
NCF	neutrophilic chemotactic factor		noncontact tonometry
			Nursing Care Technician
NCI	National Cancer Institute	NCV	nerve conduction velocity
NCIC	National Cancer Institute of Canada		nuclear venogram
NCI-CTC	National Cancer Institute Common Toxicity Criteria	ND	Doctor of Naturopathy (Naturopathic Physician)
NCIS	nursing care information sheet		nasal deformity
			nasoduodenal
NCJ	needle catheter jejunostomy		natural death
			neck dissection
NCL	neuronal ceroid lipofuscinosis		neonatal death
			neurological development
	nuclear cardiology laboratory		neurotic depression
NCM	nailfold capillary microscope		Newcastle disease
			no data
	nonclinical manager		no disease
NCNC	normochromic, normocytic		nondisabling
			nondistended
NCO	no complaints offered		none detectable
	noncommissioned officer		normal delivery
NCOG	North California Oncology Group		normal development
			nose drops
NCP	no caffeine or pepper		not detect
	nursing care plan		not diagnosed
NCPAP	nasal continuous positive airway pressure	N&D	not done
			nothing done
			Nursing Doctorate
NCPB	neurolytic celiac plexus block	N&D	nodular and diffuse
		Nd	neodymium
NcpPCu	nonceruloplasmin plasma copper	NDA	New Drug Application
			no data available
NCPR	no cardiopulmonary resuscitation		no demonstrable antibodies
			no detectable activity
NCQA	National Commission on Quality Assurance	NDC	National Drug Code
		NDD	no dialysis days
nCR	nodular complete response	NDE	near-death experience
		NDEA	no deviation of electrical axis
NCRC	nonchild-resistant container	NDF	neutral density filter (test)
			no disease found
NCS	nerve conduction studies		
	no concentrated sweets	NDGA	nordihydroguaiaretic acid

NDI	National Death Index	NEF	negative expiratory force
	nephrogenic diabetes insipidus	NEFA	nonesterified fatty acids
NDIR	nondispersive infrared	NEFG	normal external female genitalia
NDIRS	nondispersive infrared spectrometer	NEFT	nasoenteric feeding tube
Nd/NT	nondistended, nontender	NEG	negative
NDP	net dietary protein		neglect
	Nurse Discharge Planner	NEI	National Eye Institute (NIH)
NDR	neurotic depressive reaction	NEJM	*New England Journal of Medicine*
	normal detrusor reflex	NEM	neurotrophic enhancing molecule
NDS	Neurologic Disability Score		no evidence of malignancy
NDST	neurodevelopmental screening test	NEMD	nonexudative macular degeneration
NDT	nasal duodenostomy tube		nonspecific esophageal motility disorder
	neurodevelopmental techniques	NENT	nasal endotracheal tube
	neurodevelopmental treatment	NEO	necrotizing external otitis
	noise detection threshold	NEOH	neonatal high risk
NDV	Newcastle disease virus	NEOM	neonatal medium risk
Nd:YAG	neodymium:yttrium-aluminum-garnet (laser)	NEP	needle-exchange program
			no evidence of pathology
Nd:YLF	neodymium: yttrium-lithium-fluoride (laser)	NEPD	no evidence of pulmonary disease
NE	nausea and emesis	NEPHRO	nephrogram
	nephropathica epidemica	NER	no evidence of recurrence
	neurological examination	NERD	no evidence of recurrent disease
	never exposed	NES	nonepileptic seizure
	no effect		nonstandard electrolyte solution
	no enlargement		
	norethindrone		not elsewhere specified
	norepinephrine	NESP	novel erythropoiesis stimulating protein
	not elevated		
	not examined	NET	choroidal or subretinal neovascularization
NEAA	nonessential amino acids		
NEAC	norethindrone acetate		Internet
NEB	hand-held nebulizer		naso-endotracheal tube
NEC	necrotizing entercolitis		neuroectodermal tumor
	noise equivalent counts	NETA	norethisterone acetate
	nonesterified cholesterol	NETT	nasal endotracheal tube
	not elsewhere classified	NEX	nose to ear to xiphoid
NED	no evidence of disease		number of excitations
NEEG	normal electroencephalo-gram	NF	necrotizing fasciitis
			Negro female
NEEP	negative end-expiratory pressure		neurofibromatosis

	night frequency (of voiding)	NH	nursing home
		NHA	no histologic abnormalities
	none found	NHB	non-heart beating (donor)
	not found	NHC	neighborhood health center
	nursed fair		
	nursing facility		neonatal hypocalcemia
NFA	Nerve Fiber Analyzer®		nursing home care
NFALO	Nerve Fiber Analyzer laser oththalmoscope	NH_3	ammonia
		NH_4Cl	ammonium chloride
NFAR	no further action required	NHCU	nursing home care unit
NFD	no family doctor	NHD	normal hair distribution
NFFD	not fit for duty	NHL	nodular histiocytic lymphoma
NFI	no-fault insurance		
	no further information		non-Hodgkin's lymphomas
NFL	nerve fiber layer		
NFLX	norfloxacin (Noroxin)	nHL	normalized hearing level
NFP	natural family planning	NHLBI	National Heart, Lung, and Blood Institute (NIH)
	no family physician		
	not for publication	NHLPP	hereditary neuropathy with liability for pressure palsy
NFT	no further treatment		
NFTD	normal full-term delivery		
NFTs	neurofibrillary tangles	NHM	no heroic measures
NFTSD	normal full-term spontaneous delivery	NHO	notify house officer
		NHP	Nottingham Health Profile
NFTT	nonorganic failure to thrive		nursing home placement
		NHS	National Health Service (UK)
NFW	nursed fairly well		
NG	nanogram (ng)	NHT	neoadjuvant hormonal therapy
	nasogastric		
	night guard		nursing home transfer
	nitroglycerin	NHTR	nonhemolytic transfusion reaction
	no growth		
	norgestrel	NHW	non-healing wound
ng	nanogram	NI	neurological improvement
NGB	neurogenic bladder		no improvement
NGF	nerve growth factor		no information
n giv	not given		none indicated
NGJ	nasogastro-jejunostomy		not identified
NGM	norgestimate		not isolated
NGOs	nongovernmental organizations	NIA	National Institute on Aging (NIH)
NGR	nasogastric replacement		no information available
NGRI	not guilty by reason of insanity	NIAAA	National Institute on Alcohol Abuse and Alcoholism (NIH)
NGSF	nothing grown so far		
NGT	nasogastric tube	NIAID	National Institute of Allergy and Infectious Diseases (NIH)
	normal glucose tolerance		
NgTD	negative to date		
NGU	nongonococcal urethritis		

NIAL	not in active labor	NIG	NSAIA (non-steroidal anti-inflamatory agent) induced gastropathy
NIAMSD	National Institute of Arthritis and Musculoskeletal and Skin Diseases (NIH)	NIGMS	National Institute of General Medical Sciences (NIH)
NICC	neonatal intensive care center	NIH	National Institutes of Health
NICE	new, interesting, and challenging experiences	NIHD	noise-induced hearing damage
NICHHD	National Institute of Child Health and Human Development (NIH)	NIHL	noise-induced hearing loss
		NIID	neuronal intranuclear inclusion disease
NICS	noninvasive carotid studies	NIL	not in labor
NICU	neonatal intensive care unit	NIMAs	non-inherited maternal antigens
	neurosurgical intensive care unit	NIMH	National Institute of Mental Health (NIH)
NID	no identifiable disease not in distress	NIMHDIS	National Institute for Mental Health Diagnostic Interview Schedule (NIH)
NIDA five	National Institute on Drug Abuse screen for cannabinoids, cocaine metabolite, amphetamine/metham-phetamine, opiates, and phencyclidine	NINDS	National Institute of Neurological Disorders and Stroke (NIH)
		NINU	neuro intermediate nursing unit
NIDCD	National Institute of Deafness and other Communication Disorders (NIH)	NINVS	noninvasive neurovascular studies
		NIOPCs	no intraoperative complications
NIDD	noninsulin-dependent diabetes	NIOSH	National Institute of Occupational Safety and Health (NIH)
NIDDKD	National Institute of Diabetes and Digestive and Kidney Diseases (NIH)	NIP	no infection present no inflammation present
		NIPAs	noninherited paternal antigens
NIDDM	noninsulin-dependent diabetes mellitus	NIPD	nocturnal intermittent peritoneal dialysis
NIDR	National Institute of Dental Research (NIH)	NIPPV	noninvasive positive-pressure ventilation
NIEHS	National Institute of Environmental Health Sciences (NIH)	NIP/S	noninvasive programming stimulation
NIF	negative inspiratory force	NIR	near infrared
	neutrophil inhibitory factor	NIRCA	nonisotopic RNase cleavage assay
	not in file	NISS	New Injury Severity Score
NIFS	noninvasive flow studies		

NISs	no-impact sports		nursing late entry
NISV	nonionic surfactant vesicle	NLEA	Nutrition Labeling and Education Act of 1990
NITD	neuroleptic-induced tardive dyskinesia	NLF	nasolabial fold
Nitro	nitroglycerin (this is a dangerous abbreviation)	NLFGNR	nonlactose fermenting gram-negative rod
	sodium nitroprusside (this is a dangerous abbreviation)	NLM	National Library of Medicine
			no limitation of motion
NIVLS	noninvasive vascular laboratory studies	NLMC	nocturnal leg muscle cramp
NJ	nasojejunal	NLN	no longer needed
NK	natural killer (cells)	NLO	nasolacrimal occlusion
	not known	NLP	nodular liquifying panniculitis
NKA	no known allergies		
nkat	nanokatal (nanomole/sec)		no light perception
NKB	no known basis	NLS	neonatal lupus syndrome
	not keeping baby	NLT	not later than
NKC	nonketotic coma		not less than
NKD	no known diseases	NLV	nelfinavir (Viracept)
NKDA	no known drug allergies	NM	Negro male
NKFA	no known food allergies		neuromuscular
NKH	nonketotic hyperglycemia		neuronal microdysgenesis
NKHA	nonketotic hyperosmolar acidosis		nodular melanoma
			nonmalignant
NKHHC	nonketotic hyperglycemic-hyperosmolar coma		not measurable
			not measured
NKHOC	nonketotic hyperosmolar coma		not mentioned
			nuclear medicine
NKHS	nonketotic hyperosmolar syndrome		nurse manager
		N & M	nerves and muscles
NKMA	no known medication (medical) allergies		night and morning
		NMBA	neuromuscular blocking agent
NL	nasolacrimal		
	nonlatex	NMC	no malignant cells
	normal	NMD	neuromuscular disorders
NLB	needle liver biopsy		neuronal migration disorders
NLC	nocturnal leg cramps		
NLC & C	normal libido, coitus, and climax		Normosol M and 5% Dextrose®
NLD	nasolacrimal duct	NMDP	National Marrow Donor Pool
	necrobiosis lipoidica diabeticorum		
		NME	new molecular entity
	no local doctor	NMF	neuromuscular facilitation
NLDO	nasolacrimal duct obstruction	NMH	neurally mediated hypotension
NLE	neonatal lupus erythematosus	NMHH	no medical health history
		NMI	no manifest improvement

	no mental illness	NNBC	node-negative breast cancer
	no middle initial		
	no more information	NND	neonatal death
	normal male infant	NNE	neonatal necrotizing enterocolitis
NMJ	neuromuscular junction		
NMKB	not married, keeping baby	NNM	Nicolle-Novy-MacNeal (media)
NMM	nodular malignant melanoma	NNL	no new laboratory (test orders)
NMN	no middle name	NNN	normal newborn nursery
NMNKB	not married, not keeping baby	NNO	no new orders
nmol	nanomole	NNP	Neonatal Nurse Practitioner
NMOH	no medical ocular history	N:NPK	grams of nitrogen to non-protein kilocalories
NMP	normal menstrual period		
NMR	nuclear magnetic resonance (same as magnetic resonance imaging)	NNR	not necessary to return
		NNRTI	non-nucleoside reverse transcriptase inhibitor
		NNS	neonatal screen (hematocrit, total bilirubin, and total protein)
NMRS	nuclear magnetic resonance spectroscopy		
NMRT (R)	Nuclear Medicine Radiologic Technologist (Registered)		nicotine nasal spray
			nonnutritive sucking
NMS	neonatal morphine solution	NNT	number needed to treat
	neuroleptic malignant syndrome	NNU	net nitrogen utilization
		NO	nasal oxygen
NMSE	normalized mean square root		nitric oxide
			nitroglycerin ointment
NMSIDS	near-miss sudden infant death syndrome		none obtained
			nonobese
NMT	nebulized mist treatment		number (no.)
	no more than		nursing office
NMTB	neuromuscular transmission blockade	N_2O	nitrous oxide
		NOAEL	no observed adverse effect level
NMTCB	Nuclear Medicine Technology Certification Board	$N_2O:O_2$	nitrous oxide to oxygen ratio
NMT(R)	Nuclear Medicine Technologist Registered	noc.	night
		noct	nocturnal
NN	narrative notes	NOD	nonobese diabetic
	Navajo neuropathy		notice of disagreement
	neonatal		notify of death
	neural network	NOED	no observed effect dose
	normal nursery	NOFT	nonorganic failure to thrive
	nurses' notes		
N/N	negative/negative	NOFTT	nonorganic failure to thrive
NNB	normal newborn		

NOH	neurogenic orthostatic hypotension	NOT	nocturnal oxygen therapy
		NOU	not on unit
NOK	next of kin	NOV	human insulin, regular 30
NOL	not on label	70/30	units/mL with human
NOM	nonsuppurative otitis media		insulin isophane suspension 70 units/mL
NOMI	nonocclusive mesenteric infarction		(Novolin 70/30)
NOMS	not on my shift	NOV L	human insulin zinc suspension (Novolin L)
NONMEM	non-linear mixed-effects model (modeling)	NOV N	human insulin isophane suspension (Novolin N)
non pal	not palpable		
non-REM	nonrapid eye movement (sleep)	NOV R	human insulin regular (Novolin R)
non rep	do not repeat	NP	nasal prongs
NON VIZ	not visualized		nasopharyngeal
NOOB	not out of bed		near point
NOP	not on patient		neutrogenic precautions
NOR	norethynodrel		neurophysin
	normal		neuropsychiatric
	nortriptyline		newly presented
NOR-EPI	norepinephrine		nonpalpable
norm	normal		no pain
NOS	neonatal opium solution (diluted deodorized tincture of opium)		not performed
			not pregnant
			not present
	new-onset seizures		nuclear pharmacist
	nitric oxide synthase		nuclear pharmacy
	no organisms seen		nursed poorly
	not on staff		nurse practitioner
	not otherwise specified	NPA	nasal pharyngeal airway
NOSI	nitric oxide synthase inhibitors		near point of accommodation
			no previous admission
NOSIE	Nurse's Observation Scale (Schedule) for Inpatient Evaluation	NPAT	nonparoxysmal atrial tachycardia
		NPBC	node-positive breast cancer
NOSPECS	categories for classifying eye changes in Graves' ophthalmopathy: **n**o signs or symptoms, **o**nly signs, **s**oft tissue involvement with symptoms and signs, **p**roptosis, **e**xtraocular muscle involvement, **c**orneal involvement, **a**nd **s**ight loss (visual acuity)	NPC	nasopharyngeal carcinoma
			near point convergence
			Niemann-Pick disease Type C (sphingomyelin lipidosis)
			nodal premature contractions
			nonpatient contact
			nonproductive cough
			nonprotein calorie
			no prenatal care

201

	no previous complaint(s)		producing *Neisseria gonorrhoeae*
NPCC	nonprotein carbohydrate calories	NPR	normal pulse rate
			nothing per rectum
NPCPAP	nasopharyngeal continuous positive airway pressure	NPRL	normal pupillary reaction to light
NPD	Niemann-Pick disease	NPS	new patient set-up
	nonprescription drugs	NPSA	nonphysician surgical assistant
	no pathological diagnosis		
NPDL	nodular poorly differentiated lymphocytic	NPSD	nonpotassium-sparing diuretics
NPDR	nonproliferative diabetic retinopathy	NPSG	nocturnal polysomnography
NPE	neuropsychologic examination	NPT	near-patient tests
			neopyrithiamin hydrochloride
	no palpable enlargement		nocturnal penile tumescence
	normal pelvic examination		no prior tracings
NPEM	nocturnal penile erection monitoring		normal pressure and temperature
NPF	nasopharyngeal fiberscope	NPU	net protein utilization
		NPV	negative predictive value
	no predisposing factor		nothing per vagina
N-PFMSO$_4$	nebulized preservative-free morphine sulfate	NPY	neuropeptide Y
		NPZ	neuropsychologic text z
NPG	nonpregnant	NQECN	nonqueratinizing epidermoid carcinoma
NPH	isophane insulin (neutral protamine Hagedorn)	NQMI	non-Q wave myocardial infarction
	no previous history	NQWMI	non-Q wave myocardial infarction
	normal pressure hydrocephalus		
NPhx	nasopharynx	NR	do not repeat
NPI	no present illness		newly reformulated
NPJT	nonparoxysmal junctional tachycardia		nonreactive
			nonrebreathing
NPLSM	neoplasm		no refills
NPK	nonprotein kilocalories		no report
NPM	nothing per mouth		no response
NPN	nonprotein nitrogen		no return
NPNC	no prenatal care		normal range
NPNT	nonpalpable, nontender		normal reaction
NPO	nothing by mouth		not reached
NPOC	nonpurgeable organic carbon		not reacting
			not remarkable
NPOD	Neuropsychiatric Officer of the Day		not resolved
			number
NPP	normal postpartum	NRAF	nonrheumatic atrial fibrillation
NPPNG	nonpenicillinase-		

NRB	Noninstitutional Review Board		no sample
	non-rebreather (oxygen mask)		not seen
			not significant
			nuclear sclerosis
NRBC	normal red blood cell		nursing service
	nucleated red blood cell		nutritive sucking
NRBS	nonrebreathing system		nylon suture
NRC	National Research Council	NSA	normal serum albumin (albumin, human)
	normal retinal correspondence		no salt added
			no significant abnormalities
	Nuclear Regulatory Commission	NSAA	nonsteroidal antiandrogen
NREM	nonrapid eye movement	NSABP	National Surgical Adjuvant Breast Project
NREMS	nonrapid eye movement sleep		
NRF	normal renal function	NSAD	no signs of acute disease
NRI	nerve root involvement	NSAIA	nonsteroidal anti-inflammatory agent
	nerve root irritation		
	no recent illnesses	NSAID	nonsteroidal anti-inflammatory drug
N-RLX	nonrelaxed		
NRM	non rebreathing mask	NSBGP	nonspecific bowel gas pattern
	no regular medicines		
	normal range of motion	NSC	no significant change
	normal retinal movement		nonservice-connected
NRN	no return necessary	NSCC	nonsmall cell carcinoma
NRO	neurology	NSCD	nonservice-connected disability
NROM	normal range of motion		
NRP	nonreassuring patterns	NSCFPT	no significant change from previous tracing
NRPR	nonbreathing pressure relieving		
		NSCLC	nonsmall-cell lung cancer
NRS	Neurobehavioral Rating Scale		
		NSCST	nipple stimulation contraction stress test
NRT	neuromuscular reeducation techniques	NSD	nasal septal deviation
			no significant disease (difference, defect, deviation)
	nicotine-replacement therapy		
NRTs	nitron radical traps		nominal standard dose
NS	nephrotic syndrome		normal spontaneous delivery
	neurological signs		
	neurosurgery	NSDA	nonsteroid dependent asthmatic
	nipple stimulation		
	nodular sclerosis	NSDU	neonatal stepdown unit
	no-show	NSE	neuron-specific enolase
	nonsmoker		normal saline enema (0.9% sodium chloride)
	normal saline solution (0.9% sodium chloride solution)		
		N s̄ E	nausea without emesis
	normospermic	NSF	no significant findings

203

NSFTD	normal spontaneous full-term delivery	NST	nonstress test
			normal sphincter tone
NSG	nursing		not sooner than
NSGCT	nonseminomatous germ-cell tumors		nutritional support team
NSGCTT	nonseminomatous germ-cell tumor of the testis	NSTD	nonsexually transmitted disease
NSGT	nonseminomatous germ-cell tumor	NSTI	necrotizing soft-tissue infection
NSHD	nodular sclerosing Hodgkin's disease	NSTT	nonseminomatous testicular tumors
NSI	negative self-image	NSU	neurosurgical unit
	no signs of infection		nonspecific urethritis
	no signs of inflammation	NSV	nonspecific vaginitis
NSICU	neurosurgery intensive care unit	NSVD	normal spontaneous vaginal delivery
NSILA	nonsuppressible insulin-like activity	NSVT	nonsustained ventricular tachycardia
NSN	Neo-Synephrine	NSX	neurosurgical examination
	nephrotoxic serum	NSY	nursery
	nephritis	NT	nasotracheal
NSO	Neosporin® ointment		next time
NSP	neck and shoulder pain		Nordic Track®
NSPs	nonstarch polysaccharides		normal temperature
NSPVT	nonsustained polymorphic ventricular tachycardia		normotensive
			nortriptyline
NSR	nasoseptal repair		not tender
	nonspecific reaction		not tested
	normal sinus rhythm		nourishment taken
	not seen regularly		nursing technician
NSRP	nerve-sparing radical prostatectomy	N&T	nose and throat
		N Tachy	nodal tachycardia
NSS	neurological signs stable	NT-ANP	N-terminal atrial natriuretic peptide
	normal size and shape		
	not statistically significant	NTBR	not to be resuscitated
	nutritional support service	NTC	neurotrauma center
	sodium chloride 0.9% (normal saline solution)	NTCS	no tumor cells seen
1/2 NSS	sodium chloride 0.45% (1/2 normal saline solution)	NTD	negative to date
			neural-tube defects
		NTE	neutral thermal environment
NSSL	normal size, shape, and location		not to exceed
NSSP	normal size, shape, and position	NTED	neonatal toxic-shock-syndrome-like exanthematous disease
NSSTT	nonspecific ST and T (wave)		
		NTF	normal throat flora
NSST-TWCs	nonspecific ST-T wave changes	NTG	nitroglycerin
			nontoxic goiter

	nontreatment group	NV	naked vision
	normal tension glaucoma		nausea and vomiting
NTGO	nitroglycerin ointment		near vision
NTI	narrow therapeutic index		negative variation
			neovascularization
	no treatment indicated		neurovascular
NTIS	National Technical Information Service (U.S. Department of Commerce)		new vessel
			next visit
			nonvenereal
			nonveteran
			normal value
NTL	nortriptyline		not vaccinated
	no time limit		not verified
NTLE	neocortical temporal-lobe epilepsy	N&V	nausea and vomiting
		NVA	near visual acuity
NTM	nocturnal tumescence monitor	NVAF	nonvalvular atrial fibrillation
	nontuberculous mycobacterium	NVB	Navelbine (vinorelbine tartrate)
NTMB	nontuberculous myobacteria	NVC	neurovascular checks
NTMI	nontransmural myocardial infarction	nvCJD	new-variant Creutzfeldt-Jakob disease
		NVD	nausea, vomiting, and diarrhea
NTND	not tender, not distended		neck vein distention
NTP	narcotic treatment program		neovascularization of the (optic) disk
	Nitropaste® (nitroglycerin ointment)		neurovesicle dysfunction
	normal temperature and pressure		normal vaginal delivery
	sodium nitroprusside		no venereal disease
NTPD	nocturnal tidal peritoneal dialysis		no venous distention
			nonvalvular disease
NTS	nasotracheal suction	NVDC	nausea, vomiting, diarrhea, and constipation
	nicotine transdermal system	NVE	native
	nucleus tractus solitarii		native valve endocarditis
NTT	nasotracheal tube		neovascularization elsewhere
NTU	nephelometric turbidity units	NVG	neovascular glaucoma
NTX	naltrexone (ReVia)		neoviridogrisein
NTZ	nitazoxanide	NVL	neurovascular laboratory
NTZ Long-acting®	oxymetazoline nasal spray	NVP	nausea and vomiting of pregnancy
NU	name unknown		nevirapine (Viramune)
NUD	nonulcer dyspepsia	NVS	neurological vital signs
NUG	necrotizing ulcerative gingivitis		neurovascular status
		NVSS	normal variant short stature
nullip	nullipara		
NUN	nonurea nitrogen	NW	naked weight

		O	
	nasal wash		
	not weighed		
NWB	nonweight bearing		
NWBL	nonweight bearing, left		
NWBR	nonweight bearing, right		
NWC	number of words chosen		
NWD	neuroleptic withdrawal	O	eye
	normal well developed		objective findings
NWTS	National Wilms' Tumor		obvious
	Study (rating scale)		occlusal
Nx	nephrectomy		often
	next		open
NYD	not yet diagnosed		oral
NYHA	New York Heart Ass-		ortho
	ociation (classification		other
	of heart disease)		oxygen
nyst	nystagmus		pint
NZ	enzyme		zero

$\bar{o}$	negative
	no
	none
	pint
	without
O+	blood type O positive
O−	blood type O negative
Ⓞ	orally (by mouth)
$_1O_2$	singlet oxygen
O_2	both eyes
	oxygen
O_2^-	superoxide
O_3	ozone
O157	*Escherichia coli*
	O157
OA	occipital artery
	occiput anterior
	old age
	on admission
	on arrival
	ophthalmic artery
	oral airway
	oral alimentation
	osteoarthritis
	Overeaters Anonymous
O/A	on or about
O & A	observation and
	assessment
	odontectomy and
	alveoloplasty
OAA	Old Age Assistance

OAC	omeprazole, amoxicillin, and clarithromycin	OBP	office blood pressure
	oral anticoagulant(s)	OBRR	obstetric recovery room
	overaction	OBS	obstetrical service
OAD	obstructive airway disease		organic brain syndrome
	occlusive arterial disease	OBT	obtained
	overall diameter	OBTM	omeprazole, bismuth subcitrate, tetracycline, and metronidazole
OAE	otoacoustic emissions		
OAF	oral anal fistula	OBUS	obstetrical ultrasound
	osteoclast activating factor	OBW	open bed warmer
		OC	obstetrical conjugate
OAG	open angle glaucoma		office call
OAP	old age pension		on call
OAS	Older Adult Services		only child
	oral allergy syndrome		open cholecystectomy
	organic anxiety syndrome		optical chromatography
	outpatient assessment service		oral care
	overall survival		oral contraceptive
	Overt Aggression Scale		osteocalcin
OASDHI	Old Age, Survivors, Disability, and Health Insurance		osteoclast
		O & C	onset and course
		OCA	oculocutaneous albinism
OASI	Old Age and Survivors Insurance		open care area
			oral contraceptive agent
OASO	overactive superior oblique	OCAD	occlusive carotid artery disease
OASR	overactive superior rectus	OCBZ	oxcarbazepine
OATS	osteochondral autograft transfer system	OCC	occasionally
			occlusal
OAV	oculoauriculovertebral (dysplasia)		old chart called
		OCCC	open chest cardiac compression
OAW	oral airway	occl	occlusion
OB	obese	OCCM	open chest cardiac massage
	obesity		
	obstetrics	OCC PR	open chest cardiopulmonary resuscitation
	occult blood		
	osteoblast	OCC Th	occupational therapy
OB-A	obstetrics-aborted	Occup Rx	occupational therapy
OB-Del	obstetrics-delivered	OCD	obsessive-compulsive disorder
OBE	out-of-body experience		
OBE-CALP	placebo capsule or tablet		osteochondritis dissecans
		OCG	oral cholecystogram
OBG	obstetrics and gynecology	OCI	Obsessive-Compulsive Inventory
Ob-Gyn	obstetrics and gynecology		
Obj	objective	OCL®	oral colonic lavage
obl	oblique	OCN	obsessive-compulsive neurosis
OB marg	obtuse marginal		
OB-ND	obstetrics-not delivered		Oncology Certified Nurse

OCNS	Obsessive-Compulsive Neurosis Scale	(of the US Food and Drug Administration)
O-CNV	occult choroidal neovascularization	on demand analgesia computer
OCOR	on-call to operating room	ODAT	one day at a time
		ODC	oral disease control
OCP	ocular cicatricial pemphigoid		ornithine decarboxylase
	oral contraceptive pills		outpatient diagnostic center
	ova, cysts, parasites	ODCH	ordinary diseases of childhood
OCR	oculocephalic reflex		
	optical character recognition	ODD	oculodentodigital (dysplasia)
OCS	Obsessive-Compulsive Scale		opposition defiance disorder
	oral cancer screening	OD'd	overdosed
11-OCS	11-oxycorticosteroid	ODed	overdosed
OCT	optical coherence tomograph (tomography)	ODM	occlusion dose monitor
			ophthalmodynamometry
	ornithine carbamyl transferase	ODN	optokinetic nystagmus
		ODP	occipitodextra posterior
	oxytocin challenge test		offspring of diabetic parents
OCU	observation care unit	OD/P	right eye patched
OCVM	occult cerebrovascular malformations	ODQ	on direct questioning
		ODS	organized delivery system
OCX	oral cancer examination	ODSS	Office of Disability Support Services
OD	Doctor of Optometry		
	Officer-of-the-Day	ODSU	oncology day stay unit
	once daily (this is a dangerous abbreviation as it is read as right eye)		One Day Surgery Unit
		ODT	occipitodextra transerve
		OE	on examination
	on duty		orthopedic examination
	optic disk		otitis externa
	oral-duodenal	O-E	standard observed minus expected
	outdoor		
	outside diameter	O&E	observation and examination
	ovarian dysgerminoma	OEC	outer ear canal
	overdose	OEI	opioid escalation index
	right eye	O_2EI	oxygen extraction index
Δ OD 450	deviation of optical density at 450	OENT	oral endotracheal tube
		OER	oxygen extraction ratios
ODA	occipitodextra anterior	O_2ER	oxygen extraction ratio
	once-daily aminoglycoside	OERR	order entry/results-reports (Veterans Administration's physician computer order entry system)
	osmotic driving agent		
ODAC	Oncologic Drugs Advisory Committee		

OET	oral esophageal tube	OHFA	hydroxy fatty acid
OETT	oral endotracheal tube	OHFT	overhead frame and trapeze
OF	occipital-frontal		
	optic fundi	OHG	oral hypoglycemic
	osteitis fibrosa	OHI	oral hygiene instructions
OFC	occipital-frontal circumference	OHIAA	hydroxyindolacetic acid
		OHL	oral hairy leukoplakia
	orbitofacial cleft	OHNS	Otolaryngology, Head, and Neck Surgery (Dept.)
OFF	shoes off during weighing		
OFI	other febrile illness	OHP	obese hypertensive patient
OFLOX	ofloxacin (Floxin)		
OFLX	ofloxacin (Floxin)		oxygen under hyperbaric pressure
OFM	open face mask		
OFNE	oxygenated fluorocarbon nutrient emulsion	OHRP	open-heart rehabilitation program
OFPF	optic fundi and peripheral fields	OHRR	open-heart recovery room
		OHS	occupational health service
OFTT	organic failure to thrive		
OG	Obstetrics-Gynecology		ocular hypoperfusion syndrome
	orogastric (feeding)		
	outcome goal (long-term goal)		open-heart surgery
		OHSS	ovarian hyperstimulation syndrome
OGC	oculogyric crisis		
OGCT	ovarian germ cell tumor	OHT	ocular hypertension
OGD	Office of Generic Drugs (of the Food and Drug Administration)		overhead trapeze
		OHTN	ocular hypertension
		OHTx	orthotopic heart transplantation
OGT	orogastric tube		
OGTT	oral glucose tolerance test	OI	opportunistic infection
OH	occupational history		osteogenesis imperfecta
	ocular history		otitis interna
	on hand	OIF	oil-immersion field
	open-heart	OIG	Office of the Inspector General
	oral hygiene		
	orthostatic hypotension	OIH	orthoiodohippurate
	outside hospital	OIHA	orthoiodohippuric acid
17-OH	17-hydroxycorticosteroids	OINT	ointment
OHA	oral hypoglycemic agents	OIRDA	occipital intermittent rhythmical delta activity
OHC	outer hair cell (in cochlea)		
		OIS	optical intrinsic signal (imaging)
OH Cbl	hydroxycobalamine		
17-OHCS	17-hydroxycorticosteroids		optimum information size
OHD	hydroxy vitamin D	OIT	ovarian immature teratoma
	organic heart disease		
25(OH)D₃	25-hydroxy vitamin D (calcifediol, Calderol)	OIU	optical internal urethrotomy
OHF	old healed fracture	OJ	orange juice (this is a dangerous abbreviation
	Omsk hemorrhagic fever		
	overhead frame		

	as it is read as OS-left eye)	OMA	older maternal age
	orthoplast jacket	OMAC	otitis media, acute, catarrhal
OK	all right		
	approved	OMAS	otitis media, acute, suppurating
	correct		
OKAN	optokinetic after nystagmus	OMB	obtuse marginal branch
		OMB$_1$	first obtuse marginal branch
OKN	optokinetic nystagmus	OMB$_2$	second obtuse marginal branch
OKT	Ortho Kung T cell, designation for a series of antigens		
		OMC	open mitral commissuortomy
OL	left eye	OMCA	otitis media, catarrhalis, acute
	open label (study)		
OLA	occiput left anterior	OMCC	otitis media, catarrhalis, chronic
	occipitolaevoanterior		
OLB	open liver biopsy	OMD	organic mental disorder
	open lung biopsy	OME	Office of Medical Examiner
OLD	obstructive lung disease		
OLF	ouabain-like factor		otitis media with effusion
OLM	ocular larva migrans		
	ophthalmic laser microendoscope	7-OMEN	menogaril
		OMFS	oral and maxillofacial surgery
OLNM	occult lymph node metastases		
		OMG	ocular myasthenia gravis
OLP	abnormal lipoprotein	OMI	old myocardial infarct
OLR	otology, laryngology, and rhinology	OMP	oculomotor (third nerve) palsy
OLS	ouabain-like substance	OMPA	otitis media, purulent, acute
OLT	occipitolaevoposterior		
	orthotopic liver transplantation	OMPC	otitis media, purulent, chronic
OLTx	orthotopic liver transplantation	OMR	operative mortality rate
		OMS	oral morphine sulfate
OM	every morning (this is a dangerous abbreviation)		organic mental syndrome
			organic mood syndrome
	obtuse marginal	OMSA	otitis media secretory (or suppurative) acute
	ocular melanoma		
	oral motor	OMSC	otitis media secretory (or suppurative) chronic
	oral mucositis		
	organomegaly	OMT	oral mucosal transudate
	osteomalacia		Osteopathic manipulative technique
	osteomyelitis		
	otitis media	OMVC	open mitral valve commissurotomy
O$_2$M	oxygen mask		
OM$_1$	first obtuse marginal (branch)	OMVD	optimized microvessel density (analysis)
OM$_2$	second obtuse marginal (branch)	OMVI	operating motor vehicle intoxicated

ON	every night (this is a dangerous abbreviation)	OOPS	out of program status
		OOR	out of room
	optic nerve	OORW	out of radiant warmer
	optic neurophathy	OOS	out of sequence
	oronasal		out of splint
	Ortho-Novum®		out of stock
	overnight	OOT	out of town
ONC	over-the-needle catheter	OOW	out of wedlock
	vincristine (Oncovin)	OP	oblique presentation
OND	ondansetron (Zofran)		occiput posterior
	other neurologic disorder(s)		open
			operation
ONH	optic nerve head		organophosphorous
	optic nerve hypoplasia		oropharynx
ON RR	overnight recovery room		oscillatory potentials
ONSD	optic nerve sheath decompression		osteoporosis
			outpatient
ONSF	optic nerve sheath fenestration	O&P	ova and parasites (stool examination)
ONTR	orders not to resuscitate	OPA	oral pharyngeal airway
OO	ophthalmic ointment		outpatient anesthesia
	oral order	OPAC	opacity (opacification)
	other	OPAT	outpatient parenteral antibiotic therapy
	out of		
o/o	on account of	OPB	outpatient basis
O&O	off and on	OPC	operable pancreatic carcinoma
OOB	out of bed		
OOBL	out of bilirubin light		oropharyngeal candidiasis
OOBBRP	out of bed with bathroom privileges		outpatient care
			outpatient catheterization
OOC	onset of contractions		outpatient clinic
	out of cast	OPCA	olivopontocerebellar atrophy
	out of control		
OO Con	out of control	*op cit*	in the work cited
OOD	outer orbital diameter	OPD	Orphan Products Development (office)
	out of doors		
OOH&NS	ophthalmology, otorhinolaryngology, and head and neck surgery		outpatient department
		O'p'-DDD	mitotane (Lysodren)
		OPDUR	on-line prospective drug utilization review
OOI	out of isolette	OPE	outpatient evaluation
OOL	onset of labor	OPEN	vincristine (Oncovin), prednisone, etoposide, and mitoxantrone (Novantrone)
OOLR	ophthalmology, otology, laryngology, and rhinology		
OOM	onset of menarche	OPERA	outpatient endometrial resection/ablation
OOP	out of pelvis		
	out of plaster	OPG	ocular plethysmography
	out on pass		osteoprotegerin

O

211

OPL	oral premalignant lesion		(otology, rhinology and
	other party liability		laryngology)
OPM	occult primary	ORMF	open reduction metallic
	malignancy		fixation
OPN	osteopontin	ORN	operating room nurse
OPO	organ procurement		osteoradionecrosis
	organizations	OROS	ostomotic release oral
OPOC	oral pharynx, oral cavity		system
OPP	opposite	ORP	occiput right posterior
OPPG	oculopneumoplethysmog-	ORS	olfactory reference
	raphy		syndrome
OPPOS	opposition		oral rehydration salts
OPRDU	outpatient renal dialysis	ORT	oestrogen (estrogen)-
	unit		replacement therapy
OPS	Objective Pain Scores		operating room technician
	operations		oral rehydration therapy
	outpatient surgery		Registered Occupational
O PSY	open psychiatry		Therapist
OPT	optimum	OR XI	oriented to time
	outpatient treatment	OR X2	oriented to time and place
OPT c CA	Ohio pediatric tent with	OR X3	oriented to time, place,
	compressed air		and person
OPT c O₂	Ohio pediatric tent with	OR X4	oriented to time, place,
	oxygen		person, and objects
OPTN	Organ Procurement and		(watch, pen, book)
	Transplantation	OS	left eye
	Network		mouth (this is a
OPT-NSC	outpatient treatment,		dangerous abbreviation
	nonservice-connected		as it is read as left eye)
OPT-SC	outpatient treatment,		occipitosacral
	service-connected		oligospermic
OPV	oral polio vaccine		opening snap
	outpatient visit		ophthalmic solution (this
OR	odds ratio		is a dangerous
	oil retention		abbreviation as it is
	open reduction		read as left eye)
	operating room		oral surgery
	Orthodox		osmium
	own recognizance		osteosarcoma
ORA	occiput right anterior		overall survival
ORCH	orchiectomy	OSA	obstructive sleep apnea
ORD	orderly	OSAS	obstructive sleep apnea
OREF	open reduction, external		syndrome
	fixation	OSCAR	On-line Survey
OR&F	open reduction and		Certification and
	fixation		Reporting
ORIF	open reduction internal	OSCE	Objective Structured
	fixation		Clinical Examination
ORL	otorhinolaryngology	OSD	overseas duty

	overside drainage	OTS	orotracheal suction
OSESC	opening snap ejection systolic click	OTT	orotracheal tube
		OTW	off-the-wall
OSFT	outstretched fingertips	OU	each eye
OSH	outside hospital	OULQ	outer upper left quadrant
OSHA	Occupational Safety & Health Administration	OU/P	both eyes patched
		OURQ	outer upper right quadrant
OSM S	osmolarity serum	OUS	obstetric ultrasound
OSM U	osmolarity urine	OV	office visit
OSN	off service note		ovary
OSP	outside pass		ovum
OS/P	left eye patched	OVAL	ovalocytes
OSS	osseous	OVF	Octopus® visual field
	over-shoulder strap	OVR	Office of Vocational Rehabilitation
OST	optimal sampling theory	OVS	obstructive voiding symptoms (syndrome)
OT	occiput transverse		
	occupational therapy	OW	once weekly (this is a dangerous abbreviation)
	old tuberculin		
	oral transmucosal		open wound
	orotracheal		outer wall
	oxytocin (Pitocin)		out of wedlock
O/T	oral temperature		ova weight
OTA	open to air	O/W	oil in water
OTC	ornithine transcarbamoylase		otherwise
		OWL	out of wedlock
	Orthopedic Technician, Certified	OWNK	out of wedlock not keeping (baby)
	over the counter (sold without prescription)	OWR	Osler-Weber-Rendu (disease)
OTCD	ornithine-transcarbamylase deficiency	OWT	zero work tolerance
		OX	oximeter
OTD	optimal therapeutic dose	O×1	oriented to time
	organ tolerance dose	O×2	oriented to time and place
	out the door	O×3	oriented to time, place, and person
OTFC	oral transmucosal fentanyl citrate (Fentanyl Oralet)	O×4	oriented to time, place, person, and objects (watch, pen, book)
OTH	other		
OTHS	occupational therapy home service	Oxi	oximeter (oximetry)
		Ox-LDL	oxidized low-density lipoprotein
OTO	one time only		
	otolaryngology	OXPHOS	oxidative phosphorylation
	otology	OxPt	oxaliplatin
OTR	Occupational Therapist, Registered	OXM	pulse oximeter
		Oxy-5®	benzoyl peroxide
OTRL	Occupational Therapist, Registered Licensed	OXZ	oxazepam (Serax)
		OZ	optical zone
OT/RT	occupational therapy/ recreational therapy		ounce

O

P

P	para
	peripheral
	phosphorus
	pint
	plan
	poor
	protein
	Protestant
	pulse
	pupil
$\bar{p}$	after
/P	partial lower denture
P/	partial upper denture
^{32}P	radioactive phosphorus
P_2	pulmonic second heart sound
P20	Ocusert® P20
P40	Ocusert® P40
PA	panic attack
	paranoid
	periapical (x-ray)
	pernicious anemia
	phenol alcohol
	Physician Assistant
	pineapple
	posterior-anterior (posteroanterior) (x-ray)
	presents again
	professional association (similar to a corporation)
	Pseudomonas aeruginosa
	psychiatric aide
	psychoanalysis
	pulmonary artery
Pa	pascal
P&A	percussion and auscultation
	phenol and alcohol (procedure for permanent removal of toenail)
	position and alignment

$P_2 > A_2$	pulmonic second heart sound greater than aortic second heart sound
PAB	premature atrial beat
	pulmonary artery banding
PABA	aminobenzoic acid (para-aminobenzoic acid)
PAC	cisplatin (Platinol), doxorubicin (Adriamycin), and cyclophosphamide
	phenacemide
	Physical Assessment Center
	Physician Assistant, Certified
	picture archiving communication (system)
	Port-a-cath®
	premature atrial contraction
	prophylactic anticonvulsants
	pulmonary artery catheter
PACATH	pulmonary artery catheter
PACE	population-adjusted clinical epidemiology
PACH	pipers to after coming head
$PACO_2$	partial pressure (tension) of carbon dioxide, alveolar
$PaCO_2$	partial pressure (tension) of carbon dioxide, artery
PACS	picture archiving and communications systems
PACT	prism and alternate cover test
	Program of Assertive Community Treatment
PAC-V	cisplatin (Platinol), doxorubicin (Adriamycin), and cyclophosphamide
PACU	postanesthesia care unit

PAD	pelvic adhesive disease		posteroanterior and lateral
	peripheral artery disease		
	pharmacologic atrial defibrillator	PALA	N-phosphoacetate-L aspartate
	preliminary anatomic diagnosis	Pa Line	pulmonary artery line
		PALN	para-aortic lymph node
	preoperative autologous donation	PALS	pediatric advanced life support
	primary affective disorder		periarterial lymphatic sheath
PADP	pulmonary arterial diastolic pressure	PAM	potential acuity meter
	pulmonary artery diastolic pressure		primary acquired melanosis
PADS	Post Anesthesia Discharge Scoring System		primary amebic meningoencephalitis
PAE	postanoxic encephalopa-thy	2-PAM	pralidoxime (Protopam)
	postantibiotic effect	PAMP	pulmonary arterial (artery) mean pressure
	pre-admission evaluation	PAN	pancreas
	progressive assistive exercise		pancreatic
PAEDP	pulmonary artery and end-diastole pressure		pancuronium (Pavulon)
			panoral x-ray examination
PAF	paroxysmal atrial fibrillation		periodic alternating nystagmus
	platelet activating factor		polyacrylonitrile (filter)
PA&F	percussion, auscultation, and fremitus		polyarteritis nodosa
		PANENDO	panendoscopy
PAGA	premature appropriate for gestational age	PANESS	physical and neurological examination for soft signs
PAGE	polyacrylamide gel electrophoresis		
		PANSS	Positive and Negative Syndrome Scale
PAH	para-aminohippurate	PAO	peak acid output
	phenylalanine hydroxylase		peripheral arterial occlusion
	polynuclear aromatic hydrocarbon	PAO_2	alveolar oxygen pressure (tension)
	pulmonary arterial hypertension	PaO_2	arterial oxygen pressure (tension)
PAI	plasminogen activator inhibitor	PAOD	peripheral arterial occlusive disease
	platelet accumulation index	PAOP	pulmonary artery occlusion pressure
PAIDS	pediatric acquired immunodeficiency syndrome	PAP	passive aggressive personality
			peroxidase-anti-peroxidase
PAIVS	pulmonary atresia with intact ventricle septum		pokeweed antiviral protein
PAL	posterior axillary line		

P

215

	primary atypical pneumonia		peripheral anterior synechia
	prostatic acid phosphatase		physician-assisted suicide
	pulmonary alveolar proteinosis		pneumatic antiembolic stocking
	pulmonary artery pressure		postanesthesia score
Pap smear	Papanicolaou's smear		premature auricular systole
PA/PS	pulmonary atresia/ pulmonary stenosis		Professional Activities Study
PAPVC	partial anomalous pulmonary venous connection		pulmonary artery stenosis
			pulsatile antiembolism system (stockings)
PAPVR	partial anomalous pul- monary venous return	PASA	aminosalicylic acid (para-aminosalicylic acid)
PAQLQ	Pediatric Asthma Quality of Life Questionnaire		
PAR	parafin	PA/S/D	pulmonary artery systolic/diastolic
	parallel		
	perennial allergic rhinitis	Pas Ex	passive exercise
		PASG	pneumatic antishock garment
	platelet aggregate ratio		
	possible allergic reaction	PASI	Psoriasis Area and Severity Index
	postanesthetic recovery		
	procedures, alternatives, and risks	PASK	peripheral anterior stromal keratopathy
	pulmonary arteriolar resistance	PASP	pulmonary artery systolic pressure
PARA	number of pregnancies producing viable offspring	PAT	paroxysmal atrial tachycardia
			passive alloimmune thrombocytopenia
	paraplegic		patella
	parathyroid		patient
PARA 1	having borne one child		percent acceleration time
Paraflu	Parainfluenza		platelet aggregation test
PARC	perennial allergic rhinoconjunctivitis		preadmission testing
			pregnancy at term
PAROM	passive assistance range of motion	PATH	pituitary adrenotropic hormone
PARR	postanesthesia recovery room		pathology
PARS	postanesthesia recovery score	PATP	preadmission testing program
PARU	postanesthetic recovery unit	PATS	payment at time of service
PAS	aminosalicylic acid (para-aminosalicylic acid)	PAV	Pavulon (pancuronium bromide)
	periodic acid-Schiff (reagent)	PAVe	procarbazine, melphalan (Alkeran), and vinblastine (Velban)

PAVM	pulmonary arteriovenous malformation	PBL	peripheral blood lymphocyte
PAVNRT	paroxysmal atrial ventricular nodal re-entrant tachycardia		primary brain lymphoma
		PBLC	premature birth live child
PAWP	pulmonary artery wedge pressure	PBM	pharmacy benefit management (manager)
PAX	periapical x-ray	PBMC	peripheral blood mononuclear cell
PB	barometric pressure	PBMNC	peripheral blood mononuclear cell
	British Pharmacopeia		
	parafin bath	PBN	polymyxin B sulfate, bacitracin, and neomycin
	piggyback		
	powder board		
	power building	PB:ND	problem: nursing diagnosis
	premature beat		
	Presbyterian	PBNS	percutaneous bladder neck stabilization
	protein-bound		
	pudendal block	PBO	placebo
	pyridostigmine bromide	PBP	phantom breast pain
Pb	lead		protein-bound polysaccharide
	phenobarbital		
p/b	postburn	PBPC	peripheral blood progenitor cell
P&B	pain and burning		
	Papanicolaou and breast (examinations)	PBPCT	peripheral blood progenitor cell transplant
	phenobarbital and belladonna	PBPI	penile-brachial pulse index
PBA	percutaneous bladder aspiration	PBPs	penicillin-binding proteins
PBAL	protected bronchoalveolar lavage	PBS	phosphate-buffered saline
		PBSC	peripheral blood stem cells
PbB	whole blood lead		
PBC	point of basal convergence	PBT_4	protein-bound thyroxine
	prebed care	PBV	percutaneous balloon valvuloplasty
	primary biliary cirrhosis		
PBD	percutaneous biliary drainage	PBZ	phenoxybenzamine
			phenylbutazone
	postburn day		pyribenzamine
	proliferative breast disease	ΦBZ	phenylbutazone
		PC	after meals
PBE	partial breech extraction		cisplatin (Platinol) and cyclophosphamide
	power building exercise		
PBF	placental blood flow		packed cells
	pulmonary blood flow		pancreatic carcinoma
PBFS	penile blood flow study		pathologic consultation
PBG	porphobilinogen		platelet concentrate
PBI	protein-bound iodine		*Pneumocystis carinii*
PBK	pseudophakic bullous keratopathy		poor condition
			popliteal cyst

posterior chamber

premature contractions

present complaint

productive cough

professional corporation

psychiatric counselor

pubococcygeus (muscle)

PCA passive cutaneous anaphylaxis

patient care assistant (aide)

patient-controlled analgesia

penicillamine

porous coated anatomic (joint replacement)

postcardiac arrest

postciliary artery

postconceptional age

posterior cerebral artery

posterior communicating artery

procainamide

procoagulation activity

prostate cancer

PCAC Physical Care Assessment Center

PCB pancuronium bromide

para cervical block

placebo

postcoital bleeding

prepared childbirth

Pseudomonas cepacia bacteremia

PCBH personal care boarding home

PCBMN palmar cutaneous branch of the median nerve

PCBs polychlorinated biphenyls

PCBUN palmar cutaneous branch of the ulnar nerve

PCC patient care coordinator

petrous carotid canal

pheochromocytoma

pneumatosis cystoides coli

poison control center

precipitated calcium carbonate

progressive cardiac care

PCCC pediatric critical care center

PCCM primary care case management

PCCU postcoronary care unit

PCD pacer-cardioverter-defibrillator

paroxysmal cerebral dysrhythmia

plasma cell dyscrasias

postmortem cesarean delivery

primary ciliary dyskinesia

programmed cell death

PCE physical capacities evaluation

potentially compensable event

pseudophakic corneal edema

PCE® erythromycin particles in tablets

PCEA patient-controlled epidural analgesia

PCEC purified chick embryo cell (culture)

PCF pharyngeal conjunctival fever

PCFT platelet complement fixation test

PCG phonocardiogram

pubococcygeus (muscle)

PCGG percutaneous coagulation of gasserian ganglion

PCH paroxysmal cold hemoglobinuria

periocular capillary hemangioma

personal care home

PC&HS after meals and at bedtime

PCI percutaneous coronary intervention

pneumatosis cystoides intestinalis

prophylactic cranial irradiation

PCIOL posterior chamber intraocular lens

PCKD	polycystic kidney disease		pulmonary capillary pressure
PCL	pacing cycle length	PCR	percutaneous coronary revascularization
	posterior chamber lens		
	posterior cruciate ligament		polymerase chain reaction
	proximal collateral ligament		protein catabolic rate
		PCr	plasma creatinine
PCLI	plasma cell labeling index	PCRA	pure red-cell aplasia
PCLN	psychiatric consultation liaison nurse	PCR/PSA	polymerase chain reaction analysis of prostate-specific antigen
PCLR	paid claims loss ratio		
PCM	primary cutaneous melanoma	PCS	patient care system
			patient-controlled sedation
	protein-calorie malnutrition		personal care service
			portable cervical spine
PCMX	chloroxylenol		portacaval shunt
PCN	penicillin		postconcussion syndrome
	percutaneous nephrostomy	P c/s	primary cesarean section
	primary care nursing	PCT	percent
PCNA	proliferating cell nuclear antigen		porphyria cutanea tarda
			post coital test
PCNL	percutaneous nephrostolithotomy		posterior chest tube
			primary chemotherapy
PCNSL	primary central nervous system lymphoma		progestin challenge test
		PCTA	percutaneous transluminal angioplasty
PCNT	percutaneous nephrostomy tube	PCU	palliative care unit
PCO	patient complains of		primary care unit
	polycystic ovary		progressive care unit
	posterior capsular opacification		protective care unit
		PCV	packed cell volume
PCO_2	partial pressure (tension) of carbon dioxide, artery		polycythemia vera
		PCVC	percutaneous central venous catheter
PCOD	polycystic ovarian disease	PCWP	pulmonary capillary wedge pressure
P COMM A	posterior communicating artery	PCX	paracervical
		PCXR	portable chest radiograph
PCOS	polycystic ovary syndrome	PCZ	procarbazine (Matulane)
PCP	patient care plan		prochlorperazine (Compazine)
	phencyclidine (phenylcyclohexyl piperidine)	PD	interpupillary distance
			Paget's disease
	Pneumocystis carinii pneumonia		pancreaticoduodenectomy
			panic disorder
	primary care person		Parkinson's disease
	primary care physician		percutaneous drain
	prochlorperazine		peritoneal dialysis
			personality disorder

	pharmacodynamics		pyruvate dehydrogenase
	poorly differentiated	PDI	Pain Disability Index
	postural drainage		phasic detrusor instability
	prism diopter	PDIGC	patient dismissed in good
	progressive disease		condition
	pupillary distance	PDL	periodontal ligament
P/D	packs per day (cigarettes)		poorly differentiated
2PD	two point discriminatory		lymphocytic
	test		postures of daily living
103Pd	palladium 103		progressively diffused
PDA	parenteral drug abuser		leukoencephalopathy
	patent ductus arteriosus	PDL-D	poorly differentiated
	poorly differentiated		lymphocytic-diffuse
	adenocarcinoma	PDL-N	poorly differentiated
	posterior descending		lymphocytic-nodular
	(coronary) artery	PDMC	premature dead male
PDAF	platelet-derived		child
	angiogenesis factor	PDN	Paget's disease of the
PDB	preperitoneal distention		nipple
	balloon		prednisone
PDC	patient denies complaints		private duty nurse
	poorly differentiated	PDP	peak diastolic pressure
	carcinoma	PD & P	postural drainage and
	private diagnostic clinic		percussion
PD&C	postural drainage and	PDPH	postdural puncture
	clapping		headache
PDCA	Plan-Do-Check-Act	PDQ	pretty damn quick (at
	(process improvement)		once)
PDD	cisplatin	PDR	patients' dining room
	pervasive developmental		*Physicians' Desk*
	disorder		*Reference*
	premenstrual dysphoric		postdelivery room
	disorder		proliferative diabetic
	primary degenerative		retinopathy
	dementia		prospective drug review
PDE	paroxysmal dyspnea on	PDRcVH	proliferative diabetic
	exertion		retinopathy with
	pulsed Doppler		vitreous hemorrhage
	echocardiography	PDRP	proliferative diabetic
PDE 5	phosphodiesterase type 5		retinopathy
PDEGF	platelet-derived epidermal	PDS	pain dysfunction
	growth factor		syndrome
PDFC	premature dead female		polydioxanone suture
	child		Progressive Deterioration
PDGF	platelet-derived growth		Scale
	factor	PDT	percutaneous dilatational
PDGXT	predischarge graded		tracheostomy
	exercise test		photodynamic therapy
PDH	past dental history		post-disaster trauma

PDU	pulsed Doppler ultrasonography	PEC	pulmonary ejection click
		PECCE	planned extracapsular cataract extraction
PDW	platelet distribution width		
PDWHF	platelet-derived wound healing factors	PECHO	prostatic echogram
		PECHR	peripheral exudative choroidal hemorrhagic retinopathy
pDXA	peripheral dual energy x-ray absorptiometry		
PE	cisplatin (Platinol AQ) and etoposide	PECO₂	mixed expired carbon dioxide tension
	pedal edema	PED	paroxysmal exertion-induced dyskinesia
	pelvic examination		
	phenytoin equivalent (150 mg of fosphenytoin sodium is equivalent to 100 mg of phenytoin sodium)		pediatrics
			pigment epithelial detachments
		PEDD	proton-electron dipole-dipole
	physical education (gym)	PEDI-DEG	pediatric deglycerolized red blood cells
	physical examination		
	physical exercise	Peds	pediatrics
	plasma exchange	PEE	punctate epithelial erosion
	pleural effusion	PEEP	positive end-expiratory pressure
	polyethylene		
	preeclampsia	PEF	cisplatin (Platinol AQ), epirubicin, and fluorouracil
	premature ejaculation		
	pressure equalization		
	pulmonary edema		peak expiratory flow
	pulmonary embolism	PEFR	peak expiratory flow rate
P₁E₁®	epinephrine 1%, pilocarpine 1% ophthalmic solution		
		PEFSR	partial expiratory flow static recoil curve
P&E	prep and enema	PEG	pegylated
PE24	Preemie Enfamil 24		percutaneous endoscopic gastrostomy
PEA	pelvic examination under anesthesia		
			pneumoencephalogram
	pre-emptive analgesia		polyethylene glycol
	pulseless electrical activity	PEG-ELS	polyethylene glycol and iso-osmolar electrolyte solution
PEARL	physiologic endometrial ablation/resection loop		
		PEGG	Parent Education and Guidance Group
	pupils equal accommodation, reactive to light		
		PEG-J	percutaneous endoscopic gastrojejunostomy
	pupils equal and reactive to light	PEG-JET	percutaneous endoscopic gastrostomy with jejunal extension tube
PEARLA	pupils equal and react to light and accommodation		
		PEG-SOD	polyethylene glycol-conjugated superoxide dismutase (pegorgotein)
PEB	cisplatin, etoposide, and bleomycin		
		PEI	cisplatin (Platinol AQ),

etoposide, and ifosfamide

percutaneous ethanol injection

phosphate excretion index

physical efficiency index

PEJ percutaneous endoscopic jejunostomy

PEK punctate epithelial keratopathy

PEL permissible exposure limits

PELD percutaneous endoscopic lumbar diskectomy

PELV pelvimetry

PEM prescription event monitoring

protein-energy malnutrition

PEMA phenylethylmalonamide

PEMS physical, emotional, mental, and safety

PEN parenteral and enteral nutrition

Pharmacy Equivalent Name

PENS percutaneous electrical nerve stimulation

percutaneous epidural nerve stimulator

PEO progressive external ophthalmoplegia

PEP patient education program

pharmacologic erection program

postexposure prophylaxis

pre-ejection period

protein electrophoresis

PEPI pre-ejection period index

PER by

pediatric emergency room

protein efficiency ratio

PERC perceptual

percutaneous

PERF perfect

perforation

Peri Care perineum care

PERIO periodontal disease

periodontitis

peri-pads perineal pads

PERL pupils equal, reactive to light

PERLA pupils equally reactive to light and accommodation

per os by mouth (this is a dangerous abbreviation as it is read as left eye)

PERR pattern evoked retinal response

PERRL pupils equal, round, and reactive to light

PERRLA pupils equal, round, reactive to light and accommodation

PERR-LADC pupils equal, round, reactive to light and accommodation directly and consensually

PERRRLA pupils equal, round, regular, react to light and accommodation

PERT pancreatic enzyme replacement therapy

program evaluation and review technique

PERV porcine endogenous retroviruses

PES pre-excitation syndrome

programmed electrical stimulation

pseudoexfoliation syndrome

peSPL peak equivalent sound pressure level

PET poor exercise tolerance

positron-emission tomography

pre-eclamptic toxemia

pressure equalizing tubes

PETN pentaerythritol tetranitrate

PEx physical examination

PEX# 3 plasma exchange number three

PF patellofemoral

peak flow

	peripheral fields	PFRC	plasma-free red cells
	plantar flexion	PFROM	pain-free range of motion
	power factor	PFS	patellar femoral syndrome
	preservative free		prefilled syringe
	prostatic fluid		preservative-free solution
	pulmonary fibrosis		(system)
	push fluids		primary fibromyalgia
PF3	platelet factor 3		syndrome
PF4	repligen		progression-free survival
16PF	The Sixteen Personality		pulmonary function
	Factors test		studies (study)
PFA	foscarnet (phosphonofor-	PFT	parafascicular
	matic acid)		thalamotomy
	pure free acid		pulmonary function test
PFB	potential for breakdown	PFTC	primary fallopian tube
	pseudofolliculitis barbae		carcinoma
PFC	patient-focused care	PFU	plaque-forming unit
	perfluorochemical	PFW	pHisoHex® face wash
	permanent flexure	PFWB	Pall filtered whole blood
	contracture	PG	paged in hospital
	persistent fetal circulation		paregoric
	prolonged febrile		performance goal (short-
	convulsions		term goal)
$\overline{P}$ FEEDS	after feedings		phosphatidylglycerol
PFFD	proximal femoral focal		picogram (pg)
	deficiency (defect)		placental grade
PFFFP	Pall filtered fresh frozen		(biophysical profile)
	plasma		polygalacturonate
PFGE	pulsed field gel		pregnant
	electrophoresis		prostaglandin
PfHRP-2	*Plasmodium falciparum*		pyoderma gangrenosum
	histidine-rich protein 2	PGA	prostaglandin A
PFI	progression-free interval		$\underline{p}$rothrombin time,
PFJ	patellofemoral joint		$\underline{g}$amma-glutamyl
PFJS	patellofemoral joint		$\underline{t}$ranspeptidase activity,
	syndrome		and serum
PFL	cisplatin (Platinol AQ),		$\underline{a}$polipoprotein AI
	fluorouracil, and		$\underline{c}$oncentration
	leucovorin	PGCs	primordial germ cells
PFL+IFN	cisplatin (Platinol AQ),	PGE	posterior gastroen-
	fluorouracil,		terostomy
	leucovorin, and		proximal gastric exclusion
	interferon alfa 2b	PGE$_1$	alprostadil (prostaglandin
PFM	porcelain fused to metal		E$_1$)
	primary fibromyalgia	PGE$_2$	dinoprostone
PFO	patent foramen ovale		(prostaglandin E$_2$)
PFPC	Pall filtered packed cells	PGF	paternal grandfather
PFR	parotid flow rate	PGF$_{2\alpha}$	dinoprost (prostaglandin
	peak flow rate		F$_{2\alpha}$)

P

PGGF	paternal great-grandfather	PHACO OD	phacoemulsification of the right eye
PGGM	paternal great-grandmother	PHACO OS	phacoemulsification of the left eye
PGH	pituitary growth hormones	PHAL	peripheral hyperalimentation
PGI	potassium, glucose, and insulin	PHAR	pharmacist
PGI₂	epoprostenol (Prostacyclin)		pharmacy
			pharynx
PGL	persistent generalized lymphadenopathy	Pharm	Pharmacy
	primary gastric lymphoma	PharmD	Doctor of Pharmacy
PGM	paternal grandmother	PHb	pyridoxylated hemoglobin
	phosphoglucomutase	PHC	posthospital care
PGP	paternal grandparent		primary health care
Pgp	P-glycoprotein		primary hepatocellular carcinoma
PGR	pulse generated runoff	PHCA	profound hypothermic cardiac arrest
PgR	progesterone receptor		
P-graph	penile plethysmograph	PHD	paroxysmal hypnogenic dyskinesia
PGS	Persian Gulf syndrome		
PGT	play-group therapy		Public Health Department
P±GTC	partial seizures with or without generalized tonic-clonic seizures	PhD	Doctor of Philosophy
		PHE	periodic health examination
PG-TXL	poly (L-glutamic acid)-paclitaxel	PHEN-FEN	phentermine and fenfluramine
PGU	postgonococcal urethritis	PHEO	pheochromocytoma
PGW	person gametocyte week	PHF	paired helical filament
PGY-1	postgraduate year one (first year resident)	PHH	posthemorrhagic hydrocephalus
pH	hydrogen ion concentration	PHHI	persistent hyperinsulinemic hypoglycemia of infancy
PH	past history		
	personal history		
	pinhole	PHI	phosphohexose isomerase
	poor health		prehospital index
	pubic hair	PHIS	posthead injury syndrome
	public health	PHL	Philadelphia (chromosome)
	pulmonary hypertension		
P&H	physical and history	PHLS	Public Health Laboratory Service (United Kingdom)
Ph¹	Philadelphia chromosome		
PHA	arterial pH		
	passive hemagglutinating		
	peripheral hyperalimentation	PHMB	polyhexamethylene biguanide
	phenylalanine	PHMD	polyhexamethylene (Baquacil, a pool cleaner)
	phytohemagglutinin antigen		
	postoperative holding area	PHN	postherpetic neuralgia
PHACO	phacoemulsification		public health nurse

	Puritan® heated nebulizer		poison ivy
PHNC	public health nurse coordinator		postinjury
			premature infant
PHNI	pinhole no improvement		present illness
PHO	Physician/Hospital Organization		principal investigator
			protease inhibitor
PHOB	phobic anxiety		pulmonary infarction
PHP	pooled human plasma	PI-3	parainfluenza 3 virus
	postheparin plasma	P & I	probe and irrigation
	prepaid health plan	PIAT	Peabody Individual Achievement Test
	pseudohypoparathyroidism		
		PIB	professional information brochure
	pyridoxalated hemoglobin polyoxyethylene conjugate		
		PIBD	paucity of interlobular bile ducts
PHPT	primary hyperparathyroidism	PIC	peripherally inserted catheter
			postintercourse
PHPV	persistent hyperplastic primary vitreous	PICA	Porch Index of Communicative Ability
PHR	peak heart rate		posterior inferior cerebellar artery
PhRMA	Pharmaceutical Research and Manufacturers of America (Formerly the Pharmaceutical Manufacturers Association)		
			posterior inferior communicating artery
		PICC	peripherally inserted central catheter
		PICT	pancreatic islet cell transplantation
PHS	partial hospitalization program	PICU	pediatric intensive care unit
	US Public Health Service		psychiatric intensive care unit
PHT	phenytoin (Dilantin)	PICVC	peripherally inserted central venous catheter
	portal hypertension		
	primary hyperthyroidism		
	pulmonary hypertension	PID	pelvic inflammatory disease
PHVA	pinhole visual acuity		
PHVD	posthemorrhagic ventricular dilatation		prolapsed intervertebral disk
PHx	past history		proportional-integral-derivative (controller)
Phx	pharynx		
PHY	physician	PIE	pulmonary infiltration with eosinophilia
PhyO	physician's orders		
PI	package insert		pulmonary interstitial emphysema
	pallidal index		
	pancreatic insufficiency	PIEE	pulsed irrigation for enhanced evacuation
	Pearl Index		
	performance improvement	PIF	peak inspiratory flow
	peripheral iridectomy	PIFG	poor intrauterine fetal growth
	persistent illness		
	physically impaired		

PIG	pertussis immune globulin		acetanilide-iminodiacetic acid
PIGI	pregnancy-induced glucose intolerance	PIPJ	proximal interphalangeal joint
PIGN	postinfectious glomerulonephritis	PIP/TZ	piperacillin-tazobactam (Zosyn)
PIH	pregnancy induced hypertension	PIQ	Performance Intelligence Quotient (part of Wechsler tests)
	preventricular intraventricular hemorrhage	PIS	pregnancy interruption service
	prolactin inhibiting hormone	PISA	phase invariant signature algorithm
PIIID	peripheral indwelling intermediate infusion device		proximal isovelocity surface area
PIIIP	aminoterminal type three procollagen propeptide	PIT	patellar inhibition test Pitocin (oxytocin)
PIIS	posterior inferior iliac spine		Pitressin (vasopressin) (this is a dangerous abbreviation)
PILO	pilocarpine		pituitary
PIMIA	potentiometric ionophore mediated immunoassay		pulsed inotrope therapy
PIMS	programmable implantable medication system	PITP	pseudo-idiopathic thrombocytopenic purpura
PIN	pain in (the) neck (no place for such a term in a written document)	PITR	plasma iron turnover rate
		PIV	peripheral intravenous
	personal identification number	PIVD	protruded intervertebral disk
	prostatic intraepithelial neoplasia	PIVH	periventricular-intraventricular hemorrhage
PIO	pemoline	PIVKA	proteins induced in vitamin K absence
PIO$_2$	partial pressure of inspired oxygen	PIWT	partially impacted wisdom teeth
PIOK	poikilocytosis		
PIP	peak inspiratory pressure	PJ	procelin jacket (crown)
	postictal psychosis	PJB	premature junctional beat
	postinfusion phlebitis	PJC	premature junctional contractions
	proximal interphalangeal (joint)	PJRT	permanent form of junctional reciprocating tachycardia
	pulmonary insufficiency of the premature		
PIPB	performance index phonetic balance	PJS	peritoneojugular shunt Peutz-Jeghers syndrome
PI-PB	performance intensity-phonemically balanced	PJT	paroxysmal junctional tachycardia
PIPIDA	N-para-isopropyl-	PJVT	paroxysmal junctional-ventricular tachycardia

PK	penetrating keratoplasty	PLC	pityriasis lichenoides chronica
	pharmacokinetics		
	plasma potassium	PLD	partial lower denture
	pyruvate kinase		percutaneous laser diskectomy
PKB	prone knee bend		
PKC	protein kinase C	PLDD	percutaneous laser disk decompression
PKD	paroxysmal kinesigenic dyskinesia	PLE	polymorphic light eruption
	polycystic kidney disease		protein-losing enteropathy
PKND	paroxysmal nonkinesigenic dyskinesia	PLED	periodic lateralizing epileptiform discharge
PKP	penetrating keratoplasty	PLEVA	pityriasis lichenoides et varioliformis acuta
PKR	phased knee rehabilitation		
PK Test	Prausnitz-Küstner transfer test	PLFC	premature living female child
PKU	phenylketonuria	PLH	paroxysmal localized hyperhidrosis
pk yrs	pack-years (smoking one pack of cigarettes a day for one year is termed 1 pack-year of smoking, thus 2 packs a day for 20 years would be 40 pack-years)	PLIF	posterior lumbar interbody fusion
		PLL	prolymphocytic leukemia
		PLM	periodic leg movement
			Plasma-Lyte M
			polarized-light microscope
			precise lesion measuring (device)
PL	light perception		product-line manager
	palmaris longus		
	place	PLMC	premature living male child
	placebo		
	plantar	PLMD	periodic limb movement disorder
	plethoric (infant color)		
	transpulmonary pressure	PLMS	periodic limb movements during sleep
PLA	Plasma-Lyte A		
	potentially lethal arrhythmia	PLN	pelvic lymph node
			popliteal lymph node
	Product License Application	PLND	pelvic lymph node dissection
	pulpolinguoaxial	PLOSA	physiologic low stress angioplasty
PLAD	proximal left anterior descending (artery)	PLP	partial laryngopharyngec-tomy
PLAP	placental alkaline phosphatase		phantom limb pain
			protolipid protein
PLAT C	platelet concentration	PLPH	post-lumbar puncture headache
PLAT P	platelet pheresis		
PLAX	parasternal long axis	PLR	pupillary light reflex
PLB	phospholamban	PLS	plastic surgery
	placebo		Preschool Language Scale
	posterolateral branch		primary lateral sclerosis
PLBO	placebo		

P

227

PLs	premalignant lesions		pseudomembranous colitis
PLSO	posterior leafspring orthosis	PMCP	para-monochlorophenol
PLST	progressively lowered stress threshold		perinatal mortality counseling program
PLSURG	plastic surgery	PMCT	perinatal mortality counseling team
PLT	platelet		
PLT EST	platelet estimate	PMD	perceptual motor development
PLTF	plaintiff		primary myocardial disease
PLTS	platelets		
PLUG	plug the lung until it grows		primidone (Mysoline)
			private medical doctor
PLV	posterior left ventricular		progressive muscular dystrophy
PLX	plexus		
PLYO	plyometric	PMDD	premenstrual dysphoric disorder
PLZF	promyelocytic leukemia zinc finger		
		PM/DM	polymyositis and dermatomyositis
PM	afternoon		
	evening	PME	polymorphonuclear esosinophil (leukocytes)
	pacemaker		
	particulate matter		postmenopausal estrogen
	petit mal	PMEALS	after meals
	physical medicine	PMEC	pseudomembranous enterocolitis
	pneumomediastinum		
	poliomyelitis	PMF	progressive massive fibrosis
	polymyositis		
	poor metabolizers		pupils mid-position, fixed
	postmenopausal		
	postmortem	PMH	past medical history
	presents mainly	PMI	Pain Management Index
	pretibial myxedema		past medical illness
	primary motivation		patient medication instructions
	prostatic massage		
	pulpomesial		plea of mental incompetence
PMA	Pharmaceutical Manufacturers Association (see PhRMA)		point of maximal impulse
			posterior myocardial infarction
	positive mental attitude		
	premarket approval	PML	polymorphonuclear leukocytes
	premenstrual asthma		
	Prinzmetal's angina		posterior mitral leaflet
PMAA	Premarket Approval Application (medical devices)		premature labor
			progressive multifocal leukoencephalopathy
PMB	polymorphonuclear basophil (leukocytes)	PMMA	polymethyl methacrylate
	polymyxin B	PMMF	pectoralis major myocutaneous flap
	postmenopausal bleeding		
PMC	premature mitral closure	PMN	polymodal nociceptors

228

	polymorphonuclear leukocyte	PN	parenteral nutrition
	Premarket Notification (medical devices)		percussion note
			percutaneous nephrosonogram
PMNL	polymorphonuclear leukocyte		percutaneous nucleotomy
PMNN	polymorphonuclear neutrophil		periarteritis nodosa
			peripheral neuropathy
PMNS	postmalarial neurological syndrome		pneumonia
			polyarteritis nodosa
PMO	postmenopausal osteoporosis		poorly nourished
			positional nystagmus
pmol	picomole		postnasal
PMP	pain management program		postnatal
			practical nurse
	previous menstrual period		premie nipple
	psychotropic medication plan		primary nurse
			progress note
			pyelonephritis
PMPM	per member, per month	P & N	psychiatry and neurology
PMPO	postmenopausal palpable ovary	PN₂	partial pressure of nitrogen
PMR	pacemaker rhythm	PNA	Pediatric Nurse Associate
	polymorphic reticulosis		polynitroxyl albumin
	polymyalgia rheumatica	PNa	plasma sodium
	premedication regimen	PNAB	percutaneous needle aspiration biopsy
	prior medical record		
	progressive muscle relaxation	PNAC	parenteral nutrition associated cholestasis
PM&R	physical medicine and rehabilitation	PNAS	prudent no added salt
		PNB	percutaneous needle biopsy
PMS	performance measurement system		popliteal nerve block
	periodic movements of sleep		premature newborn
			premature nodal beat
	poor miserable soul		prostate needle biopsy
	postmarketing surveillance	PNC	penicillin
			peripheral nerve conduction
	postmenopausal syndrome		
	premenstrual syndrome		premature nodal contraction
PMT	pacemaker-mediated tachycardia		prenatal care
	point of maximum tenderness		prenatal course
			Psychiatric Nurse Clinician
	premenstrual tension		
PMTS	premenstrual tension syndrome	PND	paroxysmal nocturnal dyspnea
PMV	prolapse of mitral valve		pelvic node dissection
PMW	pacemaker wires		postnasal drip
PMZ	postmenopausal zest		pregnancy, not delivered

PNE	peripheral neuroepithelioma	PNT	percutaneous nephrostomy tube
	primary nocturnal enuresis	pnthx	pneumothorax
		PNU	protein nitrogen units
PNET	primitive neuroectodermal tumors	PNV	postoperative nausea and vomiting
PNET-MB	primitive neuroectodermal tumors-medulloblastoma		prenatal vitamins
		Pnx	pneumonectomy
PNEUMO	pneumothorax		pneumothorax
PNF	primary nonfunction	PO	by mouth (*per os*)
	proprioceptive neuromuscular fasciculation (reaction)		phone order
			postoperative
		P&O	parasites and ova
PNH	paroxysmal nocturnal hemoglobinuria		prosthetics and orthotics
		P_{O_2}	partial pressure (tension) of oxygen, artery
	polynitroxyl-hemoglobin	PO_4	phosphate
PNI	peripheral nerve injury	POA	pancreatic oncofetal antigen
	Prognostic Nutrition Index		power of attorney
			primary optic atrophy
PNKD	paroxysmal nonkinesigenic dyskinesia	POACH	prednisone, vincristine (Oncovin), doxorubicin (Adriamycin), cyclophosphamide, and cytarabine
PNL	percutaneous nephrolithotomy		
PNMG	persistent neonatal myasthenia gravis	POAG	primary open-angle glaucoma
PNMT	phenylethanolamine-N-methyltransferase	POB	phenoxybenzamine (Dibenzyline)
PNNP	Perinatal Nurse Practitioner		place of birth
PNP	peak negative pressure	POC	plans of care
	Pediatric Nurse Practitioner		point-of-care
			position of comfort
	progressive nuclear palsy		postoperative care
			product of conception
	purine nucleoside phosphorylase	POD	pacing on demand
			place of death
PNRB	partial non-rebreather (oxygen mask)		Podiatry
			polycystic ovarian disease
PNS	partial nonprogressing stroke	POD 1	postoperative day one
		PODx	preoperative diagnosis
	peripheral nerve stimulator	POE	point (portal, port) of entry
	peripheral nervous system		position of ease
	practical nursing student	POEMS	plasma cell dyscrasia with polyneuropathy, organomegaly, endocrinopathy,
PNSP	penicillin-nonsusceptible *S. pneumoniae*		

	monoclonal protein (M-protein), and skin changes	POMS	Profile of Mood States
		POMS-FI	Fatigue-Inertia Subscale of the Profile of Mood States
POEx	postoperative exercise		
POF	physician's order form	PONI	postoperative narcotic infusion
	position of function		
	premature ovarian failure	PONV	postoperative nausea and vomiting
P of I	proof of illness		
POG	Pediatric Oncology Group	POOH	postoperative open heart (surgery)
	Penthrane,® oxygen, and gas (nitrous oxide)	POP	pain on palpation
	products of gestation		persistent occipitoposterior
POH	personal oral hygiene		plaster of paris
	presumed ocular histoplasmosis		popiliteal
			posterior oral pharynx
POHA	preoperative holding area	POp	postoperative
POHI	physically or otherwise health impaired	poplit	popliteal
		POPs	progesterone-only pills
POHS	presumed ocular histoplasmosis syndrome	POR	physician of record
			problem-oriented record
POI	Personal Orientation Inventory	PORP	partial ossicular replacement prosthesis
	postoperative instructions	PORR	postoperative recovery room
POIB	place outpatient in inpatient bed	PORT	perioperative respiratory therapy
POIK	poikilocytosis		portable
POL	physician's office laboratory		postoperative radiotherapy
	premature onset of labor		postoperative respiratory therapy
POLS	postoperative length of stay	POS	parosteal osteosarcoma
POLY	polychromic erythrocytes		physician's order sheet
	polymorphonuclear leukocyte		point-of-service
		poss	possible
POLY-CHR	polychromatophilia	post	postmortem examination (autopsy)
POM	pain on motion	PostC	posterior chamber
	polyoximethylene	PostCap	posterior capsule
	prescription-only medication	post op	postoperative
		Post Sag D	posterior sagittal diameter
POMC	pro-opiomelanocortin		
POMP	prednisone, vincristine (Oncovin), methotrexate, and mercaptopurine (Purinthol)	post tib	posterial tibial
		PostVD	posterior vitreous detachment
		POT	peak occupancy time
POMR	problem-oriented medical record		plans of treatment
			potassium

	potential	PPAS	postpolio atrophy syndrome
POU	placenta, ovaries, and uterus	PPB	parts per billion
POV	privately owned vehicle		pleuropulmonary blastoma
POW	prisoner of war		positive pressure breathing
POX	pulse oximeter (reading)		prostate puncture biopsy
PP	near point of accommodation	PPBE	postpartum breast engorgment
	paradoxical pulse	PPBS	postprandial blood sugar
	partial upper and lower dentures	PPC	plaster of paris cast
	pedal pulse		progressive patient care
	per protocol	PPCD	posterior polymorphous corneal dystrophy
	periodontal pockets	PPCF	plasma prothrombin conversion factor
	peripheral pulses	PPD	packs per day
	pin prick		posterior polymorphous dystrophy
	pink puffer (emphysema)		postpartum day
	Planned Parenthood		probing pocket depth
	plasmapheresis		purified protein derivative (of tuberculin)
	plaster of paris		pylorus-sparing pancreaticoduodenectomy
	poor person		
	posterior pituitary		
	postpartum		
	postprandial	P & PD	percussion & postural drainage
	presenting part		
	private patient	PPD-B	purified protein derivative, Battey
	prophylactics	PPDR	preproliferative diabetic retinopathy
	protoporphyria		
	proximal phalanx	PPD-S	purified protein derivative, standard
	pulse pressure	PPE	personal protective equipment
	push pills		
P-P	probability-probability (plots)		pruritic papular eruption
P&P	pins and plaster	PPES	pedal pulses equal and strong
	policy and procedure	PPF	pellagra preventive factor
PIIIP	aminoterminal type three protocollegan propeptide		plasma protein fraction
PPIX	protoporphyrin nine	PPG	photoplethysmography
PPA	palpation, percussion, and auscultation		postprandial glucose
	phenylpropanolamine		pylorus-preserving gastrectomy
	phenylpyruvic acid	PPGI	psychophysiologic gastrointestinal (reaction)
	postpartum amenorrhea		
PP&A	palpation, percussion, and auscultation	PPH	postpartum hemorrhage
PPARs	peroxisome proliferator-activated receptors		primary postpartum hemorrhage

	primary pulmonary hypertension		protamine paracoagulation phenomenon
PPHN	persistent pulmonary hypertension of the newborn	PPPBL	peripheral pulses palpable both legs
PPHx	previous psychiatric history	PPPD	pylorus-preserving pancreatoduodenectomy
PPIX	protoporphyrin nine	PPPG	postprandial plasma glucose
PPI	patient package insert	PPPM	per patient, per month
	Present Pain Intensity	PPQ	Postoperative Pain Questionnaire
	proton pump inhibitor		
PPK	population pharmaco-kinetics	PPR	patient progress record
		PPr	periodontal prophylactics
PPL	pars plana lensectomy	PPRC	Physician Payment Review Commission
Ppl	pleural pressure		
PPLO	pleuropneumonia-like organisms	PPROM	prolonged premature rupture of membranes
PPLOV	painless progressive loss of vision	pPROM	premature rupture of the membranes before 37 weeks gestation
PPM	parts per million	PPS	peripheral pulmonary stenosis
	permanent pacemaker		
	persistent pupillary membrane		postpartum sterilization
			postperfusion syndrome
PPMA	postpoliomyelitis muscular atrophy		postpoliomyelitis syndrome
PPMS	psychophysiologic musculoskeletal (reaction)		postpump syndrome
			prospective payment system
PPN	peripheral parenteral nutrition	PPSS	peripheral protein sparing solution
PPNAD	primary pigmented nodular adrenocortical disease	PPT	person, place, and time
			Physical Performance Test
PPNG	penicillinase producing *Neisseria gonorrhoeae*	PPTL	postpartum tubal ligation
		PPU	perforated peptic ulcer
PPO	prefered provider organization	PPV	pars plana vitrectomy
			patent processus vaginalis
PPOB	postpartum obstetrics		
PPP	patient prepped and positioned		pneumococcal polysaccharide vaccine
	pedal pulse present		positive predictive value
	peripheral pulses palpable (present)		positive-pressure ventilation
	platelet-poor plasma	PPVT	Peabody Picture Vocabulary Test
	postpartum psychosis		
	preferred practice patterns	PPY	packs per year (cigarettes)
	proportional pulse pressure (SBP minus DBP)/SBP	PQ	pronator quadratus
		pQCT	peripheral quantitative computed tomography

PQOCN	Psychiatric Questionnaire Obsessive-Compulsive Neurosis		preposition
		PRERLA	pupils round, equal, react to light and accommodation
PR	far point of accommodation		
	pack removal	prev	prevent
	partial remission		previous
	patient relations	PRFD	percutaneous radio-frequency denervation
	per rectum		
	premature	PRFNB	percutaneous radio-frequency facet nerve block
	profile		
	progressive resistance		
	prolonged remission	PRG	phleborheogram
	prone	PRH	past relevant history
	Protestant		postocclusive reactive hyperemia
	Puerto Rican		
	pulmonic regurgitation		preretinal hemorrhage
	pulse rate	PRI	Pain Rating Index
P=R	pupils equal in size and reaction		Patient Review Instrument
		prim	primary
P & R	pelvic and rectal	PRIMIP	primipara (1st pregnancy)
	pulse and respiration	PR interval	part of the electrocardiographic cycle from onset of atrial depolarization on onset of ventricular depolarization
PR-2	Bennett pressure ventilator		
PRA	panel reactive antibodies (organ transplants)		
	plasma renin activity		
PRAFO	pressure relief ankle-foot orthosis	PRISM	Pediatric Risk of Mortality Score
PRAT	platelet radioactive antiglobulin test	PRK	photorefractive keratectomy
PRBC	packed red blood cells	PRL	prolactin
PRC	packed red cells	PRLA	pupils react to light and accommodation
	peer review committee		
PRCA	pure red cell aplasia	PRM	partial rebreathing mask
PRD	polycystic renal disease		phosphoribomutase
PRE	passive resistance exercises		photoreceptor membrane
			prematurely ruptured membrane
	progressive resistive exercise		
			primidone
	proton relaxation enhancement	PRMF	preretinal macular fibrosis
		PRM-SDX	pyrimethamine; sulfadoxine
Pred	prednisone	PRN	as occasion requires
PREG	Pregestimil® (infant formula)	PRO	Professional Review Organization
	pregnenolone		proline
PREMIE	premature infant		pronation
pre-op	before surgery		protein
prep	prepare for surgery		

	prothrombin		type b diphtheria
prob	probable		conjugate vaccine
PROCTO	procotoscopic	PRPP	5-phosphoribosyl-
	proctology		1-pyrophosphate
PROG	prognathism	PRP-T	polysaccharide tetanus
	prognosis		conjugate vaccine
	program	PRRE	pupils round regular, and
	progressive		equal
PROM	passive range of motion	PRRERLA	pupils round, regular,
	premature rupture of		equal; react to light and
	membranes		accommodation
ProMACE	prednisone, methotrexate,	PRS	prolonged respiratory
	calcium leucovorin,		support
	doxorubicin	PRSP	penicillinase-resistant
	(Adriamycin),		synthetic penicillins
	cyclophosphamide, and		penicillin-resistant
	etoposide		*Streptococcus*
PROMM	passive range of motion		*pneumoniae*
	machine	PRSs	positive rolandic spikes
Promy	promyelocyte	PRT	protamine response test
PRO MYELO	promyelocytes	PRTCA	percutaneous rotational
			transluminal coronary
PRON	pronation		angioplasty
PROS	prostate	PRTH-C	prothrombin time control
	prosthesis	PRV	polycythemia rubra vera
PROT REL	protrusive relationship	PRVEP	pattern reversal visual
			evoked potentials
prov	provisional	PRW	past relevant work
PROVIMI	proteins, vitamins, and		polymerized ragweed
	minerals	PRX	panoramic facial x-ray
PROX	proximal	PRZF	pyrazofurin
PRP	panretinal photocoagula-	PS	paradoxic sleep
	tion		paranoid schizophrenia
	patient recovery plan		pathologic stage
	penicllinase-resistant		patient's serum
	penicillin		performance status
	penicillin-resistant		peripheral smear
	pneumococci		physical status
	pityriasis rubra pilaris		plastic surgery (surgeon)
	platelet rich plasma		polysulfone (filter)
	polyribose ribitol		posterior synechiae
	phosphate		posterior synechiotomy
	poor progression of R		pressure support
	wave in precordial		protective services
	leads		pulmonary stenosis
	progressive rubella		pyloric stenosis
	panencephalitis		pyrimethamine
PrP	prion protein		(Daraprim); sulfadoxine
PRP-D	*Haemophilus influenzae,*		(Fansidar)

	serum from pregnant women		primary sclerosing cholangitis
P/S	polyunsaturated to saturated fatty acids ratio		pronation spring control pubosacrococcygeal (diameter)
P & S	pain and suffering paracentesis and suction	PSCC	posterior subcapsular cataract
	permanent and stationary	PSC Cat	posterior subcapsular cataract
PS I	healthy patient with localized pathological process	PSCH	peripheral stem cell harvest
PS II	a patient with mild to moderate systemic disease	PSCP	posterior subcapsular precipitates
PS III	a patient with severe systemic disease limiting activity but not incapacitating	PSCT	peripheral stem cell transplant
		PSCU	pediatric special care unit
		PSD	poststroke depression
PS IV	a patient with incapacitating systemic disease		power spectral density psychosomatic disease
PS V	moribund patient not expected to live (These are American Society of Anesthesiologists' physical status patient classifications. Emergency operations are designated by "E" after the classification.)	PSDS	palmar surface desensitization
		PSE	portal systemic encephalopathy pseudoephedrine
		PSF	posterior spinal fusion
		PSG	peak systolic gradient polysomnogram portosystemic gradient
		PSGN	post-streptococcal glomerulonephritis
PSA	polysubstance abuse product selection allowed prostate-specific antigen	PSH	past surgical history postspinal headache
		PSHx	past surgical history
PsA	psoriatic arthritis	PSI	Physiologic Stability Index
PSAD	prostate-specific antigen density		pounds per square inch
PSADT	prostate-specific antigen doubling time		punctate subepithelial infiltrate
PSAG	*Pseudomonas aeruginosa*	PSIC	pediatric surgical intensive care
PSAV	prostate-specific antigen velocity	PSIG	pounds per square inch gauge
PSBO	partial small bowel obstruction	PSIS	posterior superior iliac spine
PSC	Pediatric Symptom Checklist	PSM	presystolic murmur
	percutaneous suprapubic cystostomy	PSMA	personal self-maintenance activities
	posterior subcapsular cataract		progressive spinal muscular atrophy

	prostate-specific membrane antigen	PSVT	paroxysmal supraventricular tachycardia
PSMF	protein-sparing modified fasting (Blackburn diet)	PSW	psychiatric social worker
PSMS	Physical Self Maintenance Scale	PSY	presexual youth
		PSZ	pseudoseizures
PSNP	progressive supra-nuclear palsy	PT	cisplatin (Platinol AQ) parathormone parathyroid
PSO	pelvic stabilization orthosis		paroxysmal tachycardia patient
	physician supplemental order		phage type phenytoin (Dilantin)
	Polysporin ointment		phototoxicity
	proximal subungual onychomycosis		physical therapy pine tar
pSO₂	arterial oxygen saturation		pint
P/sore	pressure sore		posterior tibial
PSP	pancreatic spasmolytic peptide		preterm prothrombin time
	phenolsulfonphthalein	Pt	platinum
	photostimulable phosphor	P/T	piperacillin/tazobactam (Zosyn®)
	progressive supranuclear palsy	P1/2T	pressure one-half time
PSRBOW	premature spontaneous rupture of bag of waters	P&T	paracentesis and tubing (of ears) peak and trough permanent and total Pharmacy and Therapeutics (Committee)
PSRT	photostress recovery test		
PSS	painful shoulder syndrome pediatric surgical service physiologic saline solution (0.9% sodium chloride)	PTA	percutaneous transluminal angioplasty Physical Therapy Assistant
	progressive systemic sclerosis		plasma thromboplastin antecedent
PSSP	penicillin-sensitive *Streptococcus pneumoniae*		posttraumatic amnesia pretreatment anxiety prior to admission
PST	paroxysmal supraventricular tachycardia		pure-tone average
	Patient Service Technician	PTAB	popliteal-tibial artery bypass
	platelet survival time	PTB	patellar tendon bearing
	postural stress test		prior to birth
PSTT	placental site trophoblastic tumor		pulmonary tuberculosis
PSUD	psychoactive substance use disorder	PTBA	percutaneous transluminal balloon angioplasty
PSV	pressure supported ventilation	PTBD	percutaneous transhepatic biliary drain (drainage)

P

PTBD-EF	percutaneous transhepatic biliary drainage—enteric feeding		pulmonary thromboembolism
PTBS	post-traumatic brain syndrome	PTED	pulmonary thromboembolic disease
PTB-SC-SP	patellar tendon bearing-supracondylar-suprapatellar	PTER	percutaneous transluminal endomyocardial revascularization
PTC	patient to call	PTF	patient transfer form
	percutaneous transhepatic cholangiography		pentoxifylline posttetanic facilitation
	plasma thromboplastin components	PTFE	polytetrafluoroethylene
	post-tetanic count	PTG	parathyroid gland
	premature tricuspid closure	PTGBD	percutaneous transhepatic gallbladder drainage
	prior to conception	PTH	parathyroid hormone
	pseudotumor cerebri		posttransfusion hepatitis
PT-C	prothrombin time control		prior to hospitalization
PTCA	percutaneous transluminal coronary angioplasty	PTHC	percutaneous transhepatic cholangiography
PTCDLF	pregnancy, term, complicated delivered, living female	PTHrP	parathyroid hormone-related protein
PTCDLM	pregnancy, term, complicated delivered, living male	PTHS	posttraumatic hyperirritability syndrome
PTCL	peripheral T-cell lymphoma	PTI	pressure-time integral
PTCR	percutaneous transluminal coronary recanalization	PTJV	percutaneous transtracheal jet ventilation
PTCRA	percutaneous transluminal coronary rotational atherectomy	PTK	phototherapeutic keratectomy
PTD	period to discharge	PTL	preterm labor
	permanent and total disability		Sodium Pentothal®
	persistent trophoblastic disease	PTLD	posttransplantation lymphoproliferative disorder (disease)
	pharmacy to dose	PTM	patient monitored
	prior to delivery		posterior trabecular meshwork
PTDM	posttransplant diabetes mellitus	PTMC	percutaneous transvenous mitral commissurotomy
PTDP	permanent transvenous demand pacemaker	PTMDF	pupils, tension, media, disk, and fundus
PTE	pretibial edema	PT-NANB	posttransfusion non-A, non-B (hepatitis C)
	proximal tibial epiphysis	PTNB	preterm newborn
	pulmonary thromboembolectomy	pTNM	postsurgical resection-pathologic staging of cancer
		PTO	part-time occlusion (eye patch)

	please turn over		parathyroidectomy
	proximal tubal obstruction		pelvic traction
PTP	posterior tibial pulse		pentoxifylline (Trental)
	posttransfusion purpura		phototherapy
PTPM	posttraumatic progressive		pneumothorax
	myelopathy	PTZ	pentylenetetrazol
PTPN	peripheral (vein) total		phenothiazine
	parenteral nutrition	PU	pelvic-ureteric
P to P	point to point		pelviureteral
PTR	paratesticular		peptic ulcer
	rhabdomyosarcoma		pregnancy urine
	patella tendon reflex	P & U	Pharmacia & Upjohn
	patient to return		Company
	prothrombin time ratio	PUA	pelvic (examination)
PT-R	prothrombin time ratio		under anesthesia
PTRA	percutaneous transluminal	PUB	pubic
	renal angioplasty	PUBS	percutaneous umbilical
PTS	patellar tendon suspension		blood sampling
	Pediatric Trauma Score	PUC	pediatric urine
	permanent threshold shift		collector
	prior to surgery	PUD	partial upper denture
PTSD	posttraumatic stress		peptic ulcer disease
	disorder		percutaneous ureteral
PTT	partial thromboplastin		dilatation
	time	PUE	pyrexia of unknown
	platelet transfusion		etiology
	therapy	PUF	pure ultrafiltration
PTT-C	partial thromboplastin	PUFA	polyunsaturated fatty
	time control		acids
PTTW	patient tolerated traction	PUFFA	polyunsaturated free fatty
	well		acids
PTU	pain treatment unit	pul.	pulmonary
	pregnancy, term,	PULP	pulpotomy
	uncomplicated	Pulse A	pulse apical
	propylthiouracil	PULSE	pulse oximetry
PTUCA	percutaneous transluminal	OX	
	ultrasonic coronary	Pulse R	pulse radial
	angioplasty	PULSES	(physical profile) physical
PTUDLF	pregnancy, term,		condition, upper limb
	uncomplicated		functions, lower limb
	delivered, living		functions, sensory
	female		components, excretory
PTUDLM	pregnancy, term,		functions, and support
	uncomplicated		factors
	delivered, living male	PUN	plasma urea nitrogen
PTV	posterior tibial vein	PUND	pregnancy, uterine, not
PTWTKG	patient's weight in		delivered
	kilograms	PUNL	percutaneous ultrasonic
PTX	paclitaxel (Taxol)		nephrolithotripsy

P

PUO	pyrexia of unknown origin		polyethylene vacuum cup
			polyvinyl chloride
PUP	percutaneous ultrasonic pyelolithotomy		porcelain veneer crown
			postvoiding cystogram
PU/PL	partial upper and lower dentures		premature ventricular contraction
PUPPP	pruritic urticarial papules and plaque of pregnancy		pulmonary venous congestion
PUS	percutaneous ureteral stent	Pv_{CO_2}	partial pressure (tension) of carbon dioxide, vein
	preoperative ultrasound		
PUU	Puumala hantavirus	PVD	patient very disturbed
PUVA	psoralen-ultraviolet-light (treatment)		peripheral vascular disease
PUW	pick-up walker		posterior vitreous detachment
PV	papillomavirus		premature ventricular depolarization
	Parvovirus		
	per vagina		
	plasma volume	PVDA	prednisone, vincristine, daunorubicin, and asparaginase
	polio vaccine		
	polycythemia vera		
	popliteal vein	PVDF	polyvinyl difluoride
	portal vein	PVE	perivenous encephalomy-elitis
	postvoiding		
	prenatal vitamins		premature ventricular extrasystole
	projectile vomiting		
	pulmonary vein		prosthetic value endocarditis
P & V	peak and valley (this is a dangerous abbreviation, use peak and trough)		
		PVF	peripheral visual field
		PVFS	postviral fatigue syndrome
	pyloroplasty and vagotomy		
		PVGM	perifoveolar vitreoglial membrane
PVA	polyvinyl alcohol		
	Prinzmetal's variant angina	PVH	periventricular hemorrhage
			periventricular hyperintensity
PVAD	prolonged venous access devices		
			pulmonary vascular hypertension
PVAM	potential visual acuity meter		
		PVI	peripheral vascular insufficiency
PVAR	pulmonary vein atrial reversal		
			portal-vein infusion
PVB	cisplatin, (Platinol) vinblastine, and bleomycin	PVK	penicillin V potassium
		PVL	peripheral vascular laboratory
	paravertebral block		
	porcelain veneer bridge		periventricular leukomalacia
	premature ventricular beat	PVM	paraverteabral muscle
PVC	paclitaxel, vinblastine, and cisplatin		proteins, vitamins, and minerals

PVMS	paravertebral muscle spasms		previous trouble
			private
PVN	peripheral venous nutrition		proximal vein thrombosis
		PVTT	tumor thrombus in the portal vein
PVNS	pigmented villonodular synovitis	PVV	persistent varicose veins
PVO	peripheral vascular occlusion	PW	pacing wires
			patient waiting
	portal vein occlusion		plantar wart
	pulmonary venous occlusion		posterior wall
			pulse width
PVo	pulmonary valve opening		puncture wound
Pvo$_2$	partial pressure (tension) of oxygen, vein	P&W	pressures and waves
		PWA	persons with AIDS
PVOD	pulmonary vascular obstructive disease	P wave	part of the electrocardiographic cycle representing atrial depolarization
PVP	cisplatin and etoposide		
	penicillin V potassium		
	peripheral venous pressure	PWB	partial weight bearing
			psychological well-being
	polyvinylpyrrolidone	PWBL	partial weight bearing, left
	posteroventral pallidotomy	PWBR	partial weight bearing, right
P-VP-B	cisplatin (Platinol AQ), etoposide (VP-16), and bleomycin	PWD	patients with diabetes
			powder
PVR	peripheral vascular resistance	PWI	pediatric walk-in clinic
			posterior wall infarct
	perspective volume rendering	PWLV	posterior wall of left ventricle
	postvoiding residual	PWM	pokeweed mitogens
	proliferative vitreoretinopathy	PWMI	posterior wall myocardial infarction
	pulmonary vascular resistance	PWO	persistent withdrawal occlusion
	pulse-volume recording	PWP	pulmonary wedge pressure
PVRI	pulmonary vascular resistance index	PWS	port-wine stain
PVS	percussion, vibration and suction		Prader-Willi syndrome
		PWV	polistes wasp venom
	peripheral vascular surgery		pulse wave velocity
	peritoneovenous shunt	Px	physical exam
	persistent vegetative state		pneumothorax
			prognosis
	Plummer-Vinson syndrome		prophylaxis
		PXAT	paroxysmal atrial tachycardia
	pulmonic valve stenosis		
PVT	paroxysmal ventricular tachycardia	PXE	pseudoxanthoma elasticum

P

PXF	pseudoexfoliation
PXL	paclitaxel (Taxol)
PXS	dental prophylaxis (cleaning)
PY	pack years (see pk yrs)
PYE	person-years of exposure
PYHx	packs per year history
PYLL	potential years of life lost
PYP	pyrophosphate
PYP®	technetium Tc 99m pyrophosphate kit
PZ	peripheral zone
PZA	pyrazinamide pyrazoloacridine
PZD	partial zona drilling partial zonal dissection
PZI	protamine zinc insulin

Q

Q	every
	quadriceps
QA	quality assurance
QAC	before every meal (this is a dangerous abbreviation)
QALE	quality-adjusted life expectancy
QALYs	quality-adjusted life years
QAM	every morning (this is a dangerous abbreviation)
QAS	quality-adjusted survival
QB	blood flow
QC	quad cane
	quality control
	quick catheter
QCA	quantitative coronary angiography
QCT	quantitative computed tomography
QD	dialysate flow
	every day (this is a dangerous abbreviation as it is read as four times daily)
QDAM	once daily in the morning
QDPM	once daily in the evening
QDS	United Kingdom abbreviation for four times a day
QE	quinidine effect
QED	every even day (this is a dangerous abbreviation as it will be read as four times daily-QID)
	quick and early diagnosis
QEE	quadriceps extension exercise
q4h	every four hours
qh	every hour
qhs	every night (this is a dangerous abbreviation as it is read as every

	hour-QHR and four times daily-QID)	qpm	every evening (this is a dangerous abbreviation)
QIAD	Quantitative Inventory of Alcohol Disorders	QPOS	Quality Point of Service
QID	four times daily	QP/QS	ratio of pulmonary blood to systemic blood flow
QIDM	four times daily with meals and at bedtime	*QQH*	United Kingdom abbreviation for every four hours
QIG	quantitative immunoglob-ulins	QR	quiet room
QIW	four times a week (this is a dangerous abbreviation)	QRC	qualitative radiocardiography
QJ	quadriceps jerk	QRNG	quinolone-resistant *N. gonorrhoeae*
QL	quality of life	QRS	part of electrocardio-graphic wave representing ventricular depolarization
QLI	Quality of Life Index		
QM	every morning (this is a dangerous abbreviation as it will not be understood)		
		QS	every shift
			quadriceps set
			quadrilateral socket
QMB	qualified Medicare beneficiary		sufficient quantity
QMI	Q wave myocardial infarction	*qs ad*	a sufficient quantity to make
QMRP	qualified mental retardation professional	QS&L	quarters, subsistence, and laundry
QMT	quantitative muscle testing	Qs/Qt	intrapulmonary shunt fraction
q.n.	every night (this is a dangerous abbreviation as it is read as every hour)	QSP	physiological shunt fraction
		qt	quart
q.n.s.	quantity not sufficient	QTB	quadriceps tendon bearing
qod	every other day (this is a dangerous abbreviation as it is read as every day or four times a day)	QTC	quantitative tip cultures
		QTL	quantitative trait locus
		Q-TWiST	quality-adjusted time without symptoms (of disease) and toxicity
qoh	every other hour (this is a dangerous abbreviation as it is read as every day or four times a day)	QUAD	quadrant quadriceps quadriplegic
		QU	quiet
qohs	every other night (this is a dangerous abbreviation as it is not recognized)	QUART	quadrantectomy, axillary dissection, and radiotherapy
		QW	every week (this is a dangerous abbreviation)
QOL	quality of life		
QOLIE-31	quality of life in epilepsy	QWB	Quality of Well-Being (scale)
QON	every other night (this is a dangerous abbreviation)	QWE	every weekend (this is a dangerous abbreviation)

Q

QWK	once a week (this is a dangerous abbreviation)
Q4wk	every four weeks (this is a dangerous abbreviation)

R	radial
	rate
	ratio
	reacting
	rectal
	rectum
	regular
	regular insulin
	resistant
	respiration
	reticulocyte
	retinoscopy
	right
	roentgen
	rub
r	recombinant
®	registered trademark
	right
−R	Rinne's test, negative
+R	Rinne's test, positive
RA	radiographic absorptiometry
	rales
	renal artery
	repeat action
	retinoic acid
	rheumatoid arthritis
	right arm
	right atrium
	right auricle
	room air
	rotational atherectomy
RAA	renin-angiotensin-aldosterone
	right atrial abnormality
RAAS	renin-angiotensin-aldosterone system
RAB	rice (rice cereal), applesauce, and banana (diet)
RABG	room air blood gas
RAC	right atrial catheter

RACCO	right anterior caudocranial oblique	RAO	right anterior oblique
RACT	recalcified whole-blood activated clotting time	RAP	right atrial pressure
		RAPA	radial artery pseudoaneurysm
RAD	ionizing radiation unit	RAQ	right anterior quadrant
	radical	RAP	recurrent abdominal pain
	radiology		Resident Assessment Protocol
	reactive airway disease		
	right axis deviation	RAPD	relative afferent pupillary defect
RADCA	right anterior descending coronary artery	RAR	right arm, reclining
RADISH	rheumatoid arthritis diffuse idiopathic skeletal hyperostosis	RARs	retinoic acid receptors
		RAS	recurrent aphthous stomatitis
RADS	ionizing radiation units		renal artery stenosis
	rapid assay delivery systems		reticular activating system
			right arm, sitting
	reactive airway disease syndrome	RASE	rapid-acquisition spin echo
RAE	right atrial enlargement	RAST	radioallergosorbent test
RAEB	refractory anemia, erythroblastic	RAT	right anterior thigh
		RA test	test for rheumatoid factor
RAEB-T	refractory anemia with excess blasts in transition	RATG	rabbit antithymocyte globulin
		RATx	radiation therapy
RAF	rapid atrial fibrillation	RAU	recurrent aphthous ulcers
RAFF	rectus abdominis free flap	R(AW)	airway resistance
RAFT	Rehabilitative Addicted Family Treatment	RB	relieved by
			retinoblastoma
RAG	room air gas		retrobulbar
RAH	right atrial hypertrophy		right breast
RAHB	right anterior hemiblock		right buttock
rAHF	antihemophilic factor (recombinant)	R & B	right and below
		RBA	right basilar artery
RAID	radioimmunodetection		right brachial artery
RAIU	radioactive iodine uptake	RBB	right breast biopsy
RALT	routine admission laboratory tests	RBBB	right bundle branch block
RAM	radioactive material	RBBX	right breast biopsy examination
	rapid alternating movements	RBC	ranitidine bismuth citrate
			red blood cell (count)
	rectus abdominis myocutaneous	RBCD	right border cardiac dullness
RAN	resident's admission notes	RBCM	red blood cell mass
R₂AN	second year resident's admission notes	RBC s/f	red blood cells spun filtration
RANTES	regulated upon activation, normal T cell expressed and secreted	RBCV	red blood cell volume
		RBD	REM (rapid eye

	movement sleep) behavior disorder	RCF	Reiter complement fixation
	right border of dullness	RCF®	enteral nutrition product
RBE	relative biologic effectiveness	RCH	residential care home
RBF	renal blood flow	RCHF	right-sided congestive heart failure
RBG	random blood glucose		
RBL	Roche Biomedical Laboratory	RCIP	rape crisis intervention program
RBON	retrobulbar optic neuritis	RCL	range of comfortable loudness
RBOW	rupture bag of water		
RBP	retinol-binding protein	RCM	radiographic contrast media
RBRVS	Medicare resource-based relative-value scale		retinal capillary microaneurysm
RBS	random blood sugar		
RBT	rational behavior therapy		right costal margin
RBV	right brachial vein	RCP	respiratory care plan
RC	race		Royal College of Physicians
	radiocarpal (joint)	RCPM	raven colored progressive matrices
	Red Cross		
	report called	RCPT	Registered Cardiopulmonary Technician
	retrograde cystogram		
	retruded contact (position)	RCR	replication-competent retrovirus (assay)
	right coronary		
	Roman Catholic		rotator cuff repair
	root canal	RCS	repeat cesarean section
	rotator cuff		reticulum cell sarcoma
R/C	reclining chair		Royal College of Surgeons
R & C	reasonable and customary		
RCA	radiographic contrast agent	RCT	randomized clinical trial
	radionuclide cerebral angiogram		Registered Care Technologist
			root canal therapy
	right carotid artery		Rorschach Content Test
	right coronary artery	RCU	respiratory care unit
	root cause analysis	RCV	red cell volume
RCBF	regional cerebral blood flow	RCX	ramus circumflexus
		RD	radial deviation
RCC	rape crisis center		Raynaud's disease
	renal cell carcinoma		reaction of degeneration
	Roman Catholic Church		reflex decay
RCCA	right common carotid artery		Registered Dietitian
			renal disease
RCCT	randomized controlled clinical trial		respiratory disease
			respiratory distress
RCD	relative cardiac dullness		restricted duty
RCE	right carotid endarterectomy		retinal detachment
			Reye's disease

246

	right deltoid	RDW	red (cell) distribution width
	ruptured disk	RE	concerning
RDA	recommended daily allowance		Rasmussen's encephalitis
			rectal examination
	Registered Dental Assistant		reflux esophagitis
			regarding
RDB	randomized double-blind (trial)		regional enteritis
			reticuloendothelial
RDCS	Registered Diagnostic Cardiac Sonographer		retinol equivalents
			right ear
RDD	renal dose dopamine		right eye
RDE	remote data entry		rowing ergometer
RDEA	right deviation of electrical axis	^{186}Re	rhenium 186
		R & E	rest and exercise
RDG	right dorsogluteal		round and equal
RDH	Registered Dental Hygienist	R↑E	right upper extremity
		R↓E	right lower extremity
RDI	respiratory disturbance index	RE ✔	recheck
		READM	readmission
RDIH	right direct inguinal hernia	REAL	Revised European American Lymphoma (classification)
RDLBBB	rate-dependent left bundle branch block		
		REALM	Rapid Estimation of Adult Literacy in Medicine
RDM	right deltoid muscle		
RDMS	Registered Diagnostic Medical Sonographer	REC	rear end collision
			recommend
RDMs	reactive drug metabolites		record
RDOD	retinal detachment, right eye		recovery
			recreation
RDOS	retinal detachment, left eye		recur
		RECA	right external carotid artery
RDP	random donor platelets		
	right dorsoposterior	RECT	rectum
RDPE	reticular degeneration of the pigment epithelium	REDs	reproductive endocrine diseases
RDS	research diagnostic criteria	RED SUBS	reducing substances
	respiratory distress syndrome	REE	resting energy expenditure
		RE-ED	re-education
RDT	regular dialysis (hemodialysis) treatment	R-EEG	resting electroencephalo-gram
		REEGT	Registered Electroenceph-alogram Technologist
RDTD	referral, diagnosis, treatment, and discharge	REF	referred
			refused
RDU	recreational drug use		renal erythropoietic factor
RDVT	recurrent deep vein thrombosis	ref→	refer to
		REG	radioencephalogram

	regression analysis	RETRO	retrograde
Reg block	regional block anesthesia	RETRX	retractions
regurg	regurgitation	REUE	resistive exercise, upper
rehab	rehabilitation		extremities
REL	relative	REV	reverse
	religion		review
RELE	resistive exercise, lower		revolutions
	extremities	RF	radio frequency
REM	rapid eye movement		reduction fixation
	recent event memory		renal failure
	remission		respiratory failure
	roentgen equivalent unit		restricted fluids
REMS	rapid eye movement sleep		rheumatic fever
REO	respiratory and enteric		rheumatoid factor
	orphan (viruses)		right foot
REP	rapid electrophoresis		risk factor
	repair		radiofrequency
	repeat	R&F	radiographic and
	report		fluoroscopic
REP CK	rapid electrophoresis	RFA	radio frequency ablation
	creatine kinase		right femoral artery
REPL	recurrent early pregnancy		right forearm
	loss		right frontoanterior
repol	repolarization	RFB	retained foreign body
REPS	repetitions		radial flow
REPT	Registered Evoked		chromatography
	Potential Technologist		residual functional
RER	renal excretion rate		capacity
RER+	replication error positive	RFD	residue-free diet
RES	recurrent erosion	RFDT	Reach in Four Directions
	syndrome		Test
	resection	RFE	return flow enema
	resident	RFFIT	rapid fluorescent focus
	reticuloendothelial system		inhibition test
RESC	resuscitation	RFg	visual fields by
RESP	respirations		Goldmann-type
	respiratory		perimeter
REST	restoration	RFIPC	Rating Form of IBD
	restriction of		(inflammatory bowel
	environmental		disease) Patient
	stimulation therapy		Concerns
RET	retention	RFL	radionuclide functional
	reticulocyte		lymphoscintigraphy
	retina		right frontolateral
	retired	RFLF	retained fetal lung fluid
	return	RFLP	restriction fragment length
	right esotropia		polymorphism
ret detach	retinal detachment		(patterns)
retic	reticulocyte	RFM	rifampin (Rifadin)

RFP	request for payment	RHF	right heart failure
	request for proposal	RHG	right hand grip
	right frontoposterior	r-hGH(m)	mammalian-cell–derived
RFS	rapid frozen section		recombinant human
	refeeding syndrome		growth hormone
	relapse-free survival		(Serostim)
RFT	right frontotransverse	RHH	right homonymous
	routine fever therapy		hemianopsia
RFTC	radio-frequency	RHINO	rhinoplasty
	thermocoagulation	RHL	right hemisphere lesions
RFUT	radioactive fibrinogen		right heptic lobe
	uptake	rhm	roentgens per hour at one
RFV	reason for visit		meter
	right femoral vein	RHO	right heel off
RG	regurgitated (infant	Rho(D)	immune globulin to an
	feeding)		Rh-negative woman
	right (upper outer)	RhoGAM®	Rh$_o$ (D) immune globulin
	gluteus	rhPDGF	recombinant human
R/G	red/green		platelet-derived growth
RGM	recurrent glioblastoma		factor
	multiforme	RHR	resting heart rate
	right gluteus medius	RHS	right hand side
RGO	reciprocating gait orthosis	RHT	right hypertropia
RH	right hemisphere	rHuEPO	recombinant human
Rh	Rhesus factor in blood		erythropoietin
RH	reduced haloperidol	RHV	right hepatic vein
	relative humidity	RHW	radiant heat warmer
	rest home	RI	refractive index
	retinal hemorrhage		regular insulin
	right hand		renal insufficiency
	right hyperphoria		respiratory illness
	room humidifier		rooming in
Rh+	Rhesus positive	RIA	radioimmunoassay
Rh−	Rhesus negative	RIAT	radioimmune antiglobulin
RHA	right hepatic artery		test
rHA	recombinant human	RIBA	recombinant immunoblot
	albumin		assay
RHB	raise head of bed	RIC	right iliac crest
	right heart border		right internal carotid
RH/BSO	radial hysterectomy and		(artery)
	bilateral salpingo-	RICA	right internal carotid
	oophorectomy		artery
RHC	respiration has ceased	RICE	rest, ice, compression,
	right heart catheterization		and elevation
	right hemicolectomy	RICM	right intercostal margin
RHD	radial head dislocation	RICS	right intercostal space
	relative hepatic dullness	RICU	respiratory intensive care
	rheumatic heart disease		unit
rh-DNase	dornase alfa (Pulmozyme)	RID	radial immunodiffusion

R

	ruptured intervertebral disk		right kidney
		RKS	renal kidney stone
RIE	radiation induced emesis	RKT	Registered Kinesiothera-pist
	rocket immunoelectro-phoresis		
		RL	right lateral
RIF	rifampin		right leg
	right iliac fossa		right lower
	right index finger		right lung
	rigid internal fixation		Ringer's lactate
RIG	rabies immune globulin	R → L	right to left
RIGS	radioimmunoguided surgery	RLA	right lower arm
		RLB	right lateral bending
RIH	right inguinal hernia		right lateral border
RIJ	right internal jugular	RLBCD	right lower border of cardiac dullness
RIMA	reversible inhibitor of monoamine oxidase-type A		
		RLC	residual lung capacity
	right internal mammary anastamosis	RLD	related living donor
			right lateral decubitus
RIND	reversible ischemic neurologic defect		ruptured lumbar disk
		RLDP	right lateral decubital position
RIO	right inferior oblique (muscle)	RLE	right lower extremity
		RLF	retrolental fibroplasia
RIOJ	recurrent intrahepatic obstructive jaundice		right lateral femoral
		RLG	right lateral gaze
R-IOL	remove intraocular lens	RLH	reactive lymphoid hyperplasia
RIP	radioimmunoprecipitin test		
		RLL	right liver lobe
	rapid infusion pump		right lower lid
	respiratory inductance plethysmograph		right lower lobe
		RLN	recurrent laryngeal nerve
RIPA	ristocetin-induced platelet agglutination		regional lymph node(s)
		RLND	regional lymph node dissection
RIR	right inferior rectus		
RIS	responding to internal stimuli	RLQ	right lower quadrant
		RLQD	right lower quadrant defect
RISA	radioactive iodinated serum albumin		
		RLR	right lateral rectus
RIST	radioimmunosorbent test	RLS	restless legs syndrome
RIT	radioimmunotherapy		Ringer's lactate solution
	Rorschach Inkblot Test		stammerer who has difficulty in enunciating R, L, and S
RITA	right internal thoracic artery		
		RLSB	right lower scapular border
RIVD	ruptured intervertebral disk		
			right lower sternal border
RIX	radiation-induced xerostomia	RLT	right lateral thigh
		RLTCS	repeat low transverse cesarean section
RJ	radial jerk (reflex)		
RK	radial keratotomy		

RLWD	routine laboratory work done	RMS®	rectal morphine sulfate (suppository)
RLX	right lower extremity	RMSB	right middle sternal border
RM	radical mastectomy		
	repetitions maximum	RMSE	root mean square error
	respiratory movement	RMSF	Rocky Mountain spotted fever
	risk manager (management)		
	risk model	RMT	Registered Music Therapist
	room		right mentotransverse
R&M	routine and microscopic	RMV	respiratory minute volume
1-RM	single repetition maximum lift	RN	Registered Nurse
			right nostril (nare)
RMA	Registered Medical Assistant	Rn	radon
		R/N	renew
	right mentoanterior	RNA	radionuclide angiography
RMCA	right main coronary artery		ribonucleic acid
		RNC	Registered Nurse, Certified
	right middle cerebral artery		
		RNCD	Registered Nurse, Chemical Dependency
RMCAT	right middle cerebral artery thrombosis		
		RNCNA	Registered Nurse Certified in Nursing Administration
RMCL	right midclavicular line		
RMD	rapid movement disorder		
RME	resting metabolic expenditure	RNCNAA	Registered Nurse Certified in Nursing Administration Advanced
	right mediolateral episiotomy		
		RNCS	Registered Nurse Certified Specialist
RMEE	right middle ear exploration		
		RND	radical neck dissection
RMF	right middle finger	RNEF	resting (radio-) nuclide ejection fraction
RMK #1	remark number 1		
RML	right mediolateral	RNF	regular nursing floor
	right middle lobe	RNFL	retinal nerve fiber layer
RMLE	right mediolateral episiotomy	RNI	reactive nitrogen intermediates
RMO	responsible medical officer	RNLP	Registered Nurse, license pending
RMP	right mentoposterior	RNP	Registered Nurse Practitioner
RMR	resting metabolic rate		
	right medial rectus		ribonucleoprotein
RMRM	right modified radical mastectomy	RNS	replacement normal saline (0.9% sodium chloride)
RMS	red-man syndrome	RNST	reactive nonstress test
	Rehabilitation Medicine Service	RNUD	recurrent nonulcer dyspepsia
	repetitive motion syndrome	RO	reality orientation
	rhabdomyosarcoma		relative odds

R

	report of	ROS	review of systems
	reverse osmosis		rod outer segments
	routine order(s)	ROSC	restoration of spontaneous
	Russian Orthodox		circulation
R/O	rule out	ROSS	review of signs and
ROA	right occiput anterior		symptoms
ROAC	repeated oral doses of	ROT	remedial occupational
	activated charcoal		therapy
ROAD	reversible obstructive		right occipital transverse
	airway disease		rotator
ROC	receiver operating	ROU	recurrent oral ulcer
	characteristic	ROUL	rouleaux
	record of contact	RP	radial pulse
	resident on call		radical prostatectomy
	residual organic carbon		radiopharmaceutical
RODA	rapid opiate detoxification		Raynaud's phenomenon
	under anesthesia		restorative proctocolec-
ROF	review of outside films		tomy
ROG	rogletimide		retinitis pigmentosa
ROH	rubbing alcohol		retrograde pyelogram
ROI	region of interest		root plane
ROIDS	hemorrhoids	RPA	radial photon
ROIH	right oblique inguinal		absorptiometry
	hernia		Registered Physician's
ROJM	range of joint motion		Assistant
ROL	right occipitolateral		restenosis postangioplasty
ROLC	roentgenologically occult		ribonuclease protection
	lung cancer		assay
ROM	range of motion		right pulmonary artery
	right otitis media	RPAC	Registered Physician's
	rupture of membranes		Assistant Certified
Romb	Romberg	RPC	root planing and curettage
ROMCP	range of motion complete	RPCF	Reiter protein
	and painfree		complement fixation
ROMI	rule out myocardial	RPD	removable partial denture
	infarction	RPE	rating of perceived
ROMSA	right otitis media,		exertion
	suppurative, acute		retinal pigment epithelium
ROMSC	right otitis media,	RPED	retinal pigment epithelium
	suppurative, chronic		detachment
ROMWNL	range of motion within	RPEP	right pre-ejection period
	normal limits	RPF	relaxed pelvic floor
ROP	retinopathy of prematurity		renal plasma flow
	right occiput posterior		retroperitoneal fibrosis
ROR	the French acronym for	RPFT	Registered Pulmonary
	measles-mumps-rubella		Function Technologist
	vaccine	RPG	retrograde percutaneous
R or L	right or left		gastrostomy
RoRx	radiation therapy		retrograde pyelogram

RPGN	rapidly progressive glomerulonephritis	R&R	rate and rhythm
			recent and remote
RPH	retroperitoneal hemorrhage		recession and resection
			resect and recess (muscle surgery)
RPh	Registered Pharmacist		rest and recuperation
RPHA	reverse passive hemagglutination		remove and replace
RPI	resting pressure index	RRA	radioreceptor assay
	reticulocyte production index		Registered Record Administrator
			right radial artery
RPICA	right posterior internal carotid artery		right renal artery
RPICCE	round pupil intracapsular cataract extraction	RRAM	rapid rhythmic alternating movements
RPL	retroperitoneal lymphadenectomy	RRC	cohort relative risk
		RRCT, no(m)	regular rate, clear tones, no murmurs
RPLC	reversed-phase liquid chromatography	RRD	rhegmatogenous retinal detachment
RPLND	retroperitoneal lymph node dissection	RRE	round, regular, and equal (pupils)
RPN	renal papillary necrosis	RRED®	Rapid Rare Event Detection
	resident's progress notes		
R₂PN	second year resident's progress notes	RREF	resting radionuclide ejection fraction
RPO	right posterior oblique	RRI	renal resistive index
RPP	radical perineal prostatectomy	RR-IOL	remove and replace intraocular lens
	rate-pressure product	RRM	right radial mastectomy
	retropubic prostatectomy	RRMS	relapsing-remitting multiple sclerosis
RPR	rapid plasma reagin (test for syphilis)	RRNA	Resident Registered Nurse Anesthetist
	Reiter protein reagin	rRNA	ribosomal ribonucleic acid
	Rhône-Poulenc Rorer Pharmaceuticals Inc.	RRND	right radical neck dissection
RPT	Registered Physical Therapist	RROM	resistive range of motion
RPTA	Registered Physical Therapist Assistant	R rot	right rotation
		RRP	radical retropubic prostatectomy
RPU	retropubic urethropexy		
RPV	right portal vein	RRR	recovery room routine
	right pulmonary vein		regular rhythm and rate
RQ	respiratory quotient		relative risk reduction
RR	recovery room	RRRN	round, regular, and react normally
	regular rate	RRRsM	regular rate and rhythm without murmur
	regular respirations		
	relative risk	RRT	Registered Respiratory Therapist
	respiratory rate		
	retinal reflex		
R/R	rales-rhonchi		

R

RRVO	repair relaxed vaginal outlet	RSI	repetitive strain (stress) injury
RRVS	recovery room vital signs	R-SICU	respiratory-surgical intensive care unit
RRV-TV	rhesus rotavirus tetravalent (vaccine)	RSLR	reverse straight leg raise
RS	Raynaud's syndrome	RSM	remote study monitoring
	recurrent seizures	RSNI	round spermatid nuclear injection
	Reed-Sternberg (cell)		
	Reiter's syndrome	RSO	right salpingooophorec-tomy
	restart		
	Reye's syndrome		right superior oblique
	rhythm strip	rS02	regional oxygen saturation
	right side	RSOP	right superior oblique palsy
	Ringer's solution		
R/S	rest stress	RSP	rapid straight pacing
	rupture spontaneous		right sacroposterior
R & S	restraint and seclusion	RSR	regular sinus rhythm
R/S I	resuscitation status one (full resuscitative effort)		relative survival rate
			right superior rectus
		RSRI	renal:systemic renin index
R/S II	resuscitation status two (no code, therapeutic measures only)	RSS	representative sample sectioned
R/S III	resuscitation status three (no code, comfort measures only)	RSSE	Russian spring-summer encephalitis
		RST	rapid simple tests
RSA	right sacrum anterior		right sacrum transverse
	right subclavian artery	RSTs	Rodney Smith tubes
RSB	right sternal border	RSV	respiratory syncytial virus
RSC	right subclavian (artery) (vein)		right subclavian vein
		RSVC	right superior vena cava
RScA	right scapuloanterior	RSW	right-sided weakness
RSCL	Rotterdam Symptom Check List	RT	radiation therapy
			Radiologic Technologist
RScP	right scapuloposterior		recreational therapy
RSCS	respiratory system compliance score		rectal temperature
			renal transplant
rscu-PA	recombinant, single-chain, urokinase-type plasminogen activator		repetition time
			respiratory therapist
			reverse transcriptase
			right
RSD	reflex sympathetic dystrophy		right thigh
			room temperature
RSDS	reflex-sympathetic dystrophy syndrome	R/t	related to
		RTA	ready to administer
RSE	reactive subdural effusion		renal tubular acidosis
	refractory status epilepticus		road traffic accident
	right sternal edge	t-RA	tretinoin (trans-retinoic acid)

254

RTAE	right atrial enlargement	RTT	Respiratory Therapy Technician
RTAH	right anterior hemiblock		
RTAT	right anterior thigh	RT₃U	resin triiodothyronine uptake
RTB	return to baseline		
RTC	Readiness to Change (questionnaire)	RTUS	realtime ultrasound
		RTV	ritonavir (Norvir)
	return to clinic	RTW	return to ward
	round the clock		return to work
RTCA	ribavirin		Richard Turner Warwick (urethroplasty)
RTER	return to emergency room		
rt. ↑ ext.	right upper extremity	RTWD	return to work determination
RTF	ready-to-feed		
	return to flow	RTX	resiniferatoxin
RTFS	return to flying status	RTx	radiation therapy
RTI	respiratory tract infection		renal transplantation
	reverse transcriptase inhibitor	RU	residual urine
			resin uptake
RTK	rhabdoid tumor of the kidney		retrograde ureterogram
			right upper
RTL	reactive to light		routine urinalysis
RTM	regression to the mean	RU 486	mifepristone
	routine medical care	RUA	right upper arm
RTMD	right mid-deltoid		routine urine analysis
rTMS	repetitive transcranial magnetic stimulation	RUE	right upper extremity
		RUG	resource utilization group
RTN	renal tubular necrosis		retrograde urethrogram
RTNM	retreatment staging of cancer	RUL	right upper lid
			right upper lobe
RTO	return to office	RUOQ	right upper outer quadrant
RTOG	Radiation Therapy Oncology Group	rupt.	ruptured
		RUQ	right upper quadrant
RTP	renal transplant patient	RUQD	right upper quadrant defect
	return to pharmacy		
rtPA	alteplase (recombinant tissue-type plasminogen activator)	RURTI	recurrent upper respiratory tract infection
RT-PCR	reverse transcription polymerase chain reaction	RUSB	right upper scapular border
			right upper sternal border
RTR	return to room	RUT	rapid urease test
RT (R)	Radiologic Technologist (Registered)	RUV	residual urine volume
		RUX	right upper extremity
RTRR	return to recovery room	RV	rectovaginal
RTS	raised toilet seat		residual volume
	real time scan		respiratory volume
	Resolve Through Sharing		retinal vasculitis
	return to school		return visit
	return to sender		right ventricle
	Revised Trauma Score		rubella vaccine

RVA	rabies vaccine, adsorbed	RVSP	right ventricular systolic pressure
	right ventricular apex		
	right vertebral artery	RVSW	right ventricular stroke work
RVAD	right ventricular assist device		
		RVSWI	right ventricular stroke work index
RVCD	right ventricular conduction deficit	RVT	recurrent ventricular tachycardia
RVD	relative vertebral density		renal vein thrombosis
	renal vascular disease	RV/TLC	residual volume to total lung capacity ratio
RVDP	right ventricular diastolic pressure		
		RVU	relative-value units
RVE	right ventricular enlargement	RVV	rubella vaccine virus
		RVVT	Russell's viper venom time
RVEDP	right ventricular end-diastolic pressure		
		RW	radiant warmer
RVEDV	right ventricular end diastolic volume		ragweed
			red welt
RVEF	right ventricular ejection fraction		rolling walker
		R/W	return to work
RVET	right ventricular ejection time	RWM	regional wall motion
		RWP	ragweed pollen
RVF	Rift Valley fever	RWS	ragweed sensitivity
	right ventricular function	RXRs	retinoid X receptors
	right visual field	Rx	drug
RVG	radionuclide ventriculography		medication
	Radio VisioGraphy		pharmacy
	right ventrogluteal		prescription
RVH	renovascular hypertension		radiotherapy
	right ventricular hypertrophy		take
			therapy
RVHT	renovascular hypertension		treatment
RVI	right ventricle infarction	RXN	reaction
RVIDd	right ventricle internal dimension diastole	RXT	radiation therapy
			right exotropia
RVL	right vastus lateralis		
RVO	relaxed vaginal outlet		
	retinal vein occlusion		
	right ventricular outflow		
	right ventricular overactivity		
RVOT	right ventricular outflow tract		
RVOTH	right ventricular outflow tract hypertrophy		
RVP	right ventricular pressure		
RVR	rapid ventricular response		
	renal vascular resistance		
	right ventricular rhythm		

S

S sacral
 second (s)
 sensitive
 serum
 single
 sister
 son
 sponge
 subjective findings
 suicide
 suction
 sulfur
 supervision
 susceptible
/S/ signature
s̄ without (this is a
  dangerous abbreviation)
S′ shoulder
S_1 first heart sound
$S^{-1}...S^{-4}$ suicide risk classifications
S_2 second heart sound
S_3 third heart sound
  (ventricular filling
  gallop)
S_4 fourth heart sound (atrial
  gallop)
$S_1...S_5$ sacral vertebra or nerves
  1 through 5
SI to SIV symbols for the first to
  fourth heart sounds
SA sacroanterior
 salicylic acid
 semen analysis
 Sexoholics Anonymous
 sinoatrial
 sleep apnea
 slow acetylator
 Spanish American
 spinal anesthesia
 Staphylococcus aureus
 subarachnoid
 substance abuse
 suicide alert

 suicide attempt
 surface area
 surgical assistant
 sustained action
S/A same as
 sugar and acetone
S&A sugar and acetone
SAA same as above
 serum amyloid A
 Stokes-Adams attacks
 synthetic amino acids
SAAG serum-ascites albumin
  gradient
SAARDs slow-acting anti-rheumatic
  drugs
SAB serum albumin
 sino-atrial block
 Spanish American Black
 spontaneous abortion
 subarachnoid bleed
 subarachnoid block
SAC segmental antigen
  challenge
 serum aminoglycoside
  concentration
 short arm cast
 substance abuse counselor
SACC short arm cylinder cast
SACD subacute combined
  degeneration
SACH soft ankle, cushioned heel
 solid ankle, cushion heel
SACT sinoatrial conduction time
SAD seasonal affective disorder
 Self-Assessment
  Depression (scale)
 source-axis distance
 subacromial decompres-
  sion
 subacute dialysis
 sugar, acetone, and
  diacetic acid
 sugar and acetone
  determination
 superior axis deviation
SADD Students Against Drunk
  Driving
SADL simulated activities of
  daily living

SADR	suspected adverse drug reaction		self-administered medication
SADS	Schedule for Affective Disorders and Schizophrenia		sleep apnea monitor Spanish-American male systolic anterior motion
SADs	severe autoimmune diseases	SAN	side-arm nebulizer sinoatrial node
SADS-C	Schedule for Affective Disorders And Schizophrenia – Change Version	SANC sang SANS	slept all night short arm navicular cast sanguinous Schedule (Scale) for the Assessment of Negative Symptoms sympathetic autonomic nervous system
SAE	serious adverse event short above elbow (cast)		
SAEG	signal averaging electrocardiogram	SAO SaO$_2$	small airway obstruction arterial oxygen percent saturation
SAEKG	signaled average electrocardiogram	SAPD	self-administration of psychotropic drugs
SAESU	Substance Abuse valuating Screen Unit	SAPH	saphenous
SAF	Self-Analysis Form self-articulating femoral Spanish-American female	SAPHO	synovitis, acne, pustulosis, hyperostosis, and osteolysis
SAFHS	sonic accelerated fracture healing system	SAPS	short arm plaster splint Simplified Acute Physiology Score
SAG	sodium antimony gluconate	SAPS II	Simplified Acute Physiology Score version II
Sag D	sagittal diameter		
SAH	subarachnoid hemorrhage systemic arterial hypertension	SAQ	Sexual Adjustment Questionnaire short arc quad
SAHS	sleep apnea/hypopnea (hypersomnolence) syndrome	SAR	seasonal allergic rhinitis Senior Assistant Resident sexual attitudes reassessment structural activity relationships
SAI	Sodium Amytal® interview		
SAL	salicylate *Salmonella* sensory acuity level sterility assurance level	SARA	sexually acquired reactive arthritis system for anesthetic and respiratory administration analysis
SAL 12	sequential analysis of 12 chemistry constituents	SARAN	senior admitting resident's admission note
SAM	methylprednisolone sodium succinate (Solu-Medrol), aminophylline, and metaproterenol (Metaprel) selective antimicrobial modulation	SARC	seasonal allergic rhinoconjunctivitis
		S Arrh	sinus arrhythmia

SART	standard acid reflux test		Sengstaken-Blakemore (tube)
SAS	saline, agent, and saline		sick boy
	scalenus anticus syndrome		side bend
	see assessment sheet		side bending
	Self-rating Anxiety Scale		sinus bradycardia
	short arm splint		small bowel
	sleep apnea syndrome		spina bifida
	Social Adjustment Scale		sponge bath
	Specific Activity Scale		stand-by
	subarachnoid space		Stanford-Binet (test)
	sulfasalazine		sternal border
	synthetic absorbable sutures		stillbirth
SASA	Sex Abuse Survivors Anonymous		stillborn
			stone basketing
SASH	saline, agent, saline, and heparin	Sb	antimony
		SB+	wearing seat belt
SASP	sulfasalazine (salicylazo-sulfapyridine)	SB−	not wearing seat belt
		SBA	serum bactericidal activity
SAT	methylprednisolone sodium succinate (Solu-Medrol), aminophylline, and terbutaline		standby angioplasty
			standby assistant (assistance)
			Summary Basis of Approval
	saturated	SBAC	small bowel adenocarcinoma
	saturation		
	Saturday	SBB	stereotactic breast biopsy
	self-administered therapy	SBBO	small-bowel bacterial overgrowth
	Senior Apperception Test		
	speech awareness threshold	SBC	sensory binocular cooperation
	subacute thyroiditis		single base cane
SATC	substance abuse treatment clinic		standard bicarbonate
			strict bed confinement
SATL	surgical Achilles tendon lengthening		superficial bladder cancer
		SBD	straight bag drainage
SATP	substance abuse treatment program	SBE	saturated base excess
			self-breast examination
SATS	refers to oxygen saturation levels		short below elbow (cast)
			shortness of breath on exertion
SATU	substance abuse treatment unit		subacute bacterial endocarditis
SAVD	spontaneous assisted vaginal delivery	SBFT	small bowel follow through
SB	safety belt	SBG	stand-by guard
	sandbag	SBGM	self blood glucose monitoring
	scleral buckling		
	seat belt	SBH	State Board of Health
	seen by		

SBI	silicone (gel-containing) breast implants	sternoclavicular
	systemic bacterial infection	subclavian
		subclavian catheter
		subcutaneous
SBJ	skin, bones, and joints	succinylcholine
SBK	spinnbarkeit	sulfur colloid
SBL	sponge blood loss	s̄c without correction
SB-LM	Stanford-Binet	(without glasses)
	Intelligence Test-Form	S&C sclerae and conjunctivae
	LM	SCA sickle cell anemia
SBO	small bowel obstruction	subclavian artery
	specified bovine offals	subcutaneous abdominal
SBOD	scleral buckle, right eye	(block)
SBOH	State Board of Health	superior cerebellar artery
SBOM	soybean oil meal	SCa serum calcium
SBOS	scleral buckle, left eye	SCAD short chain acyl-
SBP	school breakfast program	coenzyme A
	scleral buckling procedure	dehydrogenase
	small bowel phytobezoars	SCAN suspected child abuse and
	spontaneous bacterial	neglect
	peritonitis	SCAP stem cell apheresis
	systolic blood pressure	SCARMD severe childhood
SBQC	small based quad cane	autosomal recessive
SBR	sluggish blood return	muscular dystrophy
	strict bed rest	SCAT sheep cell agglutination
SBS	shaken baby syndrome	titer
	short (small) bowel	sickle cell anemia test
	syndrome	SCB strictly confined to bed
	sick-building syndrome	SCBC small cell bronchogenic
	side-by-side	carcinoma
	small bowel series	SCBE single-contrast barium
SBT	serum bactericidal titers	enema
SBTB	sinus breakthrough beat	SCBF spinal cord blood flow
SBTT	small bowel transit time	SCC short course
SBV	single binocular vision	chemotherapy (for
SBW	seat belts worn	tuberculosis)
SBX	symphysis, buttocks, and	sickle cell crisis
	xiphoid	small cell carcinoma
SC	schizophrenia	spinal cord compression
	self-care	squamous cell carcinoma
	serum creatinine	SCCA semi-closed circle
	service connected	absorber
	sick call	squamous cell carcinoma
	sickle-cell	antigen
	small (blood pressure)	SCCa squamous cell carcinoma
	cuff	SCCE squamous cell carcinoma
	Snellen's chart	of the esophagus
	spinal cord	SCCHN squamous cell carcinoma
	sport cord	of the head and neck

SCCI	subcutaneous continuous infusion		interview for DSM-III-R
SCD	sequential compression device	SCII	Strong-Campbell Interest Inventory
	service connected disability	SCIP	Screening and Crisis Intervention Program
	sickle cell disease	SCIPP	sacrococcygeal to inferior
	spinal cord disease		pubic point
	subacute combined degeneration	SCIU	spinal cord injury unit
	sudden cardiac death	SCIV	subclavian intravenous
ScDA	scapulodextra anterior	SCI- WORA	spinal cord injury without radiographic
SCDM	soybean-casein digest medium		abnormalities
		SCL	skin conductance level
ScDP	scapulodextra posterior		symptom checklist
SCE	sister chromatid exchange	SCL-90	Symptoms Checklist—90 items
	soft cooked egg	ScLA	scapulolaeva anterior
	specialized columnar epithelium	SCLAX	subcostal long axis
		SCLC	small-cell lung cancer
SCEMIA	self-contained enzymatic membrane	SCLD	sickle cell lung disease
	immunoassay	SCLE	subacute cutaneous lupus erythematosis
SCEP	somatosensory cortical evoked potential	ScLP	scapulolaeva posterior
SCF	special care formula	SCLs	soft contact lenses
	stem cell factor		synthetic combinatorial libraries
SCFA	short-chain fatty acid	SCM	scalene muscle
SCFE	slipped capital femoral epiphysis		sensation, circulation, and motion
SCG	seismocardiography		spondylitic caudal myelopathy
	serum Chemogram		sternocleidomastoid
	sodium cromoglycate		supraclavicular muscle
SCh	succinylcholine chloride	SCMD	senile choroidal macular
SCHISTO	schistocytes		degeneration
SCHIZ	schizocytes	SCMV	serogroup C
	schizophrenia		meningococcal vaccine
SCHLP	supracricord hemilaryngopharyngec- tomy	SCN	special care nursery suprachiasmatic nucleus
SCHNC	squamous cell head and neck cancer	SCOB	Schedule-Controlled Operant Behavior
SCI	specific COX-2 inhibitor	SCOP	scopolamine
	spinal cord injury	SCOPE	arthroscopy
	subcoma insulin	SCP	sodium cellulose phosphate
SCID	severe combined immunodeficiency disorders (disease)		standardized care plan
	structured clinical		

S

SCPF	stem cell proliferation factor
S-CPK	serum creatine phosphokinase
SCR	special care room (seclusion room)
	spondylitic caudal radioculopathy
	stem cell rescue
SCr	serum creatinine
sCR	soluble complement receptor
SC/RP	scaling and root planing
SC-RNV	subcutaneous radionuclide venography
SCS	spinal cord stimulation
	splatter control shield
	suspected catheter sepsis
SCSAX	subcostal short axis
SCSIT	Southern California Sensory Integration Tests
SCT	Sertoli cell tumor
	sex chromatin test
	sickel cell trait
	stem cell transplant
	sugar coated tablet
SCTX	static cervical traction
SCU	self-care unit
	special care unit
SCUCP	small cell undifferentiated carcinoma of the prostate
SCUF	slow continuous ultrafiltration
SCUT	schizophrenia, chronic undifferentiated type
SCV	subclavian vein
	subcutaneous vaginal (block)
SD	scleroderma
	senile dementia
	severe deficit
	septal defect
	severely disabled
	shoulder disarticulation
	single dose
	skin dose

	sleep deprived
	solvent-detergent
	somatic dysfunction
	spasmodic dysphonia
	speech discrimination
	spontaneous delivery
	stable disease
	standard deviation
	standard diet
	step-down
	sterile dressing
	straight drainage
	streptozocin and doxorubicin
	sudden death
	surgical drain
S & D	seen and discussed
	stomach and duodenum
S/D	sharp/dull
	systolic-diastolic ratio
SDA	sacrodextra anterior
	same day admission
	serotonin/dopamine antagonist
	Seventh-Day Adventist
	steroid-dependent asthmatic
SDAT	senile dementia of Alzheimer's type
SDB	Sabouraud dextrose broth
	self-destructive behavior
	sleep disordered breathing
SDBP	seated diastolic blood pressure
	standing diastolic blood pressure
	supine diastolic blood pressure
SDC	serum digoxin concentration
	serum drug concentration
	Sleep Disorders Center
	sodium deoxycholate
SD&C	suction, dilation, and curettage
SDD	selective digestive (tract) decontamination
	sterile dry dressing

SDDT	selective decontamination of the digestive tract		sulfate – polyacrylamide gel electrophoresis
SDE	subdural empyema	SDT	sacrodextra transversa
SDES	symptomatic diffuse esophageal spasm		speech detection threshold
SDF	sexual dysfunction	SDU	step-down unit
	stromal-cell-derived factor	SE	saline enema (0.9% sodium chloride)
SDH	spinal detrusor hyperreflexia		self-examination
	subdural hematoma		side effect
SDI	Sandimmune (cyclosporine)		soft exudates
			spin echo
	State Disability Insurance		staff escort
			standard error
SDII	sudden death in infancy		Starr-Edwards (valve, pacemaker)
SDL	serum digoxin level		
	serum drug level		status epilepticus
	speech discrimination loss	Se	selenium
		S/E	suicidal and eloper
SDM	soft drusen maculopathy	S & E	seen and examined
	standard deviation of the mean	SEA	sheep erythrocyte agglutination (test)
S/D/M	systolic, diastolic, mean		Southeast Asia
SD/N	signal-difference-to-noise ratio		subdural electrode array
			synaptic electronic activation
SDNN	standard deviation of normal-to-normal beats	SEAR	Southease Asia refugee
SDO	surgical diagnostic oncology	SEC	second
			secondary
SDP	sacrodextra posterior		secretary
	single donor platelets		steric exclusion chromatography
	solvent-detergent plasma		
	stomach, duodenum, and pancreas	SECG	scalp electrocardiogram
		SECL	seclusion
SDR	selective dorsal rhizotomy	SECPR	standard external cardiopulmonary resuscitation
SDS	same day surgery		
	Self-Rating Depression Scale	SED	sedimentation
	sodium dodecyl sulfate		skin erythema dose
	somatropin deficiency syndrome		socially and emotionally disturbed
	Speech Discrimination Score		spondyloepiphyseal dysplasia
	standard deviation score	SED-NET	severely emotional disturbed - network
	sudden death syndrome		
	Symptom Distress Scale	sed rt	sedimentation rate
SDSO	same day surgery overnight	SEER	Surveillance, Epidemiology, and End Results (program)
SDS-PAGE	sodium dodecyl		

S

SEG	segment	SF	salt free
	sonoencephalogram		saturated fat
segs	segmented neutrophils		scarlet fever
SEH	spinal epidural		seizure frequency
	hematomas		seminal fluid
	subependymal		skull fracture
	hemorrhage		soft feces
SEI	subepithelial (comeal)		sound field
	infiltrate		spinal fluid
SELFVD	sterile elective low		sugar free
	forceps vaginal delivery		symptom-free
SEM	scanning electron		synovial fluid
	microscopy	S&F	soft and flat
	semen	SF-6	sulfahexafluoride
	slow eye movement	SF 36	36-item short form health
	standard error of mean		survey
	systolic ejection murmur	SFA	saturated fatty acids
SEMI	subendocardial		superficial femoral artery
	myocardial infarction	SFB	single frequency
SENS	sensitivity		bioimpedance
	sensorium	SFC	spinal fluid count
SEP	separate		subarachnoid fluid
	serum electrophoresis		collection
	somatosensory evoked	SFD	scaphoid fossa depression
	potential		small for dates
	systolic ejection period	SFEMG	single-fiber electromyog-
SEQ	sequela		raphy
SER	scanning equalization	SFH	schizophrenia family
	radiography		history
	sertraline (Zoloft)	SFP	simulated fluorescence
	signal enhancement ratio		process
SER-IV	supination external		simultaneous foveal
	rotation, type 4 fracture		perception
SERM	selective estrogen-receptor		spinal fluid pressure
	modulator	SFPT	standard fixation
SERO-	serosanguineous		preference test
SANG		SFS	split function studies
SERs	somatosensory evoked	SFTR	sagittal, frontal,
	responses		transverse, rotation
SES	sick euthyroid syndrome	SFUP	surgical follow-up
	socioeconomic status	SFV	simian foamy viruses
	standard electrolyte		superficial femoral vein
	solution	SFW	shell fragment wound
SET	social environmental	SFWB	social/family well-being
	therapy	SG	salivary gland
	systolic ejection time		scrotography
SEV	sevoflurane (Ultane)		serum glucose
SEWHO	shoulder-elbow-wrist-hand		side glide
	orthosis		skin graft

	specific gravity	S Hb	sickle hemoglobin screen
	Swan-Ganz (catheter)	SHBG	sex hormone-binding
SGA	small for gestational		globulin
	age	sHBO₂T	systemic hyperbaric
	subjective global		oxygen therapy
	assessment (dietary	SHC	subsequent hospital
	history and physical		care
	examination)	SHEENT	skin, head, eyes, ears,
	substantial gainful activity		nose, and throat
	(employment)	SHGT	somatic-cell human gene
SGC	Swan-Ganz catheter		therapy
SGCNB	stereotactic guided core-	SHI	standard heparin
	needle biopsy		infusion
SGD	straight gravity drainage	Shig	*Shigella*
SGE	significant glandular	SHL	sudden hearing loss
	enlargement		supraglottic horizontal
s̄ gl	without correction		laryngectomy
	(without glasses)	SHO	Senior House Officer
SGM	serum glucose monitoring	SHR	scapulohumeral rhythm
SGOT	serum glutamic oxalo-	SHS	student health service
	acetic transaminase	SHx	social history
	(same as AST)	SI	International System of
SGPT	serum glutamate pyruvate		Units
	transaminase (same as		sacroiliac
	ALT)		sagittal index
SGS	second-generation		sector iridectomy
	sulfonylurea		self-inflicted
	subglottic stenosis		sensory integration
SGTCS	secondarily generalized		seriously ill
	tonic-clonic seizures		sexual intercourse
SH	serum hepatitis		small intestine
	sexual harassment		strict isolation
	short		stress incontinence
	shoulder		stroke index
	shower		suicidal ideation
	social history	Si	silicon
	sulfhydryl (group)	S & I	suction and irrigation
	surgical history		support and interpretation
S&H	speech and hearing	SIA	small intestinal atresia
	suicidal and homicidal	SIADH	syndrome of inappropriate
S/H	suicidal/homicidal		antidiuretic hormone
	ideation		secretion
SH2	sarc homology region 2	SIAT	supervised intermittent
SHA	super heated aerosol		ambulatory treatment
SHAL	standard hyperalimenta-	SIB	self-inflating bulb
	tion		self-injurious behavior
SHAS	supravalvular	SIBC	serum iron-binding
	hypertrophic aortic		capacity
	stenosis	sibs	siblings

S

SIC	self-intermittent catherization	SIQ	stroke in progression
		SIQ	sick in quarters
	squamous intraepithelial cells	SIR	standardized incidence rate (ratio)
	Standard Industrial Classification	SIRS	systemic inflammatory response syndrome
SICD	sudden infant crib death	SIS	sister
SICT	selective intracoronary thrombolysis		Surgical Infection Stratification (system)
SICU	surgical intensive care unit	SISI	Short Increment Sensitivity Index
SIDA	French and Spanish abbreviation for AIDS	SISS	severe invasion streptococcal syndrome
SIDD	syndrome of isolated diastolic dysfunction	SIT	serum inhibitory titers
			silicon-intensified target
SIDERO	siderocyte		Slossen Intelligence Test
SIDFF	superimposed dorsiflexion of foot		sperm immobilization test
			surgical intensive therapy
SIDS	sudden infant death syndrome	SIT BAL	sitting balance
		SIT TOL	sitting tolerance
SIEP	serum immunoelectro-phoresis	SIV	simian immunodeficiency virus
SIG	let it be marked (appears on prescription before directions for patient)	SIVP	slow intravenous push
		SIW	self-inflicted wound
		SJCRH	St. Jude Children's Research Hospital
	sigmoidoscopy		
Signal 99	patient in cardiac or respiratory distress	S-JRA	systemic juvenile rheumatoid arthritis
SIJ	sacroiliac joint	SJS	Stevens-Johnson syndrome
SIJS	sacroiliac joint syndrome		
SIL	seriously ill list		Swyer-James syndrome
	sister-in-law	S_{jv02}	jugular venous oxygen saturation
	squamous intraepithelial lesion	SK	seborrheic keratosis
SILFVD	sterile indicated low forceps vaginal delivery		senile keratosis
			SmithKline
			solar keratosis
SILV	simultaneous independent lung ventilation		streptokinase
		S & K	single and keeping (baby)
SIM	selective ion monitoring	SKAO	supracondylar knee-ankle orthosis
	Similac®		
SIMCU	surgical intermediate care unit	SKB	SmithKline Beecham
		SKC	single knee to chest
Sim c̄ Fe	Similac with iron®	SK-SD	streptokinase streptodornase
SIMV	synchronized intermittent mandatory ventilation		
		SKY	spectral karyotyping
SIN	salpingitis isthmica nodose	SL	scapholunate
			secondary leukemia
SIP	Sickness Impact Profile		sensation level

	sentinel lymphadenectomy	SLND	sentinel lymph node detection
	serious list		
	shortleg	SLNM	sentinel lymph node mapping
	slight		
	sublingual	SLNTG	sublingual nitroglycerin
S/L	slit lamp (examination)	SLNWBC	short leg nonweight-bearing cast
SLA	sacrolaeva anterior		
	sex and love addictions	SLNWC	short leg non-walking cast
	slide latex agglutination	SLO	scanning laser ophthalmoscope
	The Satisfaction with Life Areas		
			second look operation
SLAA	Sex and Love Addicts Anonymous		Smith-Lemli-Opitz (syndrome)
SLAC	scapholunate advanced collapse		streptolysin O
		SLOA	short leave of absence
SLAP	serum leucine amino-peptidase	SLP	speech language pathology
SLB	short leg brace	SLPI	secretory leukocyte protease inhibitor
SLC	short leg cast		
SLCC	short leg cylinder cast	SLPMS	short-leg posterior-molded splint
SLCG	sulfolithocholyglycine		
SLCT	Sertoli-Leydig cell tumor	SLR	straight leg raising
SLD	specific language disorder	SLRT	straight leg raising tenderness
	stealth liposomal doxorubicin		straight leg raising test
		SLS	second-look sonography
SLE	slit lamp examination		short leg splint
	St. Louis encephalitis		single limb support
	systemic lupus erythematosus	SLT	sacrolaeva transversa
			scanning laser tomography
SLEX	slit lamp examination (biomicroscopy)		single lung transplantation
			swing light test
SLFVD	sterile low forceps vaginal delivery	SLT-I	Shiga-like toxin I
		SLTA	standard language test for aphasia
SLGXT	symptom limited graded exercise test		
		SLTEC	Shiga-like toxin-producing *Escherichia coli*
SLK	superior limbic keratoconjunctivitis		
SLL	second look laparotomy	sl. tr.	slight trace
	small lymphocytic lymphoma	SLUD	salivation, lacrimation, urination, and defecation
SLMFVD	sterile low mid-forceps vaginal delivery		
		SLV	since last visit
SLMMS	slightly more marked since	SLWB	severely low birth weight
		SLWC	short leg walking cast
SLMP	since last menstrual period	SM	sadomasochism
			skim milk
SLN	sentinel lymph node(s)		small
	superior laryngeal nerve		

	sports medicine	SMB	simulated moving bed
	Stairmaster®	SMBG	self-monitoring blood
	streptomycin		glucose
	systolic motion	SMC	special mouth care
	systolic murmur	SMCA	sorbitol MacConkey agar
^{153}Sm	samarium 153	SMCD	senile macular chorio-
SMA	sequential multiple		retinal degeneration
	analyzer	SMD	senile macular
	simultaneous multichannel		degeneration
	auto-analyzer	SMDA	Safe Medical Defice Act
	spinal muscular atrophy	SME	significant medical event
	superior mesenteric	SMF	streptozocin, mitomycin,
	artery		and fluorouracil
	supplementary motor area	SMFA	sodium monofluoroacetate
SMA-6	sequential multipler	SMFVD	sterile mid-forceps
	analyzer for sodium,		vaginal delivery
	potassium, CO_2,	SMG	submandibular gland
	chloride, glucose, and	SMH	state mental hospital
	BUN	SMI	sensory motor integration
SMA-7	sodium, potassium, CO_2,		(group)
	chloride, glucose,		severely mentally impaired
	BUN, and creatinine		small volume infusion
SMA-12	glucose, BUN, uric acid,		suggested minimum
	calcium, phosphorus,		increment
	total protein, albumin,		sustained maximal
	cholesterol, total		inspiration
	bilirubin, alkaline	SMIDS	suppertime mixed insulin
	phosphatase, SGOT,		and daytime
	and LDH		sulfonylureas
SMA-18	SMA-12 + SMA−6	SMILE	safety, monitoring,
SMA-23	includes the entire		intervention, length of
	SMA-12 plus sodium,		stay and evaluation
	potassium, CO_2,		sustained maximal
	chloride, direct		inspiratory lung
	bilirubin, triglycerides,		exercises
	SGPT, indirect	SMIT	standard mycological
	bilirubin, R fraction,		identification
	and BUN/creatinine		techniques
	ratio	SMN	second malignant
SMAO	superior mesenteric artery		neoplasia
	occlusion	SMO	Senior Medical Officer
SMAR	self-medication		site management
	administration record		organization(s)
SMAS	superficial musculoapo-		slip made out
	neurotic system	SMON	subacute myelo-
	superior mesenteric artery		opticoneuropathy
	syndrome	SMP	self-management program
SMAST	Short Michigan Alcohol-	SMPN	sensorimotor
	ism Screening Test		polyneuropathy

SMR	senior medical resident	SNDA	Supplemental New Drug Application
	skeletal muscle relaxant		
	standardized mortality ratio	SNE	subacute necrotizing encephalomyelopathy
	submucous resection	SNEP	student nurse extern program
SMRR	submucous resection and rhinoplasty	SnET2	tin ethyl etiopurpurin
SMS	scalded mouth syndrome	SNF	skilled nursing facility
	senior medical student	SnF_2	stannous fluoride
	somatostatin (Zecnil)	SNF/MR	skilled nursing facility for the mentally retarded
	stiff-man syndrome		
SMSA	standard metropolitan statistical area	SNGFR	single nephron glomerular filtration rate
SMV	submentovertical	SNHL	sensorineural hearing loss
	superior mesenteric vein	SNIP	silver nitrate immunoperoxidase
SMVT	sustained monomorphic ventricular tachycardia		strict no information in paper
SMX-TMP	sulfamethoxazole and tri-methoprim (SMZ-TMP)	SNM	sentinel (lymph) node mapping
SN	sciatic notch		student nurse midwife
	staff nurse	SnMp	tin-mesoporphyrin
	student nurse	SNOMED	Systematized Nomenclature of Medicine
	suprasternal notch		
	superior nasal	SNOMED-RT®	Systematized Nomenclature of Human and Veterinary Medicine—reference terminology
Sn	tin		
S/N	signal to noise ratio		
SNA	specimen not available		
	Student Nursing Assistant	SNOOP	Systematic Nursing Observation of Psychopathology
SNa	serum sodium		
SNAP	scheduled nursing activities program	SNOs	S-nitrosothiols
	Score for Neonatal Acute Physiology	SNP	simple neonatal procedure
			sodium nitroprusside
	sensory nerve action potential	SNPs	single nucleotide polymorphisms
SNAP-PE	Score for Neonatal Acute Physiology-Perinatal Extension	SNR	signal-to-noise ratio
		SNr	substantia nigra reticularis
SNAT	suspected non-accidental trauma	SNRI	serotonin norepinephrine reuptake inhibitor
SNB	scalene node biopsy	SNRT	sinus node recovery time
	sentinel (lymph) node biopsy	SNS	sterile normal saline (0.9% sodium chloride)
SNC	skilled nursing care		sympathetic nervous system
SNc	substantia nigra		
SNCV	sensory nerve conduction velocity	SNT	sinuses, nose, and throat
SND	single needle device		suppan nail technique
	sinus node dysfunction		

S

SNV	Sin Nombre virus		start of care
	skilled nursing visit		state of consciousness
	spleen necrosis virus		system organ class
SO	second opinion	S & OC	signed and on chart (e.g. permit)
	sex offender		
	shoulder orthosis	SOD	sinovenous occlusive disease
	significant other		
	special observation		sphincter of Oddi dysfunction
	sphincter of Oddi		
	standing orders		superoxide dismutase
	suboccipital		surgical officer of the day
	suggestive of	SODAS	spheriodal oral drug absorption system
	superior oblique		
	supraoptic	SOG	suggestive of good
	supraorbital	SOH	sexually oriented hallucinations
	sutures out		
	sympathetic ophthalmia	SoHx	social history
S-O	salpingo-oophorectomy	SOI	slipped on ice
S&O	salpingo-oophorectomy		surgical orthotopic implantation (implant)
SO₃	sulfite		
SO₄	sulfate		syrup of ipecac
SOA	serum opsonic activity	SOL	solution
	shortness of air		space occupying lesion
	spinal opioid analgesia	SOL I	special observations level one (there are also SOL II and SOL III)
	supraorbital artery		
	swelling of ankles		
SOAA	signed out against advice	SOM	secretory otitis media
SOAM	sutures out in the morning		serous otitis media
SOAMA	signed out against medical advice		somatization
		SOMI	sterno-occipital mandibular immobilizer
SOAP	subjective, objective, assessment, and plans	Sono	sonogram
SOAPIE	subjective, objective, assessment, plan, implementation, (intervention), and evaluation	SONP	solid organs not palpable
		SOOL	spontaneous onset of labor
		SOP	standard operating procedure
SOB	see order book	SOPM	sutures out in afternoon (or evening)
	shortness of breath (this abbreviation has caused problems)	SOR	sign own release
		SOS	if there is need
	side of bed		may be repeated once if urgently required (Latin: *si opus sit*)
SOBE	short of breath on exertion		
SOBOE	short of breath on exertion		self-obtained smear
			suicidal observation status
SOC	see old chart	SOSOB	sit on side of bed
	socialization	SOT	solid organ transplant
	standard of care		something other than

	stream of thought	SPCT	simultaneous prism and cover test
SP	sacrum to pubis		
	sequential pulse	SPD	subcorneal pustular dermatosis
	serum protein		
	shoulder press		Supply, Processing, and Distribution (department)
	spastic dysphonia		
	speech		
	Speech Pathologist		suprapubic drainage
	spinal	SPE	saw palmetto extract
	spouse		serum protein electrophoresis
	stand and pivot		
	stand pivot		solid-phase extraction
	status post		superficial punctate erosions
	Streptococcus pneumoniae		
	systolic pressure	SPEB	streptococcal pyrogenic exotoxins B
sp	species		
S/P	status post	SPEC	specimen
SP 1	suicide precautions number 1		streptococcal pyrogenic exotoxins C
SP 2	suicide precautions number 2	Spec Ed	special education
		SPECT	single photon emission computed tomography
SPA	albumin human (formerly known as salt-poor albumin)		
		SPEEP	spontaneous positive end-expiratory pressure
	serum prothrombin activity		
		SPEP	serum protein electrophoresis
	single photon absorptiometry		
		SPET	single-photon emission tomography
	Speech Pathology and Audiology	SPF	split products of fibrin
	stimulation produced analgesia		sun protective factor
		sp fl	spinal fluid
	student physician's assistant	SPG	scrotopenogram
			sphenopalatine ganglion
	subperiosteal abscess	SpG	specific gravity
	suprapubic aspiration	SPH	severely and profoundly handicapped
SPAC	satisfactory postanesthesia course		
			sighs per hour
SPAG	small particle aerosol generator		spherocytes
		SPHERO	spherocytes
SPAMM	spatial modulation of magnetization	SPI	speech processor interface
SPBI	serum protein bound iodine		surgical peripheral iridectomy
		SPIA	solid phase immunoabsorbent assay
SPBT	suprapubic bladder tap		
SPC	saturated phosphatidylcholine	SPIF	spontaneous peak inspiratory force
	statistical process control		
	suprapubic catheter	S-PIN	Steinmann pin

271

SPK	single parent keeping (baby)		status post surgery
	superficial punctate keratitis		systemic progressive sclerosis
SPL	sound pressure level	SPT	skin prick test
SPL®	Staphylococcal Phage Lysate	SP TAP	spinal tap
		SPTs	second primary tumors
SPLATTT	split anterior tibial tendon transfer	SP TUBE	suprapubic tube
		SPTX	static pelvic traction
SPM	scanning probe microscopy	SPU	short procedure unit
	second primary malignancy	SPVR	systemic peripheral vascular resistance
SPMA	spinal progressive muscle atrophy	SQ	status quo
			subcutaneous (this is a dangerous abbreviation)
SPME	solid-phase microextraction	Sq CCa	squamous cell carcinoma
SPMSQ	Short Portable Mental Status Questionnaire	SQE	subcutaneous emphysema
		SQM	square meter(s)
SPN	solitary pulmonary nodule	SQV	saquinavir (Fortovose; Invirase)
	student practical nurse	SR	screen
SPNK	single parent not keeping (baby)		sedimentation rate
			see report
SPO	status postoperative		senior resident
SpO₂	oxygen saturation by pulse oximeter		service record
			side rails
spont	spontaneous		sinus rhythm
SponVe	spontaneous ventilation		slow release
SPP	Sexuality Preference Profile		smooth-rough
			social recreation
	species (specus)		stretch reflex
	super packed platelets		superior rectus
	suprapubic prostatectomy		sustained release
SPR	surface plasmon resonance		suture removal
			system review
SPRAS	Sheehan Patient Rated Anxiety Scale	S/R	strong/regular (pulse)
		S&R	seclusion and restraint
SP-RIA	solid-phase radioimmu-noassay	⁸⁹Sr	strontium 89
		SRA	steroid-resistant asthma
SPROM	spontaneous premature rupture of membrane	SRAN	surgical resident admission note
SPS	shoulder pain and stiffness	SRBC	sheep red blood cells
			sickle red blood cells
	simple partial seizure	SRBOW	spontaneous rupture of bag of waters
	sodium polyethanol sulfonate		
	sodium polystyrene sulfonate (Kayexalate; SPS®)	SRD	service-related disability
			sodium-restricted diet

SRE	skeletal related event		surfactant replacement therapy
SRF	somatotropin releasing factor		sustained release theophylline
	subretinal fluid	SRU	side rails up
SRF-A	slow releasing factor of anaphylaxis	SRUS	solitary rectal ulcer syndrome
SRGVHD	steroid-resistant graft-versus-host disease	SR↑X2	both siderails up
SRH	signs of recent hemorrhage	SS	half
			sacrosciatic
SRI	serotonin re-uptake inhibitor		saline (sodium chloride 0.9%) soak
SRICU	surgical respiratory intensive care unit		saline solution (0.9% sodium chloride)
SRIF	somatotropin-release inhibiting factor (somatostatin; Zecnil)		saliva sample
			salt sensitivity (sensitive)
			salt substitute
SRMD	stress-related mucosal damage		serotonin syndrome
			serum sickness
SRMS	sustained-release morphine sulfate		sickle cell
			single-strength (as compared to double-strength)
SR/NE	sinus rhythm, no ectopy		
SRNV	subretinal neovasculariza-tion		Sjögren's syndrome
			sliding scale
SRNVM	subretinal neovascular membrane		slip sent
			Social Security
SRO	sagittal ramus osteotomy		social service
	single room occupancy		somatostatin
	sustained-release oral		stainless steel
SROCPI	Self-Rating Obsessive-Compulsive Personality Inventory		steady state
			step stool
			subaortic stenosis
SROM	spontaneous rupture of membrane		susceptible
			suprasciatic (notch)
SRP	septorhinoplasty		symmetrical strength
	stapes replacement prosthesis	S/S	Saturday and Sunday
SRR	surgical recovery room	SS#	Social Security number
SRS	somatostatin receptor scintigraphy	S & S	shower and shampoo
			signs and symptoms
s̄RS	without redness or swelling		sling and swathe
			soft and smooth (prostate)
SRS-A	slow-reacting substance of anaphylaxis		support and stimulation
			swish and spit
SRSV	small round structured viruses		swish and swallow
SRT	sedimentation rate test	SSA	sagittal split advancement
	sleep-related tumescence		salicylsalicylic acid (salsalate)
	speech reception threshold		

S

273

	Sjögren's syndrome antigen A		Supplemental Security Income
	Social Security Administration	SSKI	surgical site infection saturated solution of potassium iodide
SSBP	sulfasalicylic acid (test) sitting systolic blood pressure	SSL	second stage of labor subtotal supraglottic laryngectomy
SSC	sign symptom complex silver sulfadiazine and chlorhexidine	SSM	short stay medical skin surface microscopy superficial spreading melanoma
	Similac® and special care Special Services for Children	SSN	severely subnormal Social Security number
SSc	stainless steel crown systemic sclerosis	SSO	second surgical opinion short stay observation
SSCA	single shoulder contrast arthrography		(unit) Spanish speaking only
SSCP	single strand conformational polymorphism	SSOP	Second Surgical Opinion Program
	substernal chest pain	SSP	short stay procedure (unit) superior spermatic plexus
SSCr	stainless steel crown		
SSCU	surgical special care unit	SSPE	subacute sclerosing
SSCVD	sterile spontaneous controlled vaginal delivery	SSPL	panencephalitis saturation sound pressure level
SSD	serosanguineous drainage sickle cell disease	SSPU	surgical short procedure unit
	silver sulfadiazine Social Security disability	SSQ	Staring Speel Questionnaire
SSDI	source to skin distance Social Security disability income	SSR	substernal retractions sympathetic skin response
SSE	saline solution enema (0.9% sodium chloride)	SSRFC	surrounding subretinal fluid cuff
	skin self-examination soapsuds enema	SSRI	selective serotonin reuptake inhibitor
	systemic side effects	SSS	layer upon layer
SSEH	spontaneous spinal epidural hematoma		scalded skin syndrome Scandinavian Stroke Scale
SSEPs	somatosensory evoked potentials		Sepsis Severity Score Severity Scoring System
SSF	subscapular skinfold		(Dart's Snakebite)
SSG	sodium stibogluconate sublabial salivary gland		short stay service (unit) sick sinus syndrome skin and skin structures
SSI	sliding scale insulin	SSSB	sterile saline soak sagittal split setback
	sub-shock insulin superior sector iridectomy	SSSDW	significant sharp, spike, or delta waves

274

SSSE	self-sustained status epilepticus	STAI-I	State-Trait-Anxiety Index—I
SSSIs	skin and skin structure infections	STA-MCA	superficial temporary artery-middle cerebral artery (anastomosis; bypass)
SSSS	staphylococcal scalded skin syndrome		
SSSs	small short spikes (encephalography)	STAPES	stapedectomy
		staph	*Staphylococcus aureus*
SST	sagittal sinus thrombosis	stat	immediately
	somatostatin (Zecnil)	STATINS	HMG-CoA reductase inhibitors
SSU	short stay unit		
SSX	sulfisoxazole acetyl	STAXI	State-Trait Anger Expression Inventory
S/SX	signs/symptoms		
ST	esotropic	STB	stillborn
	sacrum transverse	STBAL	standing balance
	Schiotz's tonometry	ST BY	stand by
	shock therapy	STC	serum theophylline concentration
	sinus tachycardia		
	skin test		soft tissue calcification
	slight trace		special treatment center
	smokeless tobacco		stimulate to cry
	sore throat		stroke treatment center
	speech therapist		subtotal colectomy
	speech therapy		sugar tongue cast
	sphincter tone	ST CLK	station clerk
	split thickness	STD	sexually transmitted disease(s)
	spondee threshold		
	station (obstetrics)		short-term disability
	stomach		skin test dose
	straight		skin to tumor distance
	stress testing		sodium tetradecyl sulfate
	stretcher	STD TF	standard tube feeding
	subtotal	STE	ST-segment elevation
	Surgical Technologist	STEAM	stimulated-echo acquisition mode
	survival time		
	synapse time	STEM	scanning transmission electron microscopic
S & T	sulfamethoxazole and trimethoprim (SMZ-TMP or SMX-TMP)		
		Stereo	steropsis
		STET	single photon emission tomography
STA	second trimester abortion		
	superficial temporal artery		submaximal treadmill exercise test
stab.	polymorphonuclear leukocytes (white blood cells, in nonmature form)	STETH	stethoscope
		STF	special tube feeding
			standard tube feeding
		STG	short-term goals
STAI	State-Trait Anxiety Inventory		split-thickness graft
			superior temporal gyri
		STH	soft tissue hemorrhage

	somatotrophic hormone		small tandem repeat
	subtotal hysterectomy		stretcher
	supplemental thyroid hormone	Strab	strabismus
		strep	streptococcus
STHB	said to have been		streptomycin
STI	soft tissue injury	Str Post MI	strictly posterior myocardial infarction
	sum total impression		
STILLB	stillborn	STS	serologic test for syphilis
STIR	short TI (tau) inversion recovery		short-term survivors
			sodium tetradecyl sulfate
STIs	systolic time intervals		sodium thiosulfate
STJ	scapulothoracic joint		soft tissue sarcoma
	subtalar joint		soft tissue swelling
STK	streptokinase		Surgical Technology Student
STL	sent to laboratory		
	serum theophylline level	STSG	split thickness skin graft
STLE	St. Louis encephalitis	STSS	streptococcal-induced toxic shock syndrome
STLOM	swelling, tenderness, and limitation of motion		
		STT	scaphoid, trapezium trapezoid
STLV	simian T-lymphotrophic viruses		
			serial thrombin time
STM	scanning tunneling microscope		skin temperature test
			soft tissue tumor
	short-term memory	STT#1	Schirmer tear test one
	soft tissue mobilization	STT#2	Schirmer tear test two
	streptomycin	STTb	basal Schirmer tear test
STMT	Seat Movement	STTOL	standing tolerance
STN	subthalamic nucleus	STU	shock trauma unit
STNI	subtotal nodal irradiation		surgical trauma unit
STNM	surgical evaluative staging of cancer	STV	short-term variability
		STV+	short-term variability-present
STNR	symmetrical tonic neck reflex		
		STV 0	short-term variability-absent
S to	sensitive to		
STOP	sensitive, timely, and organized programs (battered spouses)	STV inter	short-term variability-intermittent
		STX	stricture
STORCH	syphilis, toxoplasmosis, other agents, rubella, cytomegalovirus, and herpes (maternal infections)	STZ	streptozocin (Zanosar)
		SU	sensory urgency
			Somogyi units
			stroke unit
STP	short-term plans		sulfonylurea
	sodium thiopental		supine
STPD	standard temperature and pressure—dry	S/U	shoulder/umbilicus
		S&U	supine and upright
STPI	State-Trait Personality Inventory	SUA	serum uric acid
			single umbilical artery
STR	sister		

SUB	Skene's urethra and Bartholin's glands	SUUD	sudden unexpected, unexplained death
Subcu	subcutaneous	SUX	succinylcholine
SUBCUT	subcutaneous		suction
Subepi M Inj	subepicardial myocardial injury	SUZI	subzonal insertion
SUBL	sublingual	SV	seminal vesical
SUB-MAND	submandibular		severe
			sigmoid volvulus
			single ventricle
sub q	subcutaneous (this is a dangerous abbreviation since the q is mistaken for every, when a number follows)		single vessel
			snake venom
			stock volume
			subclavian vein
		Sv	sievert (radiation unit)
SUCC	succinylcholine	SV40	simian virus 40
SUD	sudden unexpected death	SVA	small volume admixture
SuDBP	supine diastolic blood pressure	SVB	saphenous vein bypass
		SVBG	saphenous vein bypass graft
SUDEP	sudden unexpected death in epilepsy	SVC	slow vital capacity
SUDS	Subjective Unit of Distress (Disturbance) (Discomfort) Scale		subclavian vein compression
			superior vena cava
	sudden unexplained death syndrome	SVCO	superior vena cava obstruction
SUI	stress urinary incontinence	SVC-RPA	superior vena cava and right pulmonary artery (shunt)
	suicide		
SUID	sudden unexplained infant death	SVCS	superior vena cava syndrome
SULF-PRIM	sulfamethoxazole and trimethoprim	SVD	single vessel disease
			spontaneous vaginal delivery
SUN	serum urea nitrogen	SVE	sterile vaginal examination
SUNDS	sudden unexplained nocturnal death syndrome		*Streptococcus viridans* endocarditis
SUO	syncope of unknown origin	SV&E	suicidal, violent, and eloper
SUP	stress ulcer prophylaxis	SVG	saphenous vein graft
	superior	SVI	seminal vesicle invasion
	supination		stroke volume index
	supinator	S VISC	serum viscosity
	symptomatic uterine prolapse	SVL	severe visual loss
supp	suppository	SVN	small volume nebulizer
SUR	suramin	SVO₂	mixed venous oxygen saturation
	surgery		
	surgical	SVP	spontaneous venous pulse
Surgi	Surgigator		

277

SVPB	supraventricular premature beat	SWU	septic work-up
		Sx	signs
SVPC	supraventricular premature contraction		surgery
			symptom
SVR	supraventricular rhythm	SXA	single-energy x-ray absorptiometry
	systemic vascular resistance		
		SXR	skull x-ray
SVRI	systemic vascular resistance index	SYN	synovial
		SYN Fl	synovial fluid
SVT	supraventricular tachycardia	SYPH	syphilis
		SYR	syrup
SVVD	spontaneous vertex vaginal delivery	SYS BP	systolic blood pressure
		SZ	schizophrenic
SW	sandwich		seizure
	sea water		suction
	seriously wounded	SZN	streptozocin (Zanosar)
	short wave		
	Social Worker		
	stab wound		
	sterile water		
	swallowing reflex		
S&W	soap and water		
S/W	somewhat		
SWA	Social Work Associate		
SWD	short wave diathermy		
SWFI	sterile water for injection		
SWG	standard wire gauge		
SWI	sterile water for injection		
	surgical wound infection		
S&WI	skin and wound isolation		
SWL	shock wave lithotripsy		
SWO	superficial white onychomycosis		
SWOG	Southwest Oncology Group		
SWOT	strengths, weaknesses, opportunities, threats (analysis)		
SWP	small whirlpool		
SWR	surface wrinkling retinopathy		
	surgical waiting room		
SWS	sheltered workshop		
	slow wave sleep		
	social work service		
	student ward secretary		
	Sturge-Weber syndrome		
SWT	stab wound of the throat		
	shuttle-walk test		

T

T	inverted T wave	
	tablespoon (15 mL) (this is a dangerous abbreviation)	
	temperature	
	tender	
	tension	
	testicles	
	testosterone	
	thoracic	
	thymine	
	trace	
t	teaspoon (5 mL) (this is a dangerous abbreviation)	
T+	increase intraocular tension	
T-	decreased intraocular tension	
2,4,5-T	2,4,5-trichlorophenoxyacetic acid	
$T°$	temperature	
$T_{1/2}$	half-life	
T_1	tricuspid first sound	
T_2	tricuspid second sound	
T-2	dactinomycin, doxorubicin, vincristine, and cyclophosphamide	
T_3	triiodothyronine (liothyronine)	
T3	transurethral thermo-ablation therapy (Targis)	
	Tylenol with codeine 30 mg (this is a dangerous abbreviation)	
$T_{3/4}ind$	triiodothyronine to thyroxine index	
T_4	levothyroxine	
	thyroxine	
T4	CD4 (helper-inducer cells)	
T-7	free thyroxine factor	

T-10   methotrexate, calcium leucovorin rescue, doxorubicin, cisplatin, bleomycin, cyclophosphamide, and dactinomycin

$T_1...T_{12}$ thoracic nerve 1 through 12
thoracic vertebra 1 through 12

TA   Takayasu's arteritis
temperature axillary
temporal arteritis
therapeutic abortion
tracheal aspirate
traffic accident
tricuspid atresia
truncus arteriosus
tonometry applanation

Ta   tonometry applanation

T&A   tonsillectomy and adenoidectomy
tonsils and adenoids

T(A)   axillary temperature

TA-55   stapling device

TAA   Therapeutic Activities Aide
thoracic aortic aneurysm
total ankle arthroplasty
transverse aortic arch
triamcinolone acetonide
tumor associated antigen (antibodies)

TAAA   thoracoabdominal aortic aneursym

TAB   tablet
therapeutic abortion
total androgen blockade
triple antibiotic (bacitracin, neomycin, and polymyxin—this is a dangerous abbreviation)

TAC   tetracaine, Adrenalin® and cocaine
tibial artery catheter
total abdominal colectomy
total allergen content
triamicinolone cream

TAD   thoracic asphyxiant dystrophy

279

	transverse abdominal diameter		preperitoneal polypropylene (mesh-plasty)
TADAC	therapeutic abortion, dilation, aspiration, and curettage	T APPL	applanation tonometry
TAE	transcatheter arterial embolization	TAPVC	total anomalous pulmonary venous connection
TAF	tissue angiogenesis factor	TAPVD	total anomalous pulmonary venous drainage
TAG	tumor-associated glycoprotein		
TA-GVHD	transfusion-associated graft-versus-host disease	TAPVR	total anomalous pulmonary venous return
TAH	total abdominal hysterectomy	TAR	thrombocytopenia with absent radius
	total artificial heart		total ankle replacement
TAHBSO	total abdominal hysterectomy, bilateral salpingo-oophorectomy		total anorectal reconstruction
			treatment authorization request
TAHL	thick ascending limb of Henle's loop	TARA	total articular replacement arthroplasty
T Air	air puff tonometry	TART	tenderness, asymmetry, restricted motion, and tissue texture changes
TAL	tendon Achilles lengthening		tumorectomy plus radiotherapy
	total arm length		
T ALCON	Alcon® tonometry	TAS	therapeutic activities specialist
TAML	therapy-related acute myelogenous leukemia		turning against self
TAM	tamoxifen		typical absence seizures
	teenage mother	TAT	tandem auto-transplants
	total active motion		tell a tale
	tumor-associated macrophages		tetanus antitoxin
TAN	Treatment Authorization Number		thematic apperception test
			thrombin-antithrombin III complex
	tropical ataxic neuropathy		'til all taken
TANI	total axial (lymph) node irradiation		total adipose tissue
TAO	thromboangitis obliterans		transactivator of transcription
	troleandomycin		transplant-associated thrombocytopenia
TAP	tonometry by applanation		turnaround time
	transabdominal preperitoneal (laparoscopic hernia repair)	TAUC	time-averaged urea concentration
	transesophageal atrial paced	TAX	cefotaxime
	tumor-activated prodrug	TB	Tapes for the Blind
TAPP	transabdominal		terrible burning

	thought broadcasting	TBN	total body nitrogen
	toothbrush	TBNA	transbronchial needle aspiration
	total base		treated but not admitted
	total bilirubin	TBNa	total-body sodium
	total body	TBOCS	Tale-Brown Obsessive-Compulsive Scale
	tuberculosis		
TBA	to be absorbed	TBP	thyroxine-binding protein
	to be added		total-body phosphorus
	to be administered		total-body protein
	to be admitted		tuberculous peritonitis
	to be announced	TBPA	thyroxine-binding prealbumin
	to be arranged		
	total body (surface) area	TBR	total-bed rest
TBAGA	term birth appropriate for gestational age	TBS	tablespoon (15ml)(this is a dangerous abbreviation)
T-bar	tracheotomy bar (a device used in respiratory therapy)		total-serum bilirubin
		TBSA	total-body surface area
			total-burn surface area
TBARS	thiobarbituric acid reactive substances	tbsp	tablespoon (15 mL)
TBB	transbronchial biopsy	TBT	tolbutamide test
TBC	to be cancelled		tracheal bronchial toilet
	total-blood cholesterol		transbronchoscopic balloon tipped
	total-blood clearance		
	tuberculosis	TBV	thiotepa, bleomycin, and vinblastine
TBD	to be determined		
TBE	tick-born encephalitis		total-blood volume
T-berg	Trendelenburg (position)		transluminal balloon valvuloplasty
TBEV	tick-borne encephalitis virus		
		TBW	total-body water
TBF	total-body fat	TBZ	thiabendazole
TBG	thyroxine-binding globulin	TC	team conference
			terminal cancer
TBI	toothbrushing instruction		testicular cancer
	total-body irradiation		thioguanine and cytarabine
	traumatic brain injury		
T bili	total bilirubin		thoracic circumference
TBK	total-body potassium		throat culture
tbl	tablespoon (15 mL)		tissue culture
TBLB	transbronchial lung biopsy		tolonium chloride
TBLC	term birth, living child		total cholesterol
TBLF	term birth, living female		to (the) chest
TBLI	term birth, living infant		tracheal collar
TBLM	term birth, living male		trauma center
TBM	tracheobronchomalacia		true conjugate
	tuberculous meningitis		tubocurarine
	tubule basement membrane	Tc	technetium
TBMg	total-body magnesium	T/C	telephone call

T

	ticarcillin-clavulanic acid (Timentin)	^{99m}TcGHA	technetium Tc 99m glucceptate
	to consider	TCH	turn, cough, hyperventilate
3TC	lamivudine (Epivir)		
TC7	Interceed®	TCHRs	traditional Chinese herbal remedies
T&C	turn and cough		
	type and crossmatch	TCI	to come in
T&C#3	Tylenol with 30 mg codeine	TCID	tissue culture infective dose
TCA	thioguanine and cytarabine	TCIE	transient cerebral ischemic episode
	tissue concentrations of antibiotic(s)	TCL	tibial collateral ligament
	trichloroacetic acid	TCM	tissue culture media
	tricuspid atresia		traditional Chinese medicine
	tricyclic antidepressant		transcutaneous (oxygen) monitor
	tumor chemosensitivity assay	^{99m}Tc-MAA	technetium Tc 99m albumin microaggre-gated
	tumor clonogenic assays		
TCABG	triple coronary artery bypass graft	TCMH	tumor-direct cell-mediated hypersensitivity
TCAD	transplant-related coronary-artery disease	TCMS	transcranial cortical magnetic stimulation
	tricyclic antidepressant	TCMZ	trichlormethiazide
TCAR	tiazofurin	TCN	tetracycline
TCB	to call back		triciribine phosphate (tricyclic nucleoside)
	tumor cell burden		
TCBS agar	thiosulfate-citrate-bile salt-sucrose agar	TCNS	transcutaneous nerve stimulator
TCC	transitional cell carcinoma	TCNU	tauromustine
TCD	transcerebellar diameter	TcO$_4^-$	pertechnetate
	transcranial Doppler (ultrasonography)	TCOM	transcutaneous oxygen monitor
	transverse cardiac diameter	T Con	temporary conservatorship
TCCB	transitional cell carcinoma of bladder	TCP	transcutaneous pacing
			tranylcypromine (Parnate)
TC/CL	ticarcillin-clavulanate (Timentin)		tumor control probability
TCD	transcystic duct	TcPCO$_2$	transcutaneous carbon dioxide
TCDB	turn, cough, and deep breath	TcPO$_2$	transcutaneous oxygen
TCDD	tetrachlorodibenzo-p-dioxin	^{99m}TcPYP	technetium Tc 99m pyrophosphate
^{99m}Tc DTPA	technetium Tc 99m pentetate	TCR	T-cell receptor
		TCRE	transcervical resection of the endometrium
TCE	tetrachloroethylene	TCS	tonic-clonic seizure
	total colon examination	^{99m}TcSC	technetium Tc 99m sulfur colloid
T cell	small lymphocyte		

TCT	thyrocalcitonin	TDT	tentative discharge
	tincture		tomorrow
TCU	transitional care unit		Trieger Dot Test
TCVA	thromboembolic cerebral		tumor doubling time
	vascular accident	TdT	terminal deoxynucleotidyl
TD	Takayasu's disease		transferase
	tardive dyskinesia	TDW	target dry weight
	temporary disability	TDWB	touch down weight
	test dose		bearing
	tetanus-diphtheria toxoid	TDx®	fluorescence polarization
	(pediatric use)		immunoassay
	tidal volume	TE	echo time
	tone decay		tennis elbow
	total disability		terminal extension
	transverse diameter		tooth extraction
	travelers' diarrhea		toxoplasmic encephalitis
	treatment discontinued		trace elements
Td	tetanus-diphtheria toxoid		tracheoesophageal
	(adult type)		transesophageal
TDAC	tumor-derived activated		echocardiography
	cell (cultures)		transrectal
TDD	telephone device for the		electroejaculation
	deaf	tE	total expiratory time
	thoracic duct drainage	T/E	testosterone to
	total daily dose		epitestosterone ratio
TDE	total daily energy	T&E	testing and evaluation
	(requirement)		training and evaluation
TDF	testis determining factor		trial and error
	total-dietary fiber	TEA	thromboendarterectomy
	tumor dose fractionation		total elbow arthroplasty
TDI	tolerable daily intake	TEBG	testosterone-estradiol
	toluene diisocyanate		binding globulin
TDK	tardive diskinesia	TeBG	testeosterone binding
TDL	thoracic duct lymph		globulin
TDM	therapeutic drug	TeBIDA	99m technetium trimethyl
	monitoring		1-bromo-imono diacetic
TDMAC	tridodecylmethyl		acid
	ammonium chloride	TEC	total eosinophil count
TDN	totally digestible nutrients		toxic *Escherichia coli*
	transdermal nitroglycerin		transient
TDNTG	transdermal nitroglycerin		erythroblastopenia of
TDNWB	touchdown non-weight-		childhood
	bearing		transluminal extraction-
TdP	torsades de pointes		endarterectomy catheter
TDPWB	touchdown partial		triethyl citrate
	weight-bearing	T&EC	trauma and emergency
TdR	thymidine		center
TDS	three times a day (United	TED	thromboembolic disease
	Kingdom)		thyroid eye disease

TEDS®	anti-embolism stockings	TERT	tertiary
TEE	total energy expended	TES	therapeutic electrical
	transnasal endoscopic		stimulation
	ethmoidectomy		thoracic endometriosis
	transesophageal		syndrome
	echocardiography		treatment emergent
TEF	tracheoesophageal		symptoms
	fistula	TESE	testicular sperm
TEG	thromboelastogram		extraction
	(thromboelastography)	TESI	thoracic epidural steroid
TEI	total episode of illness		injection
	transesophageal imaging	TESS	Treatment Emergent
TEL	telemetry		Symptom Scale
	telephone	TET	transcranial electrostimu-
tele	telemetry		lation therapy
TEM	transanal endoscopic		treadmill exercise test
	microsurgery	TETE	too early to evaluate
	transmission electron	TEU	token economy unit
	microscopy	TEV	talipes equinovarus
TEMI	transient episodes of		(deformity)
	myocardial ischemia	TEVAP	transurethral
TEMP	temperature		electrovaporization of
	temporal		the prostate
	temporary	TF	tactile fremitus
TEN	tension (intraocular		tail flick (reflex)
	pressure)		tetralogy of Fallot
	toxic epidermal necrolysis		to follow
TEN®	Total Enteral Nutrition		tube feeding
TENS	transcutaneous electrical	TFA	topical fluoride
	nerve stimulation		application
TEOAE	transient evoked		trans fatty acids
	otoacoustic emission		trifluoroacetic acid
	(test)	TFB	trifascicular block
TEP	total extraperitoneal	TFBC	The Family Birthing
	(laparoscopic hernia		Center
	repair)	TFC	time to following
	tracheoesophageal		commands
	puncture	TFCC	transjugular fibrocartilage
	tubal ectopic pregnancy		complex
TER	terlipressin	TFF	tangential flow filtration
	total elbow replacement	TF-Fe	transferrin-bound iron
	total energy requirement	TFL	tensor fasciae latae
	transurethral		trimetrexate, fluorouracil,
	electroresection		and leucovorin
TERB	terbutaline	TFM	transverse friction
TERC	Test of Early Reading		massage
	Comprehension	TFPI	tissue factor pathway
TERM	full-term		inhibitor
	terminal	TFR	total fertility rate

TFT	trifluridine (trifluorothymidine)	THC	tetrahydrocannabinol (dronabinol)
TFTs	thyroid function tests		thigh circumference
TG	triglycerides		transhepatic cholangiogram
6-TG	thioguanine		
TGA	transient global amnesia	TH-CULT	throat culture
	transposition of the great arteries	tHcy	total homocysteine
		THE	transhepatic embolization
TGAR	total graft area rejected	Ther Ex	therapeutic exercise
TGB	tiagabine (Gabatril)	THF	thymic humoral factor
TGD	thyroglossal duct	THI	transient hypogammaglobinemia of infancy
TGE	transmissible gastroenteritis		
		THKAFO	trunk-hip-knee-ankle-foot orthosis
TGFA	triglyceride fatty acid		
TGF	transforming growth factor	THP	take home packs
			total hip prosthesis
TGF-$_\beta$	transforming growth factor-beta		transhepatic portography
			trihexyphenidyl (Artane)
TGGE	temperature-gradient gel electrophoresis	THR	target heart rate
			thrombin receptor
TGR	tenderness, guarding, and rigidity		total hip replacement
			training heart rate
TGS	tincture of green soap	THRL	total hip replacement, left
TGs	triglycerides		
TGT	thromboplastin generation test	THRR	total hip replacement, right
TGTL	total glottic transverse laryngectomy	THTV	therapeutic home trial visit
		THV	therapeutic home visit
TGV	thoracic gas volume	TI	terminal ileus
	transposition of great vessels		thought insertion
			transischial
TGXT	thallium-graded exercise test		transverse diameter of inlet
			tricuspid incompetence
TGZ	troglitazone (Rezulin)		tricuspid insufficiency
TH	thrill	TIA	transient ischemic attack
	thyroid hormone	TIB	tibia
	total hysterectomy	TIBC	total iron-binding capacity
T&H	type and hold	TIC	paclitaxel (Taxol), ifosfamide, and cisplain
THA	tacrine (tetrahydroacridine) Cognex		
			trypsin-inhibitor capacity
	total hip arthroplasty	TICS	diverticulosis
	transient hemispheric attack	TICU	thoracic intensive care unit
THAL	thalassemia		
THBI	thyroid hormone binding index		transplant intensive care unit
			trauma intensive care unit
THBR	thyroid hormone-binding ratio		
THAM®	tromethamine		

TID	three times a day	TJN	tongue jaw neck (dissection)
TIDM	three times daily with meals		twin jet nebulizer
TIE	transient ischemic episode	TJR	total joint replacement
TIG	tetanus immune globulin	TK	thymidine kinase
TIH	tumor-inducing hypercalcemia		toxicokinetics
TIL	tumor-infiltrating lymphocytes	TKA	total knee arthroplasty
			tyrosine kinase activity
%tile	percentile	TKD	tokodynamometer
TIMP	tissue inhibitor of metalloproteinase	TKE	terminal knee extension
		TKIC	true knot in cord
TIN	three times a night (this is a dangerous abbreviation)	TKNO	to keep needle open
		TKP	thermokeratoplasty
			total knee prosthesis
	tubulointerstitial nephritis	TKO	to keep open
tinct	tincture	TKR	total knee replacement
TIND	Treatment Investigational New Drug (application)	TKRL	total knee replacement, left
TINEM	there is no evidence of malignancy	TKRR	total knee replacement, right
		TKVO	to keep vein open
TIP	toxic interstitial pneumonitis	TL	team leader
			total laryngectomy
TIPS	transjugular intrahepatic portosystemic shunt (stent-shunt)		transverse line
			trial leave
			tubal ligation
TIPSS	transjugular intrahepatic portosystemic shunt (stent)	T/L	terminal latency
		Tl	thallium
		TLA	translumbar arteriogram (aortogram)
TIS	tumor *in situ*		
TISS	Therapeutic Intervention Scoring System	TLAC	triple lumen arrow catheter
TIT	*Treponema* (*pallidum*) immobilization test	TL BLT	tubal ligation, bilateral
		TLC	tender loving care
	triiodothyronine (liothyronine)		thin layer chromatography
			T-lymphocyte choriocarcinoma
TIUP	term intrauterine pregnancy		total lung capacity
			total lymphocyte count
TIVA	total intravenous anethesia		triple lumen catheter
TIVC	thoracic inferior vena cava	TLD	thermoluminescent dosimeter
+tive	positive	TLE	temporal lobe epilepsy
TIW	three times a week (this is a dangerous abbreviation)	TLI	total lymphoid irradiation
			translaryngeal intubation
		TLK	thermal laser keratoplasty
TJ	tendon jerk	TLNB	term living newborn
	triceps jerk	TLP	transitional living program
TJA	total joint arthroplasty		

TLR	tonic labyrinthine reflex	TMEV	Theiler's murine encephalomyelitis virus
TLS	tumor lysis syndrome		
TLSO	thoracic lumbar sacral orthosis	TMH	trainable mentally handicapped
TLSSO	thoracolumbosacral spinal orthosis	TMI	threatened myocardial infarction
TLT	tonsillectomy		transmandibular implant
TLV	total lung volume		transmural infarct
TM	temperature by mouth	T>MIC	time above minimum inhibitory concentration
	thalassemia major		
	Thayer-Martin (culture)	TMJ	temporomandibular joint
	trabecular meshwork	TMJD	temporomandibular joint dysfunction
	trademark		
	transcendental meditation	TMJS	temporomandibular joint syndrome
	treadmill		
	tropical medicine	TML	tongue midline
	tumor		treadmill
	tympanic membrane	TMM	torn medial meniscus
T & M	type and crossmatch		total muscle mass
TMA	thrombotic microangiopathy	Tmm	McKay-Marg tension
		TMNG	toxic multinodular goiter
	trained medication aid		
	transcription mediated amplification	TMP	thallium myocardial perfusion
	transmetatarsal amputation		transmembrane pressure
			trimethoprim
T/MA	tracheostomy mask	TMP/SMZ	trimethoprim and sulfamethoxazole (correct name is sulfamethoxazole and trimethoprin; SMZ-TMP)
TMAS	Taylor Manifest Anxiety Scale		
T_{max}	temperature maximum		
t_{max}	time of occurrence for maximum (peak) drug concentration		
		TMR	trainable mentally retarded
TMB	tetramethylberizidine		transmyocardial revascularization
	transient monocular blindness		
		TMS	transcranial magnetic stimulation
	trimethoxybenzoates		
TMC	transmural colitis	TMST	treadmill stress test
	triamcinolone	TMT	tarsometatarsal
TMCA	trimethylcolchicinic acid		teratoma with malignant transformation
TMCN	triamcinolone		
TMD	temporomandibular dysfunction (disorder)		treadmill test
			tympanic membrane thermometer
	treating physician		
TME	thermolysin-like metalloendopeptidase	TMTC	too many to count
		TMTX	trimetrexate
	total mesorectal excision	TMUGS	Tumor Marker Utility Grading Scale
TMET	treadmill exercise test		

T

287

TMX	tamoxifen	TOAA	to affected areas
TMZ	temazepam (Restoril)	TOB	tobacco
	temozolomide		tobramycin
TN	normal intraocular tension	TOC	total organic carbon
	team nursing	TOCE	transcatheter oily
	temperature normal		chemoembolization
T&N	tension and nervousness	TOCO	tocodynamometer
	tingling and numbness	TOD	intraocular pressure of the
TNA	total nutrient admixture		right eye
TNB	term newborn		time of death
	transnasal butorphanol		time of departure
	transrectal needle biopsy		tubal occlusion device
	(of the prostate)	TOF	tetralogy of Fallot
	Tru-Cut® needle biopsy		time of flight
TNBP	transurethral needle		total of four
	biopsy of prostate		train-of-four
TND	term, normal delivery	TOGV	transposition of the great
TNDM	transient neonatal diabetes		vessels
	mellitus	TOH	throughout hospitalization
TNF	tumor necrosis factor	TOL	tolerate
TNF-bp	tumor necrosis factor		trial of labor
	binding protein	TOLA	temporary leave of
TNG	nitroglycerin		absence
TNI	total nodal irradiation	TOLD	Test of Language
TNM	primary tumor, regional		Development
	lymph nodes, and	TOM	therapeutic outcomes
	distant metastasis (used		monitoring
	with subscripts for the		tomorrow
	staging of cancer)		transcutaneous oxygen
TNS	transcutaneous nerve		monitor
	stimulation (stimulator)	Tomo	tomography
	transient neurologic	TON	tonight
	symptoms	TOP	termination of pregnancy
	Tullie-Niebörg syndrome		Topografov (virus)
TNT	triamcinolone and nystatin		topotecan
TNTC	too numerous to count	TOPO	topotecan
TO	old tuberculin	TOPO 1	topoisermerase
	telephone order	TOPS	Take Off Pounds Sensibly
	time off	TOPV	trivalent oral polio
	tincture of opium		vaccine
	(warning: this is NOT	TOR	toremifene (Faneston)
	paregoric)	TORC	Test of Reading
	total obstruction		Comprehension
	transfer out	TORCH	toxoplasmosis, others
T(O)	oral temperature		(other viruses known to
T/O	time out		attack the fetus),
T&O	tubes and ovaries		rubella,
TOA	time of arrival		cytomegalovirus, and
	tubo-ovarian abscess		herpes simplex

	(maternal viral infections)
TORP	total ossicular replacement prosthesis
TOS	intraocular pressure of the left eye
	thoracic outlet syndrome
TOT BILI	total bilirubin
TOV	trial of void
TOWL	Test of Written Language
TP	temperature and pressure
	temporoparietal
	therapeutic pass
	thought process
	thrombophlebitis
	Todd's paralysis
	toe pressure
	toilet paper
	total protein
	"T" piece
	treating physician
	trigger point
T:P	trough-to-peak ratio
T & P	temperature and pulse
	turn and position
TPA	alteplase, recombinant (tissue plasminogen activator)
	temporary portacaval anastomosis
	third-party administrator
	tissue polypeptide antigen
	total parenteral alimentation
TPAL	term infant(s), premature infant(s), abortion(s), living children
TPC	target plasma concentration
	total patient care
TPD	tropical pancreatic diabetes
TPE	therapeutic plasma exchange
	total placental estrogens
	total protective environment
TPF	trained participating father

TPH	thromboembolic pulmonary hypertension
	trained participating husband
TPHA	*Treponema pallidum* hemagglutination
T PHOS	triple phosphate crystals
TPI	*Treponema pallidum* immobilization
TPIT	trigger point injection therapy
TPL	thromboplastin
T plasty	tympanoplasty
TPLSM	two-photon laser-scanning microscope
TPM	temporary pacemaker
	topiramate (Topamax)
TPN	total parenteral nutrition
TPO	thrombopoietin
	thyroid peroxidase
	trial prescription order
TPP	thiamine pyrophosphate
TpP	thrombus precursor protein
TP & P	time, place, and person
TPPN	total peripheral parenteral nutrition
TPPV	trans pars plana vitrectomy
TPR	temperature
	temperature, pulse, and respiration
	total peripheral resistance
TPRI	total peripheral resistance index
T PROT	total protein
TPT	time to peak tension
	topotecan (Hycamtin)
	transpyloric tube
	treadmill performance test
*t*PTEF	time to peak tidal expiratory flow
TPU	tropical phagedenic ulcer
T-putty	Theraputty
TPVR	total peripheral vascular resistance
TPZ	tirapazamine
TQM	total quality management
TR	therapeutic recreation

T

	time to repeat	TRC	tanned red cells
	tincture	TRD	tongue-retaining device
	to return		
	trace		total-retinal detachment
	transfusion reaction		traction retinal detachment
	transplant recipients		
	treatment		treatment-resistant depression
	tremor		
	tricuspid regurgitation	TRDN	transient respiratory distress of the newborn
	tumor registry		
T(R)	rectal temperature		
T & R	tenderness and rebound	Tren	Trendelenburg
	treated and released	TRH	protirelin (thyrotropin-releasing hormone) (Relefact TRH®; Thypinone®)
TRA	therapeutic recreation associate		
	to run at		
	tumor regression antigen	TRI	transient radicular irritation
TRAb	thyrotropin-receptor antibody		
			trimester
TRACH	tracheal	T₃RIA	triiodothyronine level by radioimmunoassay
	tracheostomy		
TRAFO	tone-reducing ankle/foot orthosis	TRIC	trachoma inclusion conjunctivitis
TRAM	transverse rectus abdominis myocutaneous (flap)	TRICH	*Trichomonas*
		TRIG	triglycerides
		TRISS	Trauma Related Injury Severity Score
	transverse rectus abdominum muscle	TR-LSC	time-resolved liquid scintillation counting
	Treatment Response Assessment Method	TRM	treatment related mortality
TRAMP	transversus and rectus abdominis musculo-peritoneal (flap)	TRM-SMX	trimethoprim-sulfamethoxazole (correct name is sulfamethoxazole and trimethoprin; SMZ-TMP; SMX-TMP)
Trans D	transverse diameter		
TRANS Rx	transfusion reaction		
TRAP	tartrate-resistant (leukocyte) acid phophatase	tRNA	transfer ribonucleic acid
		TRNBP	transrectal needle biopsy prostate
	thrombospondin-related anonymous protein	TRND	Trendelenburg (position)
	total radical-trapping antioxidant parameter	TRNG	tetracycline-resistant *Neisseria gonorrhoeae*
		TRO	to return to office
	trapezium	TROFO	trofosfamide
	trapezius muscle	TROM	total range of motion
TRAS	transplant renal artery stenosis	TRP	tubular reabsorption of phosphate
TRB	return to baseline	TrPs	trigger points
TRBC	total red blood cells	TRPT	transplant

TRS	Therapeutic Recreation Specialist		tyramine signal amplification
	the real symptom	TSAR®	tape surrounded Appli-rulers
TRT	tangential radiation therapy	TSAS	Total Severity Assessment Score
	thermoradiotherapy	TSB	total serum bilirubin
	thoracic radiation therapy		trypticase soy broth
	treatment-related toxicity	TSBB	transtracheal selective bronchial brushing
TR/TE	time to repetition and time to echo in spin (echo sequence of magnetic resonance imaging)	TSC	technetium sulfur colloid
			theophylline serum concentration
			total symptom complex
T₃RU	triiodothyronine resin uptake	TSD	target to skin distance
			Tay-Sachs disease
TRUS	transrectal ultrasonography	TSDP	tapered steroid dosing package
TRUSP	transrectal ultrasonography of the prostate	TSE	targeted systemic exposure
TRZ	triazolam (Halcion)		transmissible spongiform encephalopathy
TS	Tay-Sachs (disease)	T set	tracheotomy set
	telomerase	TSE	testicular self-examination
	temperature sensitive		total skin examination
	test solution	TSF	tricep skin fold (thickness)
	thoracic spine		
	thymidylate synthase	TSGs	tumor suppressor genes
	toe signs	TSH	thyroid-stimulating hormone (thyrotropin)
	Tourette's syndrome		
	transsexual	TSH-RH	thyrotropin-releasing hormone
	Trauma Score		
	tricuspid stenosis	TSIs	thymidylate synthase inhibitors
	triple strength		
	tuberous sclerosis	T-SKULL	trauma skull
	Turner's syndrome	tsp	teaspoon (5 mL)
T/S	trimethoprim/ sulfamethoxazole (correct name is sulfamethoxazole and trimethoprin)	TSP	thrombospondin
			total serum protein
			tropical spastic paraparesis
T&S	type and screen	TSPA	thiotepa
Ts	Schiotz tension	T-SPINE	thoracic spine
	T suppressor cell	TSR	total shoulder replacement
TSAb	thyroid stimulating antibodies	TSS	total serum solids
			toxic shock syndrome
TSA	toluenesulfonic acid		tumor score system
	total shoulder arthroplasty	TSST	toxic shock syndrome toxin
	tumor-specific antigen		
	type-specific antibody	TST	titmus stereocuity test

T

	trans-scrotal testosterone	TTNA	transthoracic needle
	treadmill stress test		aspiration
	tuberculin skin test(s)	TTNB	transient tachypnea of the
TSTA	tumor-specific		newborn
	transplantation antigens	TTND	time to nondetectable
T&T	tobramycin and ticarcillin	TTO	tea tree oil
	touch and tone		time trade-off
TT	Test Tape®		to take out
	tetanus toxoid		transfer to open
	thrombin time		transtracheal oxygen
	thrombolytic therapy	TTOD	tetanus toxoid outdated
	thymol turbidity	TTOT	transtracheal oxygen
	tilt table		therapy
	tonometry	TTP	thrombotic thrombocy-
	total thyroidectomy		topenic purpura
	transit time		time to pregnancy
	transtracheal		time to tumor progression
	tuberculin tested		time-to-progression
	twitch tension	TTR	transthyretin
	tympanic temperature		triceps tendon reflex
T/T	trace of ___ /trace of ___	TTS	tarsal tunnel syndrome
T&T	tympantomy and tube		temporary threshold shift
	(insertion)		through the skin
TT4	total thyroxine		transdermal therapeutic
TTA	total toe arthroplasty		system
	transtracheal aspiration		transfusion therapy service
TTAT	toe touch as tolerated	TTT	tilt table test
TTC	transtracheal catheter		tolbutamide tolerance test
TTD	tarsal tunnel		total tourniquet time
	decompression		turn-to-turn transfusion
	temporary total disability	TTUTD	tetanus toxoid up-to-date
	total tumor dose	TTV	transfusion-transmitted
	transverse thoracic		virus
	diameter	TTVP	temporary transvenous
TTDM	thallim threadmill		pacemaker
TTE	transthoracic	TTWB	touch toe weight bearing
	echocardiography	TTx	thrombolytic therapy
t test	Student's t-test	TU	Todd units
TTF	time to treatment failure		transrectal ultrasound
TTI	Teflon tube insertion		transurethral
	transfer to intermediate		tuberculin units
TTII	thyrotropin-binding	1-TU	1 tuberculin unit
	inhibitory	5-TU	5 tuberculin units
	immunoglobulins	250-TU	250 tuberculin units
TTJV	transtracheal jet	TUE	transurethral extraction
	ventilation	TUF	total ultrafiltration
TTM	total tumor mass	TUG	total urinary gonadotropin
TTN	transient tachypnea of the	TUIBN	transurethral incision of
	newborn		bladder neck

TUIP	transurethral incision of the prostate	TVI	time velocity integral
TULIP®	transurethral ultrasound-guided laser-induced prostatectomy (system)	TVN	tonic vibration response
		TVP	tensor veli palatini (muscle)
			transvenous pacemaker
TUMT	transurethral microwave thermotherapy		transvesicle prostatectomy
		TVR	tricuspid valve replacement
TUN	total urinary nitrogen	TVS	transvaginal sonography
TUNA	transurethral needle ablation		transvenous system
			trigemino-vascular system
TUPR	transurethral prostatic resection	TVSC	transvaginal sector scan
		TVU	total volume of urine
TUR	transurethral resection		transvaginal ultrasonography
T₃UR	triiodothyronine uptake ratio	TVUS	transvaginal ultrasonography
TURB	turbidity	TW	talked with
TURBN	transurethral resection bladder neck		tapwater
			test weight
TURBT	transurethral resection bladder tumor		thought withdrawal
			T-wave
TURP	transurethral resection of prostate	TW2	Tanner-Whitehouse mark 2 (bone-age assessment)
TURV	transurethral resection valves	5TW	five times a week (this is a dangerous abbreviation)
TURVN	transurethral resection of vesical neck	TWA	time-weighted average
			total wrist arthroplasty
TUU	transureteroureterostomy	TWAR	*Chlamydia psittaci*
TUV	transurethral valve	T wave	part of the electrocardiographic cycle, representing a portion of ventricular repolarization
TUVP	transurethral vaporization of the prostate		
TV	television		
	temporary visit		
	tidal volume		
	transvenous	TWD	total white and differential count
	trial visit		
	Trichomonas vaginalis	TWE	tapwater enema
	tricuspid value	TWETC	tapwater enema 'til clear
T/V	touch-verbal	TWG	total weight gain
TVC	triple voiding cystogram	TWH	transitional wall hyperplasia
	true vocal cord		
TVc	tricuspid valve closure	TWHW ok	toe walking and heel walking all right
TVD	triple vessel disease		
TVDALV	triple vessel disease with an abnormal left ventricle	TWI	T-wave inversion
		TWiST	time without symptoms of progression or toxicity
TVF	tactile vocal fremitus		
	true vocal fold	TWR	total wrist replacement
TVH	total vaginal hysterectomy	T1WT	T1 weighted image

T

TWWD	tap water wet dressing
Tx	therapy
	traction
	transcription
	transfuse
	transplant
	transplantation
	treatment
	tympanostomy
T & X	type and crossmatch
TXA$_2$	thromboxane A$_2$
TXB$_2$	thromboxane B$_2$
TXE	Timoptic-XE®
TXL	paclitaxel (Taxol) (this is a dangerous abbreviation as it can be read as TXT)
TXM	type and crossmatch
TXS	type and screen
TXT	docetaxel (Taxotere) (this is a dangerous abbreviation as it can be read as TXL)
TYCO #3	Tylenol with 30 mg of codeine (#1=7.5 mg, #2=15 mg and #4=60 mg of codeine present)
Tyl	Tylenol (acetaminophen)
	tyloma (callus)
TYMP	tympanogram
TZ	temozolomide
	transition zone
TZD	thiazolidinedione
TZDs	thiazolidinediones

U	Ultralente Insulin®
	units (this is the most dangerous abbreviation —spell out "unit")
	unknown
	upper
	urine
Ⓤ	Kosher
U/1	1 finger breadth below umbilicus
1/U	1 finger over umbilicus
U/	at umbilicus
24U	24 hour urine (collection)
U100	100 units per milliliters
UA	umbilical artery
	unauthorized absence
	uncertain about
	unstable angina
	upper airway
	upper arm
	uric acid
	urinalysis
UAC	umbilical artery catheter
	under active
	upper airway congestion
UA/C	uric acid to creatinine (ratio)
UAD	upper airway disease
UADT	upper aerodigestive tract
UAE	urinary albumin excretion
UAL	umbilical artery line
	up *ad lib*
UA&M	urinalysis and microscopy
UAO	upper airway obstruction
UAPD	Union of American Physicians and Dentists
UAPF	upon arrival patient found
U-ARM	upper arm
UAS	upstream activating sequence
UASA	upper airway sleep apnea
UAT	up as tolerated

			urethral closure pressure
UAVC	univentricular atrioventricular connection	UCR	unconditioned reflex unconditioned response usual, customary, and reasonable
UBC	University of British Columbia (brace)	UCRE	urine creatinine
UBD	universal blood donor	UCRP	universal coagulation reference plasma
UBF	unknown black female uterine blood flow	UCS	unconscious
UBI	ultraviolet blood irradiation	UC&S	urine culture and sensitivity
UBM	unknown black male	UCX	urine culture
UBO	unidentified bright object	UD	as directed
UBT	urea breath test		ulnar deviation
UBW	usual body weight		urethral dilatation
UC	ulcerative colitis		urethral discharge
	umbilical cord		urodynamics
	unchanged		uterine distension
	unconscious	UDC	uninhibited detrusor (muscle) capacity
	Unit clerk		usual diseases of childhood
	United Church of Christ		
	urea clearance	UDCA	ursodeoxycholic acid
	urinary catheter	UDN	updraft nebulizer
	urine culture	UDO	undetermined origin
	usual care	UDP	unassisted diastolic pressure
	uterine contraction		
U&C	urethral and cervical usual and customary	UDPGT	uridinediphospho-glucuronyl transferase
UCB	umbilical cord blood unconjugated bilirubin (indirect)	UDS	unconditioned stimulus urine drug screen
UCBT	unrelated cord blood transplant	UDT	undescended testicle(s)
UCD	urine collection device usual childhood diseases	UE	under elbow undetermined etiology upper extremity
UCE	urea cycle enzymopathy	U & E	urea and electrolytes
UCG	urinary chorionic gonadotropins	UEDs	unilateral epileptiform discharges
UCHD	usual childhood diseases	UES	undifferentiated embryonal sarcoma upper esophageal sphincter
UCHI	usual childhood illnesses		
UCHS	uncontrolled hemorrhagic shock	UESEP	upper extremity somatosensory evoked potential
UCI	urethral catheter in usual childhood illnesses		
UCL	uncomfortable loudness level	UESP	upper esophageal sphincter pressure
UCLP	unilateral cleft lip and palate	UF	ultrafiltration until finished
UCO	urethral catheter out		
UCP	umbilical cord prolapse		

U

UFC	urine-free cortisol	UI	urinary incontinence
UFF	unusual facial features	UIB	Unemployment Insurance Benefits
UFFI	urea formaldehyde foam insulation	UIBC	unbound iron binding capacity
UFH	unfractionated heparin		unsaturated iron binding capacity
UFN	until further notice		
UFO	unflagged order	UID	once daily (this is a dangerous abbreviation, spell out "once daily")
	unidentified foreign object		
UFOV	useful field of view		
UFR	ultrafiltration rate		
UFT	uracil and tegafur	UIEP	urine (urinary) immunoelectrophoresis
UFV	ultrafiltration volume		
UG	until gone	UIP	usual interstitial pneumonitis (pneumonia)
	urinary glucose		
	urogenital		
UGA	under general anesthesia	UIQ	upper inner quadrant
	urogenital atrophy	UJ	universal joint (syndrome)
UGCR	ultrasound-guided compression repair	UK	United Kingdom
			unknown
UGDP	University Group Diabetes Project		urine potassium
			urokinase
UGH	uveitis, glaucoma, and hyphema (syndrome)	UK IC	urokinase intracoronary
		UKO	unknown origin
UGI	upper gastrointestinal series	UL	Unit Leader
			upper left
UGIB	upper gastrointestinal bleeding		upper lid
			upper limb
UGIH	upper gastrointestinal (tract) hemorrhage		upper lobe
		U/L	upper and lower
UGIS	upper gastrointestinal series	U & L	upper and lower
		ULLE	upper lid, left eye
UGIT	upper gastrointestinal tract	ULN	upper limits of normal
		ULPA	ultra-low particulate air
UGI w/SBFT	upper gastrointestinal (series) with small bowel follow through	ULQ	upper left quadrant
		ULRE	upper lid, right eye
		ULSB	upper left sternal border
UGK	urine, glucose, and ketones	ULYTES	electrolytes, urine
UGP	urinary gonadotropin peptide	UM	unmarried
		Umb A Line	umbilical artery line
UGVA	ultrasound-guided vascular access		
		Umb V Line	umbilical venous line
UH	umbilical hernia		
	unfavorable history	umb ven	umbilical vein
	University Hospital	UMCD	uremic medullary cystic disease
UHBI	upper hemibody irradiation		
		UMN	upper motor neuron (disease)
UHDDS	Uniform Hospital Discharge Data Set		
		UN	undernourished
UHP	University Health Plan		urinary nitrogen

UNA	urinary nitrogen appearance	U/P ratio	urine to plasma ratio
UNa	urine sodium	UPSC	uterine papillary serous carcinoma
unacc	unaccompanied		
UNC	uncrossed	UPT	uptake
UNDEL	undelivered		urine pregnancy test
UNG	ointment	UR	unrelated
UNK	unknown		upper respiratory
UNL	upper normal levels		upper right
UNOS	United Network for Organ Sharing		urinary retention
			utilization review
UN/P	unpatched eye	URAC	Utilization Review Accreditation Commission
UN/P OD	unpatched right eye		
UN/P OS	unpatched left eye		
UNS	unsatisfactory	UR AC	uric acid
UNSAT	unsatisfactory	URD	undifferentiated respiratory disease
UO	under observation		
	undetermined origin	URG	urgent
	ureteral orifice	URI	upper respiratory infection
	urinary output	URIC A	uric acid
UOP	urinary output	url	unrelated
UOQ	upper outer quadrant	UR&M	urinalysis, routine and microscopic
Uosm	urinary osmolality		
✔ up	check up	URO	urology
UP	unipolar	UROD	ultra-rapid opiate detoxification [under anesthesia]
	ureteropelvic		
U/P	urine to plasma (creatinine)		
UPC	unknown primary carcinoma	UROL	Urologist
			urology
		UROB	urobilinogen
UPDRS	Unified Parkinson's Disease Rating Scale	URQ	upper right quadrant
		URR	urea reduction ratio
UPEP	urine protein electrophoresis	URS	ureterorenoscopy
		URSB	upper right sternal border
UPG	uroporphyrinogen	URT	uterine resting tone
UPIN	unique physician identification number	URTI	upper respiratory tract infection
UPJ	ureteropelvic junction	US	ultrasonography
UPLIF	unilateral posterior lumbar interbody fusion		unit secretary
		USA	unit services assistant
			United States Army
UPN	unique patient number		unstable angina
UPO	metastatic carcinoma of unknown primary origin	USAF	United States Air Force
		USAN	United States Adopted Names
UPOR	usual place of residence	USAP	unstable angina pectoris
UPP	urethral pressure profile	USB	upper sternal border
UPPP	uvulopalatopharyngo-plasty	U-SCOPE	ureteroscopy
		USCVD	unsterile controlled vaginal delivery

U

USDA	United States Department of Agriculture	
USED-CARP	**u**reterosigmoidostomy, **s**mall bowel fistula, **e**xtra chloride, **d**iarrhea, **c**arbonic anhydrase inhibitors, **a**drenal insufficiency, **r**enal tubular acidosis, and **p**ancreatic fistula (common causes of nonanion gap metabolic acidosis)	
USG	ultrasonography	
USH	United Services for Handicapped	
	usual state of health	
USI	urinary stress incontinence	
USM	ultrasonic mist	
USMC	United States Marine Corps	
USN	ultrasonic nebulizer	
	United States Navy	
USOGH	usual state of good health	
USOH	usual state of health	
USP	unassisted systolic pressure	
	United States Pharmacopeia	
USPHS	United States Public Health Service	
USUCVD	unsterile uncontrolled vaginal delivery	
USVMD	urine specimen volume measuring device	
UTD	unable to determine	
	up to date	
ut dict	as directed	
UTF	usual throat flora	
UTI	urinary tract infection	
UTL	unable to locate	
UTM	urinary-tract malformations	
UTMDACC	University of Texas M.D. Anderson Cancer Center	
UTO	unable to obtain	
	upper tibial osteotomy	

UTS	ulnar tunnel syndrome
	ultrasound
U/U−	uterine fundus at umbilicus (usually modified as number of finger breadths below)
U/U+	uterine fundus at umbilicus (usually modified as number of finger breadths above)
UUD	uncontrolled unsterile delivery
UUN	urinary urea nitrogen
UUTI	uncomplicated urinary tract infections
UV	ultraviolet
	ureterovesical
	urine volume
UVA	ultraviolet A light
	ureterovesical angle
UVB	ultraviolet B light
UVC	umbilical vein catheter
UVH	univentricular heart
UVJ	ureterovesical junction
UVL	ultraviolet light
	umbilical venous line
UVR	ultraviolet radiation
UVT	unsustained ventricular tachycardia
U/WB	unit of whole blood
UW	unilateral weakness
UWF	unknown white female
UWM	unknown white male
	unwed mother

V

V	five
	gas volume
	minute volume
	vaccinated
	vagina
	vein
	ventricular
	verb
	verbal
	vertebral
	very
	viral
	vitamin
	vomiting
$\dot{V}$	ventilation (L/min)
+V	positive vertical divergence
V1	fifth cranial nerve, ophthalmic division
V2	fifth cranial nerve, maxillary division
V3	fifth cranial nerve, mandibular division
V_1 to V_6	precordial chest leads
VA	vacuum aspiration
	valproic acid
	Veterans Administration
	visual acuity
V_A	alveolar gas volume
V&A	vagotomy and antrectomy
VAB	vinblastine, dactinomycin (actinomycin D), bleomycin
VAC	ventriculo-arterial connections
	vincristine, dactinomycin (actinomycin D), and cyclophosphamide
	vincristine, doxorubicin (Adriamycin), and cyclophosphamide
VA cc	distance visual acuity with correction
VA ccl	near visual acuity with correction
VAC EXT	vacuum extractor
VACO	Veterans Administration Central Office
VACTERL	vertebral, anal, cardiac, tracheal, esophageal, renal, and limb anomalies
VAD	vascular (venous) access device
	ventricular assist device
	Veterans Administration Domiciliary
	vincristine, doxorubicin (Adriamycin), and dactinomycin
VaD	vascular dementia
VADCS	ventricular atrial distal coronary sinus
VADRIAC	vincristine, doxorubicin (Adriamycin), and cyclophosphamide
VAERS	Vaccine Adverse Events Reporting System
VAFD	vascular access flush device
VAG	vagina
VAG HYST	vaginal hysterectomy
VAH	Veterans Administration Hospital
VAHBE	ventricular atrial His bundle electrocardiogram
VAHRA	ventricular atrial height right atrium
VAIN	vaginal intraepithelial neoplasia
VALE	visual acuity, left eye
VAMC	Veterans Affairs Medical Center
VAMP®	venous arterial management protection system
VAMS	Visual Analogue Mood Scale
VANCO/P	vancomycin-peak
VANCO/T	vancomycin-trough
VAOD	visual acuity, right eye

V

VAOS	visual acuity, left eye	VB₃	voided bladder specimen after expression of prostatic secretions
VA OS LP with P	visual acuity, left eye, left perception with projection		
		VBAC	vaginal birth after cesarean
VAP	venous access port		
	ventilator-associated pneumonia	VBAI	vertebrobasilar artery insufficiency
	vincristine, asparaginase, and prednisone	VBAP	vincristine, carmustine (BiCNU), doxorubicin (Adriamycin), and prednisone
VAPCS	ventricular atrial proximal coronary sinus		
VAPP	vaccine-associated paralytic poliomyelitis	VBC	vinblastine, bleomycin, and cisplatin
VAR	variant	VBG	venous blood gas
	varicella vaccine		vertical banded gastroplasty
VARE	visual acuity, right eye		
VAS	vasectomy	VBGP	vertical banded gastroplasty
	vascular		
	Visual Analogue Scale (Score)	VBI	vertebrobasilar insufficiency
VASC	Visual-Auditory Screen Test for Children	VBL	vinblastine
		VBM	vinblastine, bleomycin, and methotrexate
VA sc	distance visual acuity without correction		
VA scl	near visual acuity without correction	VBP	vinblastine, bleomycin, and cisplatin
		VBR	ventricular brain ratio
VASPI	Visual Analogue Self Assessment Scales For Pain Intensity	VBS	vertebral-basilar system
		VC	color vision
			etoposide and carboplatin
VAS RAD	vascular radiology		pulmonary capillary blood volume
VAT	video-assist thoracoscopy		
	visceral adipose tissue		vena cava
VATER	vertebral, anal, tracheal, esophageal, and renal anomalies		verbal cues
			vincristine
			vital capacity
VATH	vinblastine, doxorubicin (Adriamycin), thiotepa, and fluoxymesterone (Halotestin)		vocal cords
		V&C	vertical and centric (a bite)
		VCA	vasoconstrictor assay
VATS	video assisted thoracic surgery	VCAM	vascular cell adhesion molecule
VB	Van Buren (catheter)	VCAP	vincristine, cyclophospha-mide, doxorubicin (Adriamycin), and prednisone
	venous blood		
	vinblastine		
	vinblastine and bleomycin		
VB₁	first voided bladder specimen	Vcc	vision with correction
		VCCA	velocity common carotid artery
VB₂	second midstream bladder specimen		
		VCD	vocal cord dysfunction

VCE	vaginal cervical endocervical (smear)	VD or M	venous distention or masses
VCF	Vaginal Contraception Film™	VDP	vinblastine, dacarbazine, and cisplatin (Platinol AQ)
VCG	vectorcardiography voiding cystogram	VDRF	ventilator dependent respiratory failure
vCJD	variant Creutzfeldt-Jakob disease	VDRL	Venereal Disease Research Laboratory (test for syphilis)
VCO	ventilator CPAP oxyhood		
VCR	video cassette recorder vincristine sulfate	VDRR	vitamin D-resistant rickets
VCT	venous clotting time	VDRS	Verdun Depression Rating Scale
VCTS	vitreal corneal touch syndrome	VDS	vasodepressor syncope venereal disease—syphilis
VCU	voiding cystourethrogram		vindesine
VCUG	vesicoureterogram voiding cystourethrogram	VDT	video display terminal
VD	venereal disease	VD/VT	dead space to tidal volume ratio
	viral diarrhea	VE	vaginal examination
	voided		vertex
	volume of distribution		Vietnam era
V_D	deadspace volume		virtual endoscopy
V_d	volume of distribution		visual examination
V&D	vomiting and diarrhea		vitamin E
VDA	venous digital angiogram visual discriminatory acuity		vocational evaluation
		V_E	minute volume (expired)
		V/E	violence and eloper
VDAC	vaginal delivery after cesarean	VEA	ventricular ectopic activity
VDC	vincristine, doxorubicin, and cyclophosphamide		viscoelastic agent
		VEB	ventricular ectopic beat
VDD	atrial synchronous ventricular inhibited pacing	VEC	vecuronium velocity-encoded cine
		VECG	vector electrocardiogram
VDDR I	vitamin D dependency rickets type I	VED	vacuum erection device vacuum extraction delivery
VDDR II	vitamin D dependency rickets type II		ventricular ectopic depolarization
VDG	venereal disease–gonorrhea	VEE	Venezuelan equine encephalitis
Vdg	voiding	VEF	visually evoked field
VDH	valvular disease of the heart	VEG	vegetation (bacterial)
VDJ	variable diversity joining	VEGF	vascular endothelial growth factor
VDL	vasodepressor lipid visual detection level	VeIP	vinblastine (Velban), ifosfamide, and cisplatin (Platinol AQ)
VDO	varus derotational osteotomy		

V

VENT	ventilation		von Herrick (grading
	ventilator		system)
	ventral	VH I	very narrow anterior
	ventricular		chamber angles
VEP	visual evoked potential	VH II	moderately narrow
VER	ventricular escape rhythm		anterior chamber angles
	visual evoked responses	VH III	moderately wide open
VES	ventricular extrasystoles		anterior chamber angles
VET	veteran	VH IV	wide open anterior
	Veterinarian		chamber angles
	veterinary	VHD	valvular heart disease
VF	left leg (electrode)	VHL	von Hippel-Lindau
	ventricular fibrillation		disease (complex)
	visual field	VI	six
	vocal fremitus		volume index
VFC	Vaccines for Children	*via*	by way of
	(program)	vib	vibration
VFD	visual fields	VIBS	Victim's Information
VFFC	visual fields full to		Bureau Service
	confrontation	VICA	velocity internal carotid
VFI	visual fields intact		artery
	Visual Functioning index	VICP	Vaccine Injury
V. Fib	ventricular fibrillation		Compensation Program
VFL	vinflunine	VID	videodensitometry
VFP	vitreous fluorophotometry	VIG	vaccinia immune globulin
VFPN	Volu-feed premie nipple		vinblastine, ifosfamide,
VFRN	Volu-feed regular nipple		and gallium nitrate
VFT	venous filling time	VIH	Spanish and French
	ventricular fibrillation		abbreviation for human
	threshold		immunodeficiency
VG	vein graft		virus
	ventricular gallop	VIN	vulvar intraepithelial
	ventrogluteal		neoplasm
	very good	VIP	etopside (VePesid),
V&G	vagotomy and		ifosfamide, and
	gastroenterotomy		cisplatin (Platinol AQ)
VGAD	vein of Galen aneurysmal		vasoactive intestinal
	dilatation		peptide
VGAM	vein of Galen aneurysmal		vasoactive intracorporeal
	malformation		pharmacotherapy
VGH	very good health		very important patient
VGM	vein graft myringoplasty		vinblastine, ifosfamide,
VGPO	volume-guaranteed		and cisplatin (Platinol)
	pressure option		voluntary interruption of
VH	vaginal hysterectomy		pregnancy
	Veterans Hospital	VIPomas	vasoactive intestinal
	viral hepatitis		peptide-secreting
	visual hallucinations		tumors
	vitreous hemorrhage	VIQ	Verbal Intelligence

	Quotient (part of Wechsler tests)		Venturi mask
			vestibular membrane
VIS	Visual Impairment Service	VM 26	teniposide (Vumon)
		VMA	vanillylmandelic acid
VISC	vitreous infusion suction cutter	VMCP	vincristine, melphalan, cyclophosphamide, and prednisone
VISI	volar intercalated segmental instability	VMD	Doctor of Veterinary Medicine (DVM)
VIT	venom immunotherapy		vertical maxillary deficiency
	vital		
	vitamin	VME	vertical maxillary excess
VIT CAP	vital capacity	VMH	ventromedial hypothalamus
VIU	visual internal urethrotomy	VMO	vastus medalis oblique
VIZ	namely	VMR	vasomotor rhinitis
V-J	ventriculo-jugular (shunt)	VMS	vanilla milkshake
VKC	vernal keratoconjunctivitis	VN	visiting nurse
VKDB	vitamin K deficiency bleeding	VNA	Visiting Nurses' Association
VKH	Vogt-Koyanagi-Harada's disease	VNB	vinorelbine
VL	left arm (electrode)	VNC	vesicle neck contracture
	vial	VNS	vagus nerve stimulation
VLA	very-late antigen	VNTR	variable number of tandem repeats
VLAD	variable life-adjusted display	VO	verbal order
VLAP	vaporization laser ablation of the prostate	VO₂	oxygen consumption
VLBW	very low birth weight (less than 1500 g)	VOCAB	vocabulary
		VOCOR	void on-call to operating room
VLBWPN	very low birth weight preterm neonate	VOCs	volatile organic compounds
VLCAD	very-long-chain acyl coenzyme A dehydrogenase deficiency	VOCTOR	void on-call to operating room
		VOD	veno-occlusive disease
			vision right eye
VLCD	very low calorie diet	VOE	vascular occlusive episode
VLCFA	very long chain fatty acids	VO₂I	oxygen consumption index
VLDL	very low density lipoprotein	VOL	volume
			voluntary
VLE	vision left eye	VOM	vomited
VLH	ventrolateral nucleus of the hypothalamus	VOO	continuous ventricular asynchronous pacing
VLM	visceral larva migrans	VOR	vestibular ocular reflex
VLP	virus-like particle	VOS	vision left eye
VLR	vastus lateralis release	VOSS	visual observation shivering score
VM	ventilated mask	VOT	Visual Organization Test
	ventimask	VOU	vision both eyes

Note: VO_2 oxygen consumption; VO_2I oxygen consumption index.

V

VP	etoposide (VePesid) and cisplatin (Platinol AQ)	V_3R to V_6R	right sided precordial leads
	variegate porphyria	VRA	visual reinforcement audiometry
	venipuncture		
	venous pressure		visual response audiometry
	ventriculo-peritoneal		
	visual perception	VRB	vinorelbine (Navelbine)
V & P	vagotomy and pyloroplasty	VRC	vocational rehabilitation counselor
	ventilation and perfusion	VRE	vancomycin-resistant enterococci
VP-16	etoposide		
VPA	valproic acid		vision right eye
	ventricular premature activation	VREF	vancomycin-resistant *Enterococcus faecium*
V-Pad	sanitary napkin	VRI	viral respiratory infection
VPB	ventricular premature beat	VRL	ventral root, lumbar
VPC	ventricular premature contractions	VRP	vocational rehabilitation program
VPD	ventricular premature depolarization	VRS	viral rhinosinusitis
		VRSA	vancomycin-resistant *Staphylococcus aureus*
VPDC	ventricular premature depolarization contraction	VRT	variance of resident time
VPDF	vegetable protein diet plus fiber		ventral root, thoracic
			vertical radiation topography
VPDs	ventricular premature depolarizations		Visual Retention Test
VPI	velopharyngeal incompetence		vocational rehabilitation therapy
	velopharyngeal insufficiency	VRTA	Vocational Rehabilitation Therapy Assistant
VPL	ventro-posterolateral	VRU	ventilator rehabilitation unit
VPLS	ventilation-perfusion lung scan	VS	vagal stimulation
			vegetative state
VPM	venous pressure module		versus *(vs)*
VPR	volume pressure response		very sensitive
VPS	valvular pulmonic stenosis		visit
			visited
VPT	vascularized patellar tendon		vital signs (temperature, pulse, and respiration)
	vibration perception threshold	VSADP	vocational skills assessment and development program
VQ	ventilation perfusion		
VR	right arm (electrode)	VSBE	very short below elbow (cast)
	valve replacement		
	venous resistance	VSD	ventricular septal defect
	ventricular rhythm	VSI	visual motor integration
	verbal reprimand	VSMC	vascular smooth muscle cell
	vocational rehabilitation		

VSN	vital signs normal	VVD	vaginal vertex delivery
VSO	vertical subcondylar oblique	VVETP	Vietnam Veterans Evaluation and Treatment Program
VSOK	vital signs normal	VVFR	vesicovaginal fistula repair
VSQOL	Vital Signs Quality of Life	V/VI	grade 5 on a 6 grade basis
VSR	venous stasis retinopathy	VVI	ventricular demand pacing
VSS	vital signs stable	VVL	varicose veins ligation
V_{ss}	apparent volume of distribution		verruca vulgaris of the larynx
VSSAF	vital signs stable, afebrile	VVOR	visual-vestibulo-ocular-reflex
VST	visual search task		
VSV	vesicular stomatitis virus	VVR	ventricular response rate
VT	validation therapy	VVT	ventricular synchronous pacing
	ventricular tachycardia	VW	vessel wall
V_t	tidal volume	VWD	ventral wall defect
VTA	ventral tegmentum area		von Willebrand disease
VTBI	volume to be infused	vWF	von Willebrand factor
v. tach.	ventricular tachycardia	VWM	ventricular wall motion
VTE	venous thromboembolism	V_x	vitrectomy
VTEC	verotoxin-producing *Escherichia coli*	V-XT	V-pattern exotropia
VTED	venous thromboembolic disease	VY	surgical replacement flap
		VZ	varicella zoster
VT-NS	ventricular tachycardia non-sustained	VZIG	varicella zoster immune globulin
VTOP	voluntary termination of pregnancy	VZV	varicella zoster virus
VTP	voluntary termination of pregnancy		
VTS	Volunteer Transport Service		
VT-S	ventricular tachycardia sustained		
VTSRS	Verdun Target Symptom Rating Scale		
VT/VF	ventricular tachycar-dia/fibrillation		
VTX	vertex		
VU	vesicoureteral (reflux)		
V/U	verbalize understanding		
VUJ	vesico ureteral junction		
VUR	vesicoureteric reflux		
VV	varicose veins		
V-V	ventriculovenous (shunt)		
V&V	vulva and vagina		
V/V	volume to volume ratio		
VVB	venovenous bypass		
VVC	vulvovaginal candidiasis		

V

W

W	wash	WAP	wandering atrial pacemaker
	wearing glasses	WARI	wheezing associated respiratory infection
	week	WAS	whiplash-associated disorders
	weight		
	well		Wiskott-Aldrich syndrome
	white	WASO	wakefulness after sleep onset
	widowed		
	wife	WASS	Wasserman test
	with	WAT	word association test
	work	WB	waist belt
W-1	insignificant (allergies)		weight bearing
W-3	minimal (allergies)		well baby
W-5	moderate (allergies)		Western blot
W-7	moderate-severe (allergies)		whole blood
W-9	severe (allergies)	WBACT	whole blood activated clotting time
WA	when awake	WBAT	weight bearing as tolerated
	while awake		
	White American	WBC	weight bearing with crutches
	wide awake		
	with assistance		well baby clinic
W-A	Wyeth-Ayerst Laboratories		white blood cell (count)
		WBCT	whole blood clotting time
W or A	weakness or atrophy		
WACH	wedge adjustable cushioned heel	WBD	weeks by dates (for gestational age)
WAF	weakness, atrophy, and fasciculation	WBE	weeks by examination (for gestational age)
	white adult female	WBH	weight-based heparin (dosing)
WAGR	Wilms' tumor, aniridia, genitourinary malformations, and mental retardation (syndrome)		whole-body hyperthermia
		WBI	whole bowel irrigation
		W Bld	whole blood
		WBN	wellborn nursery
		WBOS	wide base of support
		WBPTT	whole blood partial thromboplastin time
WAIS	Wechsler Adult Intelligence Scale	WBQC	wide base quad cane
WAIS-R	Wechsler Adult Intelligence Scale-Revised	WBR	whole body radiation
		WBRT	whole brain radiotherapy
		WBS	weeks by size (for gestational age)
WALK	weight activated locking knee (prosthesis)		whole body scan
		WBTF	Waring Blender tube feeding
WAM	white adult male	WBTT	weight bearing to tolerance

WBUS	weeks by ultrasound	WDWN-BM	well-developed, well-nourished black male
WBV	whole blood volume		
WC	ward clerk	WDWN-WF	well-developed, well-nourished white female
	ward confinement		
	warm compress		
	wet compresses	WE	weekend
	wheelchair	W/E	weekend
	when called	WEE	Western equine encephalitis
	white count		
	whooping cough	WEP	weekend pass
	will call	WESR	Westergren erythrocyte sedimentation rate
	workers' compensation		
WCA	work capacity assessment		Wintrobe erythrocyte sedimentation rate
WCC	well child care		
	white cell count	WEUP	willful exposure to unwanted pregnancy
WCE	white coat effect		
WCH	white coat hypertension	WF	well flexed
WC/LC	warm compresses and lid scrubs		wet film
			white female
WCM	whole cow's milk	W/F	weakness and fatigue
WCS	work capacity specialist	WFE	Williams flexion exercises
WD	ward		
	well developed	W FEEDS	with feedings
	well differentiated	WFH	white-faced hornet
	wet dressing	WFI	water for injection
	Wilson's disease	WFL	within full limits
	word		within functional limits
	working distance	WFLC	white female living child
	wound	WF-O	will follow in office
W/D	warm and dry	WFR	wheel-and-flare reaction
	withdrawal	WG	Wegener's granulomatosis
W → D	wet to dry	WGA	wheat germ agglutinin
W4D	Worth four-dot (test for fusion)	WH	walking heel (cast)
			well healed
WDCC	well-developed collateral circulation		well hydrated
		WHA	warmed humidified air
WDF	white divorced female	WHNR	well healed, no residuals
WDHA	watery diarrhea, hypokalemia, and achlorhydria	WHNS	well healed, no sequelae
			well healed, nonsymptomatic
WDHH	watery diarrhea, hypokalemia, and hypochlorhydria		well healed, no sequelae
		WHO	World Health Organization
WDLL	well-differentiated lymphocytic lymphoma		wrist-hand orthosis
		WHOART	World Health Organization Adverse Reaction Terms (Terminology)
WDM	white divorced male		
WDS	word discrimination score		

W

307

WHP	whirlpool	WMLC	white male living child
WHPB	whirlpool bath	WMM	white married male
WHR	ratio of waist to hip circumference	WMP	warm moist packs (unsterile) weight management program
WHV	woodchuck hepatitis virus		
WHVP	wedged hepatic venous pressure	WMS	Wechsler Memory Scale Wilson-Mikity syndrome
WHZ	wheezes	WMX	whirlpool, massage, and exercise
WI	ventricular demand pacing walk-in		
		WN	well nourished
W/I	within	WND	wound
W+I	work and interest	WNF	well-nourished female West Nile fever
WIA	wounded in action		
WIC	Women, Infants, and Children (program)	WNL	within normal limits
		WNM	well-nourished male
WID	widow widower	WNLS	weighted nonlinear least squares
WIED	walk-in emergency department	WNt^{50}	Wagner-Nelson time 50 hours
WIS	Ward Incapacity Scale	WO	weeks old wide open written order
WISC	Wechsler Intelligence Scale for Children		
WISC-R	Wechsler Intelligence Scale for Children-Revised	W/O	water in oil without
WK	week work	WOB	work of breathing
		WOCN	wound ostomy continence nurse
WKI	Wakefield Inventory		
WKS	Wernicke-Korsakoff Syndrome	WOP	without pain
		WP	whirlpool
WL	waiting list wave length weight loss	WPBT	whirlpool, body temperature
		WPCs	washed packed cells
WLE	wide local excision	WPFM	Wright peak flow meter
WLM	working level months	WPOA	wearing patch on arrival
WLS	wet lung syndrome	WPP	Wechsler Preschool Primary Scale of Intelligence
WLT	waterload test		
WM	wall motion warm, moist wet mount white male whole milk	WPPSI	Wechsler Preschool Primary Scale of Intelligence
		WPPSI-R	WPPSI revised
WMA	wall motion abnormality	WPW	Wolff-Parkinson-White (syndrome)
WMD	warm moist dressings (sterile)		
		WR	Wassermann reaction wrist
WMF	white married female		
WMI	wall motion index	WRA	with-the-rule astigmatism
WML	white matter lesions (cerebral)	WRAT	Wide Range Achievement Test

WRAT-R	The Wide Range Achievement Test, Revised		**X**
WRBC	washed red blood cells		
WRC	washed red (blood) cells		
WRIOT	Wide Range Interest-Opinion Test (for career planning)	X	break
			cross
WRT	weekly radiation therapy		crossmatch
WRUED	work-related upper-extremity disorder		exophoria for distance
			extra
WS	walking speed		female sex chromosome
	ward secretary		start of anesthesia
	watt seconds		ten
	Williams syndrome		times
	work simplification		xylocaine
	work simulation	$\bar{x}$	except
	work status	X'	exophoria at 33 cm
W&S	wound and skin	X^2	chi-square
WSepF	white separated female	X+#	xyphoid plus number of fingerbreadths
WSepM	white separated male		
WSF	white single female	$\bar{x}$	mean
WSM	white single male	X3	orientation as to time, place and person
WSP	wearable speech processor		
WT	walking tank	XBT	xylose breath test
	weight (wt)	XC	excretory cystogram
	wild type (strains of infection)	XCF	aortic cross clamp off
		XCO	aortic cross clamp on
	Wilms' tumor	XD	times daily
	wisdom teeth	X&D	examination and diagnosis
0WT	zero work tolerance	X2d	times two days
W-T-D	wet to dry	XDP	xeroderma pigmentosum
WTP	willingness to pay	Xe	xenon
WTS	whole tomography slice	^{133}Xe	xenon, isotope of mass 133
W/U	workup		
WV	whispered voice	XeCT	xenon-enhanced computed tomography
W/V	weight-to-volume ratio		
WW	Weight Watchers	X-ed	crossed
	wheeled walker	XEM	xonics electron mammography
WWI	World War One		
WWII	World War Two	XES	x-ray energy spectrometer
W/W	weight-to-weight ratio	XFER	transfer
W→W	wet to wet	XGP	xanthogranulomatous pyelonephritis
WWAC	walk with aid of cane		
WW Brd	whole wheat bread	XI	eleven
WWidF	white widowed female	XII	twelve
WWidM	white widowed male	XIP	x-ray in plaster
WWW	World Wide Web	XKO	not knocked out
WYOU	women years of usage	XL	extended release (once a

X

	day oral solid dosage form)	XY	normal male sex chromosome type
	extra large	XYL	Xylocaine®
	forty		xylose
XLA	X-linked infantile agammaglobulinemia	XYLO	Xylocaine®
X-leg	cross leg		
XLFDP	cross-linked fibrin degradation products		
XLH	X-linked hypophos-phatemia		
XLJR	X-linked juvenile retinoschisis		
XLMR	X-linked mental retardation		
XM	crossmatch		
X-mat.	crossmatch		
XMM	xeromammography		
XNA	xenoreactive natural antibodies		
XOM	extraocular movements		
XOP	x-ray out of plaster		
XP	xeroderma pigmentosum		
XR	x-ray		
XRT	radiation therapy		
XS	excessive		
X-SCID	X-linked severe combined immunodeficiency disease		
XS-LIM	exceeds limits of procedure		
XT	exotropia		
	extract		
	extracted		
X(T')	intermittent exotropia at 33 cm		
X(T)	intermittent exotropia		
XTLE	extratemporal-lobe epilepsy		
XU	excretory urogram		
XULN	times upper limit of normal		
XV	fifteen		
3X/WK	three times a week		
XX	normal female sex chromosome type		
	twenty		
XX/XY	sex karyotypes		
XXX	thirty		

Y

Y	male sex chromosome
	year
	yellow
YAC	yeast artificial chromosome
YACs	yeast artificial chromosomes
YACP	young adult chronic patient
YAG	yttrium aluminum garnet (laser)
YAS	youth action section (police)
Yb	ytterbium
YBOCS	Yale-Brown Obsessive-Compulsive Scale
Yel	yellow
YF	yellow fever
YFH	yellow-faced hornet
YFI	yellow fever immunization
YHL	years of healthy life
YJV	yellow jacket venom
Y2K	year 2,000
YLC	youngest living child
YLD	years of life with disability
YLL	years of life lost
YMC	young male Caucasian
YMRS	Young Mania Rating Scale
Y/N	yes/no
YO	years old
YOB	year of birth
YOD	year of death
YORA	younger-onset rheumatoid arthritis
YPC	YAG (yttrium aluminum garnet) posterior capsulotomy
YPLL	years of potential life lost before age 65

Y

Z

Z	impedance
ZDV	zidovudine (Retrovir)
Z-E	Zollinger-Ellison (syndrome)
ZEEP	zero end-expiratory pressure
ZES	Zollinger-Ellison syndrome
Z-ESR	zeta erythrocyte sedimentation rate
ZIFT	zygote intrafallopian (tube) transfer
ZIG	zoster serum immune globulin
ZIP	zoster immune plasma
ZMC	zygomatic zygomatic maxillary compound (complex)
Zn	zinc
ZnO	zinc oxide
ZnOE	zinc oxide and eugenol
ZnPc	zinc phthalocyanine
ZNS	zonisamide
ZOT	zonula occludens toxin
ZPC	zero point of charge zopiclone
z-Plasty	surgical relaxation of contracture
ZPO	zinc peroxide
ZPP	zinc protoporphyrin
ZPT	zinc pyrithione
ZSB	zero stools since birth
ZSR	zeta sedimentation rate
ZSRDS	Zung Self-Rating Depression Scale

Chapter 4

Symbols and Numbers

↑	above alive elevated greater than high improved increase rising up upper	↔	same as stable to and from unchanging
		⇊	flexor plantar response (Babinski) testes descended
		⇈	extensor
↑g	increasing		extensor response (positive Babinsky)
↓	dead decrease depressed diminished down falling lower lowered normal plantar reflex restricted		testes undescended
		‖	parallel parallel bars
		√	check flexion
		√'d	checked
		√'ing	checking
↓g	decreasing	#	fracture number pound weight
→	causes to greater than progressing results in showed to the right transfer to	∴	therefore
		∵	because
		Δ scan	delta scan (computed tomography scan)
←	less than resulted from to the left	+	plus positive present

–	absent minus negative	~	about approximately difference
		≈	approximately equal to
/	slash mark signifying per, and, or with (this is a dangerous symbol as it is mistaken for a one)	≡	identical
		×	left ear-air conduction threshold ten
		]	left ear-masked bone conduction threshold
±	either positive or negative no definite cause plus or minus very slight trace	△	right ear-masked air conduction threshold change
└ ┌	right lower quadrant right upper quadrant	[	right ear-masked bone conduction threshold
┐ ┘	left upper quadrant left lower quadrant	⊖	reversible
		?	questionable not tested
>	greater than left ear-bone conduction threshold	∅	no none without
≥	greater than or equal to	@	at
<	caused by less than right ear-bone conduction threshold	1/2 and 1/2	half Dakin's solution and half glycerin
		1°	first degree primary
		1:1	one-to-one (individual session with staff)
≤	less than or equal to		
≮	not less than		
≯	not more than	2°	second degree secondary
∧	above diastolic blood pressure increased	2×2	gauze dressing folded 2″×2″
∨	below systolic blood pressure	3°	tertiary third degree
≠	not equal to	3×	three times
≅	approximately equal to	4×4	gauze dressing folded 4″×4″
=	equal equal to	5+2	cytarabine and daunorubicin

24°	twenty-four hours (24 hr is safer as the ° is seen as a zero)	■	deceased male
		●	deceased female
		□	living male
			left ear-masked air conduction threshold
777	Ortho Novum 777® (a triphasic oral contraceptive)		
		○	living female respiration
1,000	one thousand (1^3)		right ear-air conduction threshold
10,000	ten thousand (1^4)		
100,000	one hundred thousand (1^5)	◇	sex unknown
1,000,000	one million (1^6)		
10,000,000	ten million (1^7)	(□)	adopted living male
100,000,000	one hundred million (1^8)	*	birth
		†	dead
1,000,000,000	one billion (1^9)		death
i	one (Roman numerals are dangerous expressions and should not be used)	♀	standing
		○—<	recumbent position
ii	two	♀,	sitting position
iii	three		
iiii	four	♥	heart
iv	four (this is a dangerous abbreviation as it is read as intravenous, use 4)	A α	alpha
		β B	beta
		Γ γ	gamma
		Δ δ	anion gap
v	five		change
vi	six		delta
vii	seven		delta gap
viii	eight		prism diopter
ix	nine		temperature
			trimester
x	ten		
xi	eleven	E ε	epsilon
xii	twelve	Z ζ	zeta
XL	forty	H η	eta
	extended release dosage form	Θ θ	negative
			theta
i̇	one		
ɪ̇ɪ	two	I ι	iota
♂	male	K κ	kappa
♀	female	Λ λ	lambda
♂̈	gay	M μ	micro
♀̈	lesbian		mu

N ν	nu		phi
Ξ ξ	xi		thyroid
O o	omicron	X χ	chi
Π π	pi	Ψ ψ	psi
P ρ	rho		psychiatric
Σ σ	sigma	Ω ω	omega
	sum of	'	feet
	summary		minutes (as in 30')
		"	inches
T τ	tau		seconds
Y υ	upsilon	⊙	start of an operation
Φ φ	phenyl	⊗	end of anesthesia

Numbers and letters for teeth

Two adult numbering systems and a deciduous system are shown. The adult systems are shown as numbers, whereas deciduous teeth are lettered. The system commonly used in the U.S. is 1 to 32 (shown in bold face type).

1 (18) upper right 3rd molar
2 (17) (A) upper right 2nd molar
3 (16) (B) upper right 1st molar
4 (15) upper right 2nd bicuspid
5 (14) upper right 1st bicuspid
6 (13) (C) upper right canine (eyetooth)
7 (12) (D) upper right lateral incisor
8 (11) (E) upper right central incisor
9 (21) (F) upper left central incisor
10 (22) (G) upper left lateral incisor
11 (23) (H) upper left canine
12 (24) upper left 1st bicuspid
13 (25) upper left 2nd bicuspid
14 (26) (I) upper left 1st molar
15 (27) (J) upper left 2nd molar
16 (28) upper left 3rd molar

17 (38) lower left 3rd molar
18 (37) (K) lower left 2nd molar
19 (36) (L) lower left 1st molar
20 (35) lower left 2nd bicuspid
21 (34) lower left 1st bicuspid
22 (33) (M) lower left canine
23 (32) (N) lower left lateral incisor
24 (31) (O) lower left central incisor
25 (41) (P) lower right central incisor
26 (42) (Q) lower right lateral incisor
27 (43) (R) lower right canine
28 (44) lower right 1st bicuspid
29 (45) lower right 2nd bicuspid
30 (46) (S) lower right 1st molar
31 (47) (T) lower right 2nd molar
32 (48) lower right 3rd molar

UPPER																UPPER
	1	**2**	**3**	**4**	**5**	**6**	**7**	**8**	**9**	**10**	**11**	**12**	**13**	**14**	**15**	**16**
	18	17	16	15	14	13	12	11	21	22	23	24	25	26	27	28
Right	A	B			C	D	E		F	G	H			I	J		**Left**
	T	S			R	Q	P		O	N	M			L	K	
	48	47	46	45	44	43	42	41	31	32	33	34	35	36	37	38
	32	**31**	**30**	**29**	**28**	**27**	**26**	**25**	**24**	**23**	**22**	**21**	**20**	**19**	**18**	**17**
LOWER																LOWER

Shorthand for laboratory test values

See text for meaning of the abbreviations shown

Complete Blood Count

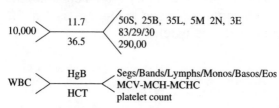

Electrolytes

142	99	sodium	chloride
4.7	25	potassium	bicarbonate

SMA 6 (Astra 7)

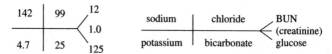

Blood Gases
7.4/80/48/98/25   pH/PO$_2$/PCO$_2$/% O$_2$ saturation/bicarbonate

Obstetrical shorthand

$$\frac{2 \text{ cm} \mid 80\%}{-2 \text{ Vtx}}$$ 2 cm = dilation of cervix

80% = degree of cer-   Vtx = vertex; presen-
vix effacement   tation of fetus,
                                      (breech = Br)

−2 = station; distance
       above (−) or
       below (+) the
       spine of the ischium measured in cm

318

Reflexes[1]

Reflexes are usually graded on a 0 to 4+ scale

4+ may indicate disease
    often associated with clonus
    very brisk, hyperactive (or ++++)
3+ brisker than average
    possibly but not necessarily indicative of disease
      (or +++)
2+ average
    normal (or ++)
1+ low normal
    somewhat diminished (or +)
0   may indicate neuropathy
    no response

Muscle strength[1]

0—No muscular contraction detected
1—A barely detectable flicker or trace of contraction
2—Active movement of the body part with gravity eliminated
3—Active movement against gravity
4—Active movement against gravity and some resistance
5—Active movement against full resistance without evident
    fatigue. This is normal muscle strength

Pulse[1]

 0 completely absent
+1 markedly impaired (or 1+, or +)
+2 modererately impaired (or 2+, or ++)
+3 slightly impaired (or 3+, or +++)
+4 normal (or 4+, or ++++)

Gradation of intensity of heart murmurs[1]

1/6 or I/VI   may not be heard in all positions
                very faint, heard only after the listener has
                  "tuned in"
2/6 or II/VI   quiet, but heard immediately upon placing
                  the stethoscope on the chest
3/6 or III/VI   moderately loud
4/6 or IV/VI   loud
5/6 orV/VI   very loud, may be heard with a stethoscope
                  partly off the chest (thrills are associated)
6/6 or VI/VI   may be heard with the stethoscope entirely
                  off the chest (thrills are associated)

Tonsil Size

0 no tonsils
1 less than normal
2 normal
3 greater than normal
4 touching

Apothecary symbols (Should never be used)

The symbols presented below are for informational use. The apothecary system should *not* be used. Only the metric system should be used. The methods of expressing the symbols, the meanings, and the equivalence are not the classic ones, nor are they accurate, but reflect the usual intended meanings when used by some older physicians in writing prescription directions.

ℨ or ℨ i̇	dram, teaspoonful, (5 mL)	℥ or ℥ i̇	ounce, (30 mL)
		gr	grain (approximately 60 mg)
ℨ ii̇	two drams, 2 teaspoonfuls, (10 mL)	ℳ	minim (approximately 0.06 mL)
ℨ ss	half ounce, tablespoonful, (15 mL)	gtt	drop

Reference

1. Bates B. A guide to physical examinations and history taking, 6th ed. Philadelphia: J.B. Lippincott; 1995.

Chapter 5

Pharmaceutical Generic Name and Trademark Cross-Reference Index

Listed below is a cross-referenced index of generic and trademark drug names. Generic names begin with a lower case letter while trademarks begin with a capital letter. This partial list consists of frequently prescribed and new drugs.

The meanings of abbreviated and coded drug names can be found in Chapter 3 (Lettered Abbreviations and Acronyms).

Complete indices of United States drug names can be found in current editions of Drug Facts and Comparisons[1], the American Drug Index[2], and Physicians GenRx[3]. A complete list of world-wide names may be found in Martindales.[4] These and other references should be used to determine the equivalence of products, strengths, and dosage forms. Although several products may be listed under one generic name they may differ in strength, dosage form, or concentration available, as is the case with estradiol transdermal (Climara, Estraderm, and Vivelle).

Some products are marketed without a trademark, as in the case of thioguanine. In such cases only the generic names are listed. When a product is often prescribed and/or labeled generically, the generic name is shown in italics.

The following abbreviations are used in this listing:

EC	enteric coated	SR	sustained release tablets or capsules
HCl	hydrochloride		(and other forms of extended
IM	intramuscular		release)
IV	intravenous	susp	suspension
inj	injection	(W)	withdrawn or discontinued from
oint	ointment		US market
ophth	ophthalmic	(WA)	withdrawn or discontinued from
soln	solution		US market but available under
			different name from another
			manufacturer

A

Abbokinase	urokinase
abciximab	ReoPro
Abelcet	amphotericin B lipid complex
acarbose	Precose
Accolate	zafirlukast
Accupril	quinapril HCl
Accutane	isotretinoin
acebutolol HCl	Sectral
Acel-Imune	diphtheria & tetanus toxoids & acellular pertussis vaccine
acetaminophen	paracetamol Tylenol
acetaminophen 300 mg with Codeine Phosphate (15, 30, and 60 mg)	Phenaphen with Codeine (#2, 3, and 4) Tylenol with Codeine (#2, 3, and 4)
acetazolamide	Diamox
acetohexamide	Dymelor
acetohydroxamic acid	Lithostat
acetylcholine ophth	Miochol E
acetylcysteine	Mucomyst
Achromycin (WA)	tetracycline HCl
acitretin	Soriatane
Acthar	corticotropin
ActHIB/Tripedia	*Haemophilus b* conjugate vaccine reconstituted with diphtheria and tetanus toxoids and acellular pertussis vaccine adsorbed
Acthrel	corticorellin ovine triflutate
Actifed	triprolidine HCl; pseudo-ephedrine HCl
Actigall	ursodiol
Activase	alteplase, recombi-nant
Actonel	risedronate sodium
Acular	ketorolac tromethamine ophth
acyclovir	Zovirax
Adalat	nifedipine
Adalat CC	nifedipine SR
adapalene	Differin
Adapin	doxepin HCl
Adderall	amphetamine; dextroamphet-amine mixed salts
adefovir dipivoxil	Preveon
Adenocard	adenosine
adenosine	Adenocard
Adrenalin	epinephrine
Adriamycin	doxorubicin HCl
Advil	ibuprofen
AeroBid	flunisolide
Afrin nasal spray	oxymetazoline HCl
Aggrastat	tirofiban HCl
Agrylin	anagrelide HCl
Akineton	biperiden
alatrovafloxacin mesylate IV	Trovan inj
albendazole	Albenza
Albenza	albendazole
albumin human	Albuminar Albutein Buminate

	Plasbumin	alprostadil	Caverject
albumin	Albunex		Edex
(human),			Prostin VR
sonicated		alprostadil	Muse
Albuminar	albumin human	urethral	
Albunex	albumin	suppository	
	(human),	Alrex	loteprednol
	sonicated		etabonate
Albutein	albumin human		ophth susp
albuterol	Proventil	Altace	ramipril
	salbutamol	alteplase,	Activase
	Ventolin	recombinant	
albuterol SR	Proventil	altretamine	Hexalen
	Repetabs	aluminum	Domeboro
	Volmax	acetate	
albuterol sulfate	Proventil HFA	aluminum	Basaljel
inhalation		carbonate	
aerosol		aluminum	Amphojel
Aldactazide	spironolactone;	hydroxide	
	hydrochloro-	aluminum	Maalox
	thiazide	hydroxide;	
Aldactone	spironolactone	magnesium	
Aldara	imiquimod	hydroxide	
	cream	Alupent	metaproterenol
aldesleukin	Proleukin		sulfate
Aldomet	methyldopa	amantadine HCl	Symmetrel
Aldoril	methyldopa;	Amaryl	glimepiride
	hydrochloro-	Ambien	zolpidem
	thiazide		tartrate
alendronate	Fosamax	AmBisome	liposomal
sodium			amphotericin
Alesse	levonorgestrel;		B
	ethinyl	amcinonide	Cyclocort
	estradiol	Amerge	naratriptan
Alfenta	alfentanil HCl		HCl
alfentanil HCl	Alfenta	Amicar	aminocaproic
alglucerase	Ceredase		acid
Allegra	fexofenadine	Amidate	etomidate
	HCl	amifostine	Ethyol
Alkeran	melphalan	amikacin sulfate	Amikin
allopurinol	Zyloprim	Amikin	amikacin
Alomide	lodoxamide		sulfate
	tromethamine	amiloride HCl	Midamor
	ophth soln	amiloride; hydro-	Moduretic
Alphagan	brimonidine	chlorothiazide	
	tartrate	amino acid inj	Aminosyn
	ophth		Travasol
alprazolam	Xanax		TrophAmine

amino acid with electrolytes in dextrose with calcium inj (various concentrations)	Clinimix E		cholesteryl sulfate
		amphotericin B	Fungizone
		amphotericin B cholesteryl sulfate	Amphotec
aminocaproic acid	Amicar	amphotericin B lipid complex	Abelcet
aminocaproic acid gel	Caprogel	*ampicillin*	Principen
aminogluteth-imide	Cytadren	ampicillin sodium; sulbactam sodium	Unasyn
aminophylline	aminophylline		
Aminosyn	amino acid inj	amrinone lactate	Inocor
amiodarone HCl	Cordarone		
amitriptyline HCl	Elavil Endep	amsacrine	Amsidyl
		Amsidyl	amsacrine
AmLactin	ammonium lactate lotion	Amvisc	sodium hyaluronate
amlexanox oral paste	Aphthasol	Amytal	amobarbital sodium
amlodipine besylate	Norvasc	Anadrol-50	oxymetholone
		Anafranil	clomipramine HCl
amlodipine besylate; benazepril HCl	Lotrel	anagrelide HCl	Agrylin
		Anaprox	naproxen sodium
ammonium lactate lotion	AmLactin	anastrozole	Arimidex
		Anbesol	benzocaine
amobarbital sodium	Amytal	Ancef	cefazolin sodium
amoxapine	Asendin	Ancobon	flucytosine
amoxicillin	Amoxil Trimox Wymox	Androderm	testosterone transdermal system
amoxicillin; clavulanic acid	Augmentin	Androgel-DHT	dihydrotestosterone transdermal
Amoxil	amoxicillin	Anectine	succinylcholine chloride
amphetamine resins (W)	Biphetamine (W)	Anexsia	hydrocodone bitartrate; acetamino-phen
amphetamine; dextroamphet-amine mixed salts	Adderall		
		Ansaid	flurbiprofen
		Antabuse	disulfiram
Amphojel	aluminum hydroxide	Antilirium	physostigmine salicylate
Amphotec	amphotericin B	antipyrine otic	Auralgan

Antivert	meclizine	aspirin 325 mg	Empirin with
Antizol	fomepizole	with codeine	codeine #3
Anturane	sulfinpyrazone	phosphate (30	and #4
Anzemet	dolasetron	and 60 mg)	
	mesylate	aspirin buffered	Bufferin
Aphthasol	amlexanox oral	*aspirin EC*	Ecotrin
	paste	Astelin	azelastine HCl
A.P.L.	chorionic		nasal spray
	gonadotropin	astemizole	Hismanal
apligraf	Graftskin	Atacand	candesartan
Aplisol	tuberculin skin		cilexetil
	test		hydroxyzine HCl
Apresazide	hydralazine HCl;	Atarax	
	hydrochloro-	*atenolol*	Tenormin
	thiazide	atenolol;	Tenoretic
		chlorthalidone	
Apresoline	hydralazine HCl	Atgam	lymphocyte
aprotinin	Trasylol		immune
AquaMEPHY-	phytonadione		globulin
TON		Ativan	lorazepam
Aquasol A	vitamin A	atorvastatin	Lipitor
Aralen	chloroquine	calcium	
	phosphate	atovaquone	Mepron
Aramine	metaraminol	atracurium	Tracrium
	bitartrate	besylate	
Arava	leflunomide	Atridox	doxycycline
arbutamine HCl	GenEsa		hyclate gel
arcitumomab	CEA-Scan	Atromid-S	clofibrate
ardeparin sodium	Normiflo	atropine sulfate	Sal-Tropine
Arduan	pipecuronium	tablets	
	bromide	Atrovent	ipratropium
Aredia	pamidronate		bromide
	disodium	Augmentin	amoxicillin;
Arfonad	trimethaphan		clavulanic acid
	camsylate	Auralgan	antipyrine otic
arginine HCl	R-Gene	auranofin	Ridaura
Aricept	donepezil HCl	Aurolate	gold sodium
Arimidex	anastrozole		thiomalate
Aristocort	triamcinolone	aurothioglucose	Solganal
	acetonide	Avapro	irbesartan
Arlidin (W)	nylidrin HCl (W)	Aventyl	nortriptyline HCl
Artane	trihexyphenidyl	Avita	tretinoin cream
	HCl		0.025%
Arthrotec	diclofenac	Avitene	collagen
	sodium;		hemostat
	misoprostol	Avonex	interferon
Asacol	mesalamine		beta-la
Asendin	amoxapine	Axid	nizatidine
asparaginase	Elspar	Azactam	aztreonam

azatadine maleate	Optimine	beclomethasone dipropionate	Beclovent
azathioprine	Imuran		Beconase AQ Nasal
azelaic acid cream	Azelex		Vancenase
azelastine HCl nasal spray	Astelin		Vancenase AQ Nasal
Azelex	azelaic acid cream		Vanceril
azithromycin	Zithromax	Beclovent	beclomethasone dipropionate
Azmacort	triamcinolone acetonide aerosol	Beconase AQ Nasal	beclomethasone dipropionate
Azopt	brinzolamide ophth susp	belladonna alkaloids; phenobarbital	Donnatal
aztreonam	Azactam	Bellergal-S	phenobarbital; ergotamine; belladonna
Azulfidine	sulfasalazine	Benadryl	diphenhydramine HCl
		benazepril HCl	Lotensin
		BeneFix	factor IX, concentrate

B

		Benemid	probenecid
		bentoquatam	IvyBlock
		Bentyl	dicyclomine HCl
Baciguent	bacitracin ointment	benzocaine	Anbesol
bacitracin ointment	Baciguent		Hurricaine
baclofen	Lioresal		Orabase
Bactrim	sulfamethoxazole; trimethoprim		Orajel
		benzocaine; tetracaine HCl	Cetacaine
Bactroban	mupirocin nasal ointment	benztropine mesylate	Cogentin
BAL in Oil	dimercaprol	bepridil	Vascor
Basaljel	aluminum carbonate	beractant	Survanta
		Berroca	vitamin B complex; folic acid; vitamin C
balsalazide disodium	Colazide		
basiliximab	Simulect	Betadine	povidone iodine
Baycol	cerivastatin sodium	Betagan	levobunolol HCl
BCG intravesical	TheraCys TICE BCG	betaine anhydrous	Cystadane
		betamethasone	Celestone
		betamethasone dipropionate	Diprosone
becaplermin gel	Regranex	betamethasone; clotrimazole cream	Lotrisone

Betapace	sotalol	fumarate; hydrochlorothiazide	
Betaseron	interferon beta-1b		
betaxolol	Kerlone	bitolterol mesylate	Tornalate
betaxolol HCl ophth soln	Betoptic	Blenoxane	bleomycin sulfate
betaxolol HCl ophth susp	Betoptic S	bleomycin sulfate	Blenoxane
betaxolol HCl; pilocarpine HCl ophth soln	Betoptic Pilo	Blocadren	timolol maleate
		B & O Supprettes	opium; belladonna suppositories
bethanechol chloride	Urecholine		
Betoptic	betaxolol HCl ophth soln	Botox	botulinum toxin type A
Betoptic Pilo	betaxolol HCl; pilocarpine HCl, ophth soln	botulinum toxin type A	Botox
		Brethaire	terbutaline sulfate aerosol
Betoptic S	betaxolol HCl ophth suspension	Brethine	terbutaline sulfate tablets and inj
Biaxin	clarithromycin	bretylium tosylate	Bretylol
bicalutamide	Casodex		
Bicillin C-R	penicillin G benzathine; penicillin G procaine (for IM use only)	Bretylol	bretylium tosylate
		Brevibloc	esmolol HCl
		Brevital Sodium	methohexital sodium
Bicillin L-A	penicillin G benzathine (for IM use only)	Bricanyl	terbutaline sulfate tablets and inj
Bicitra	sodium citrate; citric acid	brimonidine tartrate ophth	Alphagan
BiCNU	carmustine	brinzolamide ophth suspension	Azopt
Bilopaque	tyropanoate sodium		
biperiden	Akineton	bromfenac sodium (W)	Duract (W)
Biphetamine (W)	amphetamine resins (W)	bromocriptine mesylate	Parlodel
bisacodyl	Dulcolax		
bismuth subsalicylate; metronidazole; tetracycline HCl	Helidac	brompheniramine maleate	Dimetane
		brompheniramine maleate; phenylpropanolamime	Dimetapp Extentabs
bisoprolol	Ziac		

Bronkometer	isoetharine HCl aerosol	Cafergot	ergotamine tartrate; caffeine
Bronkosol	isoetharine HCl soln	Cafcit	caffeine citrate inj
Bucladin-S	buclizine HCl	caffeine citrate inj	Cafcit
buclizine HCl	Bucladin-S	Calan SR	verapamil HCl SR
budesonide inhalation powder	Pulmicort Turbuhaler	Calciferol	ergocalciferol
budesonide nasal inhaler	Rhinocort	Calcimar calcipotriene cream	calcitonin Dovonex
Bufferin	aspirin buffered	calcitonin	Calcimar
bumetanide	Bumex	calcitonin-salmon	Miacalcin
Bumex	bumetanide	calcium carbonate	Os-Cal 500 Tums
Buminate	albumin human	calfactant intratracheal susp	Infasurf
Buphenyl	phenylbutyrate sodium		
bupivacaine HCl	Marcaine HCl	camphorated tincture of opium	paregoric
bupropion HCl	Wellbutrin		
bupropion HCl SR	Wellbutrin SR Zyban	Camptosar	irinotecan HCl
BuSpar	buspirone HCl	candesartan cilexetil	Atacand
buspirone HCl	BuSpar	Capastat Sulfate	capreomycin sulfate
busulfan	Myleran		
Busulfanex	busulfan inj	capecitabine	Xeloda
busulfan inj	Busulfanex	Capital w/ Codeine Suspension	codeine phosphate; acetaminophen suspension
butabarbital sodium	Butisol		
butalbital; acetaminophen; caffeine	Fioricet	Capitrol	chloroxine
		Capoten	captopril
butalbital; aspirin; caffeine	Fiorinal	capreomycin sulfate	Capastat Sulfate
butenafine HCl	Mentax	Caprogel	aminocaproic acid gel
Butisol	butabarbital sodium		
butorphanol tartrate inj	Stadol	capromab pendetide	ProstaScint
butorphanol tartrate nasal spray	Stadol NS	captopril	Capoten
		Carafate	sucralfate
		carbachol	Isopto Carbachol
C			
		carbamazepine	Tegretol
cabergoline	Dostinex	carbamazepine SR	Carbatrol Tegretol-XR

carbamide peroxide otic	Debrox	Cefizox	ceftizoxime sodium
Carbatrol	carbamazepine SR	Cefobid	cefoperazone sodium
carbenicillin	Geocillin	cefonicid sodium	Monocid
Carbex	selegiline	cefoperazone sodium	Cefobid
Carbocaine	mepivacaine HCl	Cefotan	cefotetan
carboplatin	Paraplatin	cefotaxime sodium	Claforan
Cardene	nicardipine HCl	cefotetan	Cefotan
Cardiotec	technetium Tc-99m teboroxime kit	cefoxitin sodium	Mefoxin
		cefpodoxime proxetil	Vantin
Cardizem	diltiazem HCl	cefprozil	Cefzil
Cardizem CD	diltiazem HCl SR	ceftazidime	Ceptaz
			Fortaz
Cardura	doxazosin mesylate		Tazicef
			Tazidime
carisoprodol	Soma	ceftibuten	Cedax
carmustine	BiCNU	Ceftin	cefuroxime axetil
carmustine implantable wafer	Gliadel	ceftizoxime sodium	Cefizox
Carnitor	levocarnitine	ceftriaxone sodium	Rocephin
Cartia XR	diltiazem HCl SR	cefuroxime axetil	Ceftin
carvedilol	Coreg	cefuroxime sodium	Kefurox
Casodex	bicalutamide		Zinacef
Cataflam	diclofenac potassium	Cefzil	cefprozil
		Celestone	betamethasone
Catapres	clonidine HCl	Celexa	citalopram hydrobromide
Caverject	alprostadil		
CEA-SCAN	arcitumomab	CellCept	mycophenolate mofetil
Ceclor	cefaclor		
Cedax	ceftibuten	Centrum	vitamins; minerals
CeeNu	lomustine		
cefaclor	Ceclor	cephalexin	Keflex
cefadroxil	Duricef	cephalexin HCl	Keftab
Cefadyl	cephapirin sodium	cephalothin sodium (W)	Keflin (W)
cefamandole nafate	Mandol	cephapirin sodium	Cefadyl
cefazolin sodium	Ancef	cephradine	Velosef
	Kefzol	Cephulac	lactulose
cefdinir	Omnicef	Ceptaz	ceftazidime
cefepime HCl	Maxipime		
cefixime	Suprax		

C
Rx

329

Cerebyx	fosphenytoin sodium	chlorprothixene (W)	Taractan (W)
Ceredase	alglucerase	chlorthalidone	Hygroton
Cerezyme	imiglucerase	chlorthalidone;	Regroton
cerivastatin sodium	Baycol	reserpine	
Cerubidine	daunorubicin HCl	Chlor-Trimeton	chlorpheniramine maleate
Cervidil	dinoprostone vaginal insert	chlorzoxazone 250 mg	Paraflex
Cetacaine	benzocaine; tetracaine HCl	chlorzoxazone 500 mg	Parafon Forte DSC
		Cholebrine	iocetamic acid
cetirizine HCl	Zyrtec	Choledyl	oxtriphylline
chloral hydrate	chloral hydrate	cholestyramine	Questran
chlorambucil	Leukeran	choline chloride inj	Intrachol
chloramphenicol	Chloromycetin		
chloramphenicol ophth	Chloroptic ophth	choline magnesium trisalicylate	Trilisate
chlordiazepoxide HCl	Librium	Choloxin	dextrothyroxine sodium
chlordiazepoxide HCl; amitriptyline HCl	Limbitrol	chorionic gonadotropin	A.P.L.
		Chronulac	lactulose
		Chymodiactin	chymopapain
chlorhexidine gluconate	Hibiclens PerioChip	chymopapain	Chymodiactin
		Cibalith-S	lithium citrate
chlorhexidine gluconate mouth rinse	Peridex	cidofovir	Vistide
		cilostazol	Pletal
		Ciloxan	ciprofloxacin ophth soln
Chloromycetin	chloramphenicol	cimetidine HCl	Tagamet
chloroprocaine HCl	Nesacaine	Cipro	ciprofloxacin HCl
Chloroptic ophth	chloramphenicol ophth	ciprofloxacin HCl	Cipro
chloroquine phosphate	Aralen	ciprofloxacin; hydrocortisone otic	Cipro HC Otic
chlorothiazide	Diuril		
chlorotrianisene (W)	TACE (W)	ciprofloxacin ophth soln	Ciloxan
chloroxine	Capitrol	Cipro HC Otic	ciprofloxacin; hydrocortisone otic
chlorpheniramine maleate	Chlor-Trimeton		
chlorpheniramine maleate SR	Teldrin	cisapride	Propulsid
		cisatracurium besylate	Nimbex
chlorpromazine	Thorazine		
chlorpropamide	Diabinese	cisplatin	Platinol AQ

citalopram hydrobromide	Celexa	clorazepate dipotassium	Tranxene
cladribine	Leustatin	Clorpactin WCS-90	oxychlorosene sodium
Claforan	cefotaxime sodium	clotrimazole	Gyne-Lotrimin
clarithromycin	Biaxin		Lotrimin
Claritin	loratadine		Mycelex
Claritin D	loratadine; pseudoephed-rine sulfate	clozapine	Clozaril
		Clozaril	clozapine
		coal tar product	Zetar
clemastine fumarate	Tavist	codeine phosphate; acetaminophen suspension	Capital w/ Codeine Suspension
Cleocin	clindamycin HCl		
clidinium bromide	Quarzan	Cogentin	benztropine mesylate
clidinium; chlordiaze-poxide	Librax	Cognex	tacrine HCl
		Colace	docusate sodium
Climara	estradiol transdermal	Colazide	balsalazide disodium
		ColBENEMID (W)	probenecid; colchicine (W)
clindamycin HCl	Cleocin	colchicine	colchicine
clindamycin phosphate pledgets	Clindets	Colestid	colestipol HCl
		colestipol HCl	Colestid
Clindets	clindamycin phosphate pledgets	colistimethate sodium	Coly-Mycin M
Clinimix E	amino acid with electrolytes in dextrose with calcium inj (various concentrations)	colistin sulfate; hydrocortisone, and neomycin otic soln	Coly-Mycin S
		collagen hemostat	Avitene
		collagenase	Santyl
Clinoril	sulindac	Collyrium	tetrahydrozoline HCl ophth
clioquinol	Vioform		
clofibrate	Atromid-S	Colomed	short chain fatty acids enema
Clomid	clomiphene citrate	Coly-Mycin M	colistimethate sodium
clomiphene citrate	Clomid	Coly-Mycin S	colistin sulfate; hydrocortisone, and neomycin otic soln
clomipramine HCl	Anafranil		
clonazepam	Klonopin		
clonidine HCl	Catapres	CoLyte	polyethylene glycol-electrolyte soln
clonidine HCl inj	Duraclon		
clopidogrel bisulfate	Plavix		

C
Rx

CombiPatch	norethindrone acetate; estradiol transdermal	Coumadin	warfarin sodium
		Covera HS	verapamil HCl SR bedtime formulation
Combivent	ipratropium bromide; albuterol sulfate	Cozaar	losartan potassium
		Crinone	progesterone gel
Combivir	lamivudine; zidovudine	Crixivan	indinavir
		cromolyn sodium	Gastrocrom
Compazine	prochlorperazine		Intal
Comvax	*Haemophilus b* conjugate; Hepatitis B vaccine		Nasalcrom
			Opticrom
		crotamiton	Eurax
Condylox	podofilox gel	Crystodigin	digitoxin
Copaxone	glatiramer acetate	Cuprimine	penicillamine
		Curosurf	poractant alpha intratracheal susp
Cordarone	amiodarone HCl		
		Cutivate	fluticasone propionate cream & ointment
Coreg	carvedilol		
Corgard	nadolol		
Corlopam	fenoldopam mesylate	cyanocobalamin nasal gel	Nascobal
Cortef	hydrocortisone	cyclobenzaprine HCl	Flexeril
corticorellin ovine triflutate	Acthrel		
		Cyclocort	amcinonide
corticotropin	Acthar	Cyclogyl	cyclopentolate HCl
cortisone acetate	Cortone Acetate		
Cortone Acetate	cortisone acetate	cyclopentolate HCl	Cyclogyl
Cortrosyn	cosyntropin		
Corvert	ibutilide fumarate	cyclophospha-mide	Cytoxan Neosar
Cosmegen	dactinomycin		
Cosopt	dorzolamide HCl; timolol maleate ophth soln	cycloserine	Seromycin
		cyclosporine	Sandimmune
		cyclosporine microemulsion capsules and oral soln	Neoral
cosyntropin	Cortrosyn		
Cotazym	pancrelipase		
Cotazym-S	pancrelipase EC	Cycrin	medroxyproges-terone acetate
Cotrim	sulfamethoxazole; trimethoprim		
		Cylert	pemoline
co-trimoxazole	Bactrim Cotrim Septra sulfamethoxa-zole; trimetho-prim	cyproheptadine HCl	Periactin
		Cystadane	betaine anhydrous
		Cystospaz-M	hyoscyamine sulfate SR

Cytadren	aminogluteth-imide	DaunoXome	daunorubicin citrate liposomal
cytarabine	Cytosar-U	Daypro	oxaprozin
Cytomel	liothyronine sodium	DDAVP	desmopressin acetate
Cytosar-U	cytarabine	Debrox	carbamide peroxide otic
Cytotec	misoprostol		
Cytovene	ganciclovir	Decadron	dexamethasone
Cytoxan	cyclophosphamide	Deca-Durabolin	nandrolone decanoate
		Declomycin	demeclocycline HCl
D		deferoxamine mesylate	Desferal
		delavirdine mesylate	Rescriptor
dacarbazine	DTIC-Dome	Delestrogen	estradiol valerate
daclizumab	Zenapax	Deltasone	prednisone
dactinomycin	Cosmegen	Demadex	torsemide
Dalmane	flurazepam HCl	demecarium bromide	Humorsol
dalteparin sodium	Fragmin	demeclocycline HCl	Declomycin
danaparoid sodium	Orgaran	Demerol	meperidine HCl
danazol	Danocrine	Demser	metyrosine
Danocrine	danazol	Demulen	ethynodiol diacetate; ethinyl estradiol
Dantrium	dantrolene sodium		
dantrolene sodium	Dantrium	Denavir	penciclovir cream
dapsone	dapsone	denileukin diftitox	Ontak
Daranide	dichlorphena-mide	Depacon	valproate sodium inj
Daraprim	pyrimethamine	Depakene	valproic acid
Darvocet-N 100	propoxyphene napsylate; acetaminophen	Depakote	divalproex sodium
Darvon	propoxyphene HCl	Depo-Medrol	methylprednis-olone acetate SR
Darvon Compound 65	propoxyphene HCl; aspirin; caffeine	Depo-Provera	medroxyproges-terone acetate SR
daunorubicin citrate liposomal	DaunoXome	Depo-Testosterone	testosterone cypionate SR
daunorubicin HCl	Cerubidine		

D
Rx

Desferal	deferoxamine mesylate	diazepam rectal gel	Diastat
desflurane	Suprane	diazoxide	Hyperstat
desipramine HCl	Norpramin	Dibenzyline	phenoxybenz-amine HCl
desmopressin acetate	DDAVP	dibucaine	Nupercainal
Desogen	desogestrel; ethinyl estradiol	dichlorphena-mide	Daranide
desogestrel; ethinyl estradiol	Desogen Ortho-Cept	diclofenac potassium	Cataflam
desogestrel and ethinyl estradiol; ethinyl estradiol	Mircette	diclofenac sodium	Voltaren
		diclofenac sodium; misoprostol	Arthrotec
desonide	Tridesilon	diclofenac sodium SR	Voltaren-XR
desoximetasone	Topicort	dicloxacillin sodium	Dynapen
Desoxyn	methamphet-amine HCl	dicyclomine HCl	Bentyl
Desyrel	trazodone HCl	didanosine	Videx
Detrol	tolterodine tartrate	Didronel	etidronate disodium
dexamethasone	Decadron Hexadrol	diethylpropion HCl	Tenuate
dexchlorphenir-amine maleate SR	Polaramine Repetabs	diethylstilbestrol diphosphate	Stilphostrol
dexfenfluramine HCl (W)	Redux (W)	Differin	adapalene
		diflorasone diacetate	Florone
Dexferrum	iron dextran inj	Diflucan	fluconazole
dexrazoxane	Zinecard	diflunisal	Dolobid
dextrothyroxine sodium	Choloxin	Digibind	digoxin immune fab
		digitoxin	Crystodigin
D.H.E. 45	dihydroergot-amine mesylate inj	digoxin	Lanoxin
		digoxin capsules	Lanoxicaps
DiaBeta	glyburide	digoxin immune fab	Digibind
Diabinese	chlorpropamide	dihydroergota-mine mesylate inj	D.H.E. 45
Diamox	acetazolamide		
Diapid	lypressin		
Diastat	diazepam rectal gel	dihydroergota-mine mesylate nasal spray	Migranol
diazepam	Valium	dihydrotestoster-one transdermal	Androgel-DHT
diazepam emulsified inj	Dizac		

Dilacor XR	diltiazem HCl SR	conjugate vaccine	
Dilantin	phenytoin	dipivefrin	Propine
Dilaudid	hydromorphone HCl	Diprivan	propofol
diltiazem HCl	Cardizem	Diprosone	betamethasone dipropionate
diltiazem HCl SR	Cardizem CD	dipyridamole	Persantine
	Cartia XR	dirithromycin	Dynabac
	Dilacor XR	Disalcid	salsalate
	Tiazac	disopyramide phosphate	Norpace
diltiazem maleate SR	Tiamate	disulfiram	Antabuse
dimenhydrinate	Dramamine	Ditropan	oxybutynin chloride
dimercaprol	BAL in Oil		
Dimetane	brompheniramine maleate	Diulo	metolazone
		Diuril	chlorothiazide
dinoprostone gel	Prepidil	divalproex sodium	Depakote
dinoprostone vaginal insert	Cervidil	Dizac	diazepam emulsified inj
dinoprostone vaginal suppositories	Prostin E2	dobutamine HCl	Dobutrex
		Dobutrex	dobutamine HCl
Diovan	valsartan	docetaxel	Taxotere
Dipentum	olsalazine sodium	docusate calcium	Surfak
diphenhydramine HCl	Benadryl	docusate calcium; phenolphthalein	Doxidan
diphenoxylate HCl; atropine sulfate	Lomotil	docusate sodium	Colace
		docusate sodium; casanthranol	Peri-Colace
diphtheria and tetanus toxoids and acellular pertussis vaccine	Acel-Imune Tripedia	dolasetron mesylate	Anzemet
		Dolobid	diflunisal
		Dolophine	methadone HCl
diphtheria and tetanus toxoids and pertussis vaccine, adsorbed	DTwP Tri-Immunol	Domeboro	aluminum acetate
		donepezil HCl	Aricept
		Donnatal	belladonna alkaloids; phenobarbital
diphtheria and tetanus toxoids; pertussis vaccine, adsorbed and haemophilus b	Tetramune	dopamine HCl	Intropin
		Dopar	levodopa
		Dopram	doxapram HCl
		dornase alpha	Pulmozyme
		dorzolamide HCl	Trusopt
		dorzolamide	Cosopt

HCl; timolol maleate ophth soln	
Dostinex	cabergoline
Dovonex	calcipotriene cream
doxacurium chloride	Nuromax
doxapram HCl	Dopram
doxazosin mesylate	Cardura
doxepin HCl	Adapin Sinequan
Doxidan	docusate calcium; phenolphthalein
Doxil	doxorubicin, liposomal
doxorubicin HCl	Adriamycin Rubex
doxorubicin, liposomal	Doxil
doxycycline hyclate	Vibramycin
doxycycline hyclate gel	Atridox
Dramamine	dimenhydrinate
Drisdol	ergocalciferol
Dristan Long Lasting	oxymetazoline HCl
Drixoral Syrup	pseudoephedrine HCl; brompheniramine maleate
dronabinol	Marinol
droperidol	Inapsine
Droxia	hydroxyurea
DTIC-Dome	dacarbazine
Dulcolax	bisacodyl
Durabolin	nandrolone phenpropionate
Duraclon	clonidine HCl inj
Duract (W)	bromfenac sodium (W)
Duragesic	fentanyl transdermal

Duramorph	morphine sulfate inj
Duranest	etidocaine HCl
Duricef	cefadroxil
Dyazide	triamterene 37.5 mg; hydrochlorothiazide 25 mg
Dymelor	acetohexamide
Dynabac	dirithromycin
DynaCirc	isradipine
Dynapen	dicloxacillin sodium
dyphylline	Lufyllin
Dyrenium	triamterene

E

EchoGen	perflenapent emulsion
echothiophate iodide	Phospholine Iodide
Ecotrin	aspirin EC
Edecrin	ethacrynic acid
edetate disodium	Endrate
Edex	alprostadil inj
edrophonium chloride	Tensilon
E.E.S. 400	erythromycin ethylsuccinate
efavirenz	Sustiva
Effexor	venlafaxine HCl
Effexor XR	venlafaxine HCl SR
Elavil	amitriptyline HCl
Eldepryl	selegiline HCl
Eldisine	vindesine sulfate
Elixophyllin	theophylline
Elmiron	pentosan polysulfate sodium

Elocon	mometasone furoate topical
Elspar	asparaginase
Emadine	emedastine difumarate opthth soln
Emcyt	estramustine phosphate sodium
emedastine difumarate opthth soln	Emadine
EMLA Cream	lidocaine; prilocaine cream
Empirin with codeine #3 and #4	aspirin 325 mg with codeine phosphate (30 and 60 mg)
E-Mycin	erythromycin
enalapril maleate	Vasotec
enalapril maleate; diltiazem malate	Teczem
enalapril maleate; felodipine SR	Lexxel
enalapril maleate; hydrochlorothi-azide	Vaseretic
Enbrel	etanercept
encainide HCl	Enkaid
Endep	amitriptyline HCl
Endocet	oxycodone HCl; acetaminophen
Endrate	edetate disodium
Enduron	methyclothiazide
enflurane	Ethrane
Engerix-B	hepatitis B vaccine
Enkaid	encainide HCl
enoxaparin sodium	Lovenox
Entex LA	phenylpropanol-amine HCl; guaifenesin SR
epinephrine	Adrenalin
epinephrine racemic	Vaponefrin
Epivir	lamivudine
epoetin alfa	Epogen Procrit
Epogen	epoetin alfa
epoprostenol sodium	Flolan
eprosartan mesylate	Teveten
eptifibatide	Integrilin
Equanil	meprobamate
Ergamisol	levamisole HCl
ergocalciferol	Calciferol Drisdol
ergoloid mesylates	Hydergine
ergotamine tartrate; caffeine	Cafergot
ergotamine tartrate	Ergostat
Ergotrate	ergonovine maleate
Ery-Tab	erythromycin EC
Erythrocin Stearate	erythromycin stearate
erythromycin	E-Mycin
erythromycin base coated particles	PCE Dispertab
erythromycin EC	Ery-Tab
erythromycin estolate	Ilosone
erythromycin ethylsuccinate	E.E.S. 400
erythromycin ethylsuccinate; sulfisoxazole	Pediazole
erythromycin stearate	Erythrocin Stearate

Esclim	estradiol transdermal	estrogens, esterified; methyltestoster-one	Estratest
Eserine Sulfate	physostigmine ophth ointment		
Esidrix	hydrochlorothi-azide	estrogens, esterified methyltestost-erone, half strength	Estratest H.S.
Esimil	guanethidine monosulfate; hydrochloro-thiazide		
Eskalith	lithium carbonate	estropipate	Ogen
esmolol HCl	Brevibloc	Estrostep	norethindrone acetate; ethinyl estradiol
estazolam	ProSom		
Estinyl	ethinyl estradiol	etanercept	Enbrel
Estrace	estradiol	ethacrynic acid	Edecrin
Estraderm	estradiol transdermal	ethambutol HCl	Myambutol
		ethchlorvynol	Placidyl
estradiol	Estrace	ethinyl estradiol	Estinyl
estradiol transdermal	Climara	ethionamide	Trecator-SC
	Esclim	Ethmozine	moricizine
	Estraderm	ethopropazine HCl	Parsidol
	FemPatch		
	Vivelle	ethosuximide	Zarontin
estradiol vaginal ring	Estring	Ethrane	enflurane
		ethyl chloride	ethyl chloride
estradiol valerate	Delestrogen	ethynodiol diacetate; ethinyl estradiol	Demulen
estramustine phosphate sodium	Emcyt		
		Ethyol	amifostine
Estratest	estrogens, esterified; methyltestos-terone	etidocaine HCl	Duranest
		etidronate disodium	Didronel
		etodolac	Lodine
Estratest H.S.	estrogens, esterified; methyltestos-terone, half strength	etodolac SR	Lodine XL
		etomidate	Amidate
		Etopophos	etoposide phosphate diethanolate
Estring	estradiol vaginal ring	etoposide	VePesid
		etoposide phosphate diethanolate	Etopophos
estrogens, conjugated	Premarin		
		Etrafon	perphenazine; amitriptyline HCl
estrogens, conjugated; medroxyproges-terone acetate	Premphase Prempro		
		Eulexin	flutamide

Eurax	crotamiton	fentanyl transdermal	Duragesic
Euthroid (WA)	liotrix	fentanyl transmucosal	Fentanyl Oralet
Eutonyl	pargyline HCl		
Evista	raloxifene HCl	Feosol	ferrous sulfate
Ex-Lax	senna	Fer-In-Sol	ferrous sulfate
		Fergon	ferrous gluconate
		Feridex	ferumoxide HCl
		ferrous gluconate	Fergon
F		*ferrous sulfate*	Feosol
			Fer-In-Sol
		ferrous sulfate SR	SlowFe
factor IX, concentrate	BeneFix	Fertinex	urofollitropin for inj
Factrel	gonadorelin HCl	ferumoxetil oral suspension	Gastromark
famciclovir	Famvir	ferumoxide HCl	Feridex
famotidine	Pepcid	fexofenadine HCl	Allegra
famotidine, oral disintegrating tablet	Pepcid RPD	filgrastim	Neupogen
Famvir	famciclovir	finasteride	Propecia 1 mg tablet
Fareston	toremifene citrate		Proscar 5 mg tablet
Fastin	phentermine HCl	Fioricet	butalbital; acetamino-phen; caffeine
fat emulsion	Intralipid Liposyn II and III	Fiorinal	butalbital; aspirin; caffeine
felbamate	Felbatol		
Felbatol	felbamate	Flagyl	metronidazole
Feldene	piroxicam	Flagyl ER	metronidazole SR
felodipine	Plendil		
Femara	letrozole	flavoxate HCl	Urispas
FemPatch	estradiol transdermal	Flaxedil	gallamine triethiodide
fenfluramine HCl (W)	Pondimin (W)	flecainide acetate	Tambocor
fenofibrate	Tricor	Flexeril	cyclobenzaprine HCl
fenoldopam mesylate	Corlopam	Flolan	epoprostenol sodium
fenoprofen calcium	Nalfon	Flomax	tamsulosin HCl
fentanyl citrate	Sublimaze	Flonase	fluticasone propionate spray
fentanyl citrate; droperidol	Innovar		
Fentanyl Oralet	fentanyl transmucosal	Florinef	fludrocortisone acetate

F
Rx

339

Florone	diflorasone diacetate	fluvastatin sodium	Lescol
Floropryl	isoflurophate	fluvoxamine maleate	Luvox
Flovent	fluticasone propionate spray	FML	fluorometholone
Floxin	ofloxacin	Folex PFS	methotrexate inj
Floxin Otic	ofloxacin otic soln	*folic acid*	Folvite
floxuridine	FUDR	Follistim	follitropin beta
fluconazole	Diflucan	follitropin alfa	Gonal-F
flucytosine	Ancobon	follitropin beta	Follistim
Fludara	fludarabine phosphate	Folvite	folic acid
		fomepizole	Antizol
fludarabine phosphate	Fludara	fomivirsen sodium inj	Vitravene
fludrocortisone acetate	Florinef	Forane	isoflurane
		Fortaz	ceftazidime
Flumadine	rimantadine	Fortovase	saquinavir soft gel capsule
flumazenil	Romazicon		
flunisolide	Aero Bid	Fosamax	alendronate sodium
fluocinolone acetonide	Synalar		
		foscarnet	Foscavir
fluocinonide	Lidex	Foscavir	foscarnet
Fluor-I-Strip	fluorescein sodium strips	fosfomycin tromethamine	Monurol
fluorescein sodium soln	Fluorescite	fosinopril sodium	Monopril
fluorescein sodium strips	Fluor-I-Strip	fosphenytoin sodium	Cerebyx
Fluorescite	fluorescein sodium soln	Fragmin	dalteparin sodium
		FUDR	floxuridine
fluorometholone	FML	Fulvicin P/G	griseofulvin
Fluothane	halothane	Fungizone	amphotericin B
fluoxetine HCl	Prozac	Furacin	nitrofurazone
fluoxymesterone	Halotestin	*furosemide*	Lasix
fluphenazine HCl	Permitil		
	Prolixin		
flurazepam HCl	Dalmane		
flurbiprofen	Ansaid		
flutamide	Eulexin	**G**	
fluticasone propionate spray	Flonase Flovent		
		gabapentin	Neurontin
fluticasone propionate cream & ointment	Cutivate	Gabitril	tiagabine HCl
		gadoteridol	ProHance
		gallamine triethiodide	Flaxedil
		gallium nitrate	Ganite
		Galzin	zinc acetate

Gamimune N	immune globulin intravenous	Glucophage	metformin HCl
		Glucotrol	glipizide
gamma hydroxybutyrate	Xyrem	Glucotrol XL	glipizide SR
		glyburide	DiaBeta
Gammagard S/D	immune globulin intravenous		Micronase
			Glynase
Gammar-P IV	immune globulin intravenous	glyburide micronized	
		glycerin ophth soln	Ophthalgan
ganciclovir	Cytovene		
ganciclovir ophthalmic implant	Vitrasert	glycopyrrolate	Robinul
		Glynase	glyburide micronized
Ganite	gallium nitrate	gold sodium thiomalate	Aurolate
Gantanol	sulfamethoxazole		
Garamycin	*gentamicin sulfate*	GoLYTELY	polyethylene glycol-electrolyte soln
Gastrocrom	cromolyn sodium		
Gastromark	ferumoxetil oral suspension	gonadorelin HCl	Factrel
		Gonal-F	follitropin alfa
gemcitabine HCl	Gemzar	goserelin acetate implant	Zoladex
gemfibrozil	Lopid	graftskin	Apligraf
Gemzar	gemcitabine HCl	granisetron HCl	Kytril
GenEsa	arbutamine HCl	grepafloxacin HCl	Raxar
Genora	norethindrone; mestranol	Grifulvin V	griseofulvin
		griseofulvin	Fulvicin P/G
Genotropin	somatropin for inj		Grifulvin V
gentamicin sulfate	Garamycin	guaifenesin	Organidin NR
			Robitussin
Geocillin	carbenicillin	guaifenesin; codeine phosphate	Robitussin A-C
Geref	sermorelin acetate		Tussi-Organidin NR
glatiramer acetate	Copaxone	guaifenesin; dextromethor-phan	Robitussin-DM
Gliadel	carmustine implantable wafer		
		guanabenz acetate	Wytensin
glimepiride	Amaryl	guanadrel sulfate	Hylorel
glipizide	Glucotrol	guanethidine monosulfate	Ismelin
glipizide SR	Glucotrol XL		
GlucaGen	glucagon (rDNA origin)	guanethidine monosulfate; hydrochlorothi-azide	Esimil
glucagon	glucagon		
glucagon (rDNA origin)	GlucaGen	guanfacine	Tenex

G
Rx

HCl	
Gyne-Lotrimin	clotrimazole

H

Habitrol	nicotine transdermal system
Haemophilus b conjugate vaccine reconstituted with diphtheria and tetanus toxoids and acellular pertussis vaccine adsorbed	ActHIB/Tripedia
Haemophilus b conjugate; Hepatitis B vaccine	Comvax
haemophilus b vaccine	Hib-Immune HibTITER PedvaxHIB ProHIBiT
halcinonide	Halog
Halcion	triazolam
Haldol	haloperidol
Halfan	halofantrine HCl
halofantrine HCl	Halfan
Halog	halcinonide
haloperidol	Haldol
haloprogin	Halotex
Halotestin	fluoxymesterone
Halotex	haloprogin
halothane	Fluothane
Havrix	hepatitis A vaccine, inactivated
H-BIG	hepatitis B

	immune globulin
Healon	sodium hyaluronate
Helidac	bismuth subsalicylate; metronidazole; tetracycline HCl
heparin sodium	Liquaemin Sodium
hepatitis A vaccine, inactivated	Havrix Vaqta
hepatitis B immune globulin	H-BIG
hepatitis B vaccine	Engerix-B Recombivax HB
Herceptin	trastuzumab
Herplex	idoxuridine
Hespan	hetastarch
hetastarch	Hespan
Hexadrol	dexamethasone
Hexalen	altretamine
Hib-Immune	haemophilus b vaccine
Hibiclens	chlorhexidine gluconate
HibTITER	haemophilus b vaccine
Hiprex	methenamine hippurate
Hismanal	astemizole
Hivid	zalcitabine
homatropine hydrobromide ophth	Isopto Homatropine
Humalog	insulin, lispro (human)
Humatin	paromomycin sulfate
Humatrope	somatropin
Humorsol	demecarium bromide
Humulin 70/30	isophane insulin suspension

H
Rx

Hyzaar	losartan potassium; hydrochlorothiazide	Inapsine	droperidol
		indapamide	Lozol
		Inderal	propranolol HCl
		Inderide	propranolol HCl; hydrochlorothiazide
		indinavir	Crixivan
		indium In-111 pentetreotide	OctreoScan

I-J

		Indocin	indomethacin
		indomethacin	Indocin
		Infasurf	calfactant intratracheal susp
ibuprofen	Advil Motrin Nuprin		
		INFeD	iron dextran inj
ibutilide fumarate	Corvert	Infergen	interferon alfacon-1
Idamycin	idarubicin	infliximab	Remicade
idarubicin	Idamycin	Innovar	fentanyl citrate; droperidol
idoxuridine	Herplex		
IFEX	ifosfamide	Inocor	amrinone lactate
ifosfamide	IFEX	insulin inj (human)	Humulin R Novolin R Velosulin Human
Ilosone	erythromycin estolate		
		insulin lispro (human)	Humalog
Imagent GI	perflubron		
imciromab pentetate	Myoscint	insulin zinc suspension (Lente) (human)	Humulin L Novolin L
Imdur	isosorbide mononitrate SR		
		insulin zinc suspension, extended (beef)	Ultralente U
imiglucerase	Cerezyme		
imipenem-cilastatin sodium	Primaxin		
		insulin zinc suspension, extended, (human)	Humulin U Ultralente
imipramine HCl	Tofranil		
imiquimod cream	Aldara		
Imitrex	sumatriptan	Intal	cromolyn sodium
immune globulin intravenous	Gamimune N Gammagard S/D Gammar-P IV Sandoglobulin	Integrilin	eptifibatide
		interferon alfa-2a	Roferon-A
		interferon alfa-2b	Intron A
Imodium	loperamide HCl	interferon alfacon-1	Infergen
Imogam	rabies immune globulin, human	interferon beta-la	Avonex
		interferon beta-1b	Betaseron
Imuran	azathioprine		

Intrachol	choline chloride inj	isoniazid; rifampin	Rifamate
Intralipid	fat emulsion	isophane insulin suspension (NPH) (human)	Humulin N Novolin N
Intron A	interferon alfa-2b		
Intropin	dopamine HCl	isophane insulin suspension (NPH) 70%, insulin inj 30% (human)	Humulin 70/30 Novolin 70/30
Inversine	mecamylamine HCl		
Invirase	saquinavir mesylate		
iocetamic acid	Cholebrine	isoproterenol HCl	Isuprel
iodamide meglumine	Renovue 65	Isoptin	verapamil HCl
iodixanol	Visipaque	Isopto Carbachol	carbachol ophth
iohexol	Omnipaque	Isopto Carpine	pilocarpine HCl ophth
Ionamin	phentermine resin	Isopto Homatropine	homatropine hydrobromide ophth
iopamidol	Isovue		
iopanoic acid	Telepaque	Isopto Hyoscine	scopolamine hydrobromide ophth
iopromide	Ultravist		
iotrolan	Osmovist		
ioversol	Optiray	Isordil	isosorbide dinitrate
ioxilan	Oxilan		
Ipol	poliovirus vaccine inactivated	isosorbide dinitrate	Isordil
ipratropium bromide	Atrovent	isosorbide mononitrate	ISMO
ipratropium bromide; albuterol sulfate	Combivent	isosorbide mononitrate SR	Imdur
irbesartan	Avapro	isotretinoin	Accutane
irinotecan HCl	Camptosar	Isovue	iopamidol
iron dextran inj	INFeD Dexferrum	isoxsuprine HCl	Vasodilan
		isradipine	DynaCirc
Ismelin	guanethidine monosulfate	Isuprel	isoproterenol HCl
ISMO	isosorbide mononitrate	itraconazole	Sporanox
		ivermectin	Stromectol
isocarboxazid	Marplan	IvyBlock	bentoquatam
isoetharine HCl aerosol	Bronkometer		
isoetharine HCl soln	Bronkosol	**K**	
isoflurane	Forane		
isoflurophate	Floropry l		
isoniazid	Nydrazid	Kadian	morphine sulfate SR

kanamycin sulfate	Kantrex		potassium bicarbonate effervescent
Kantrex	kanamycin sulfate	Kolyum	potassium chloride; potassium gluconate
Kaon	potassium gluconate		
Kaon-Cl	potassium chloride SR		
Kayexalate	polystyrene sulfonate sodium	Konsyl-D	psyllium
		Kwell (WA)	lindane
		Kytril	granisetron HCl
K-Dur	potassium chloride SR		
Keflex	cephalexin		
Keflin (W)	cephalothin sodium (W)		
Keftab	cephalexin HCl		**L**
Kefurox	cefuroxime sodium		
Kefzol	cefazolin sodium	labetalol HCl	Normodyne
Kemadrin	procyclidine HCl		Trandate
Kenalog	triamcinolone acetonide	lactulose	Cephulac
			Chronulac
Kerlone	betaxolol	Lamictal	lamotrigine
Ketalar	ketamine HCl	Lamisil	terbinafine HCl
ketamine HCl	Ketalar	lamivudine	Epivir
		lamivudine; zidovudine	Combivir
ketoconazole	Nizoral		
ketoprofen	Orudis	lamotrigine	Lamictal
ketoprofen SR	Oruvail	Lanoxicaps	digoxin capsules
ketorolac tromethamine	Toradol	Lanoxin	digoxin
		lansoprazole	Prevacid
ketorolac tromethamine ophth	Acular	lansoprazole; amoxicillin; clarithromycin	Prevpac
Klaron	sodium sulfacetamide lotion	Lariam	mefloquine HCl
		Larodopa	levodopa
		Lasix	furosemide
Klonopin	clonazepam	latanoprost	Xalatan
Klor-Con 10	potassium chloride SR	leflunomide	Arava
		lepirudin	Refludan
K-Lyte	potassium bicarbonate; potassium citrate effervescent	Lescol	fluvastatin sodium
		letrozole	Femara
		leucovorin calcium	Wellcovorin
K-Lyte/Cl	potassium chloride	Leukeran	chlorambucil
		Leukine	sargramostim

leuprolide acetate	Lupron	Librax	clidinium; chlordiaz-epoxide
Leustatin	cladribine		
levamisole HCl	Ergamisol	Librium	chlordiazepoxide HCl
Levaquin	levofloxacin		
Levbid	hyoscyamine sulfate SR	Lidex	fluocinonide
		lidocaine HCl	Xylocaine HCl
Levlite	levonorgestrel; ethinyl estradiol	lidocaine; prilocaine cream	EMLA Cream
levocabastine HCl ophth susp	Livostin	Limbitrol	chlordiazepoxide HCl; amitrip-tyline HCl
Levo-Dromoran	levorphanol tartrate	Lincocin	lincomycin HCl
		lincomycin HCl	Lincocin
levobunolol HCl	Betagan	lindane	Kwell (WA) lindane
levocarnitine	Carnitor	Lioresal	baclofen
levodopa	Dopar Larodopa	liothyronine sodium	Cytomel
levodopa; carbidopa	Sinemet	liothyronine sodium inj	Triostat
levodopa; carbidopa SR	Sinemet CR	liotrix	Thyrolar
		Lipitor	atorvastatin calcium
levofloxacin	Levaquin	liposomal amphotericin B	AmBisome
levonorgestrel implant	Norplant		
levonorgestrel; ethinyl estradiol	Alesse Levlite Nordette Preven Emergency Contraceptive Kit Tri-Levlen Triphasil	Liposyn II and III	fat emulsion
		Liquaemin Sodium	heparin sodium
		lisinopril	Prinivil Zestril
		lisinopril; hydrochloro-thiazide	Zestoretic
Levophed	norepinephrine bitartrate	lithium carbonate	Eskalith Lithobid
levorphanol tartrate	Levo-Dromoran	lithium citrate	Cibalith-S
		Lithobid	lithium carbonate
levothyroxine sodium	Levoxyl Synthroid	Lithostat	acetohydroxamic acid
Levoxyl	levothyroxine sodium	Livostin	levocabastine HCl ophth susp
Lexxel	enalapril maleate; felodipine SR	Lodine	etodolac
		Lodine XL	etodolac SR

L
Rx

Iodoxamide tromethamine ophth soln	Alomide
Loestrin	norethindrone acetate; ethinyl estradiol
lomefloxacin	Maxaquin
Lomotil	diphenoxylate HCl; atropine sulfate
lomustine	CeeNu
Loniten	minoxidil tablets
Lo/Ovral	norgestrel; ethinyl estradiol
loperamide HCl	Imodium
Lopid	gemfibrozil
Lopressor	metoprolol tartrate
Lorabid	loracarbef
loracarbef	Lorabid
loratadine	Claritin
loratadine; pseudoephedrine sulfate	Claritin D
lorazepam	Ativan
Lorcet	hydrocodone bitartrate; acetaminophen
Lortab	hydrocodone bitartrate; acetaminophen
losartan potassium	Cozaar
losartan potassium; hydrochlorothiazide	Hyzaar
Lotemax	loteprednol etabonate ophth susp
Lotensin	benazepril HCl
loteprednol etabonate ophth susp	Alrex
	Lotemax
Lotrel	amlodipine besylate; benazepril HCl
Lotrimin	clotrimazole
Lotrisone	betamethasone; clotrimazole cream
lovastatin	Mevacor
Lovenox	enoxaparin sodium
loxapine succinate	Loxitane
Loxitane	loxapine succinate
Lozol	indapamide
Ludiomil	maprotiline HCl
Lufyllin	dyphylline
LumenHance	manganese chloride
Lupron	leuprolide acetate
Luride	sodium fluoride
Luvox	fluvoxamine maleate
lymphocyte immune globulin	Atgam
lypressin	Diapid
Lysodren	mitotane

M

Maalox	aluminum hydroxide; magnesium hydroxide
Macrobid	nitrofurantoin macrocrystals and monohydrate
Macrodantin	nitrofurantoin macrocrystals
magaldrate	Riopan

manganese chloride	LumenHance	meclocycline sulfosalicylate	Meclan
magnesium chloride SR	Slow-Mag	meclofenamate sodium	Meclomen
magnesium sulfate	magnesium sulfate	Meclomen	meclofenamate sodium
Mandol	cefamandole nafate	Medrol	methylprednisolone
mangofodipir trisodium	Teslascan	medroxyprogesterone acetate	Cycrin Provera
maprotiline HCl	Ludiomil	medroxyprogesterone acetate SR	Depo-Provera
Marcaine HCl	bupivacaine HCl	mefenamic acid	Ponstel
Marinol	dronabinol	mefloquine HCl	Lariam
Marplan	isocarboxazid	Mefoxin	cefoxitin sodium
Matulane	procarbazine HCl	Megace	megestrol acetate
Mavik	trandolapril	megestrol acetate	Megace
Maxalt	rizatriptan benzoate	Mellaril	thioridazine HCl
Maxalt-MLT	rizatriptan oral disintegrating tablet	melphalan	Alkeran
		menadiol sodium diphosphate	Synkayvite
Maxaquin	lomefloxacin	menotropins	Pergonal Repronex
Maxipime	cefepime HCl	Mentax	butenafine HCl
Maxzide	triamterene 75 mg; hydrochlorothiazide 50 mg	meperidine HCl	Demerol
		mephentermine sulfate	Wyamine
Maxzide-25MG	triamterene 37.5 mg; hydrochlorothiazide 25 mg	mephenytoin	Mesantoin
		mephobarbital	Mebaral
		mepivacaine HCl	Carbocaine
		meprobamate	Equanil Miltown
mazindol	Sanorex	Mepron	atovaquone
measles, mumps, rubella vaccines, combined	M-M-R II	mercaptopurine	Purinethol
		Meridia	sibutramine HCl monohydrate
		meropenem	Merrem
Mebaral	mephobarbital	Merrem	meropenem
mebendazole	Vermox	Meruvax II	rubella virus vaccine live attenuated
mecamylamine HCl	Inversine		
mechlorethamine HCl	Mustargen	mesalamine	Asacol Rowasa
Meclan	meclocycline sulfosalicylate	Mesantoin	mephenytoin
		mesna	Mesnex
meclizine	Antivert	Mesnex	mesna
		mesoridazine	Serentil

Mestinon	pyridostigmine bromide	methylprednisolone	Medrol
Metamucil	psyllium	methylprednisolone acetate SR inj	Depo-Medrol
Metaprel	metaproterenol sulfate		
metaproterenol sulfate	Alupent	methylprednisolone sodium succinate inj	Solu-Medrol
	Metaprel		
metaraminol bitartrate	Aramine	methyltestosterone	Oreton Methyl
metformin HCl	Glucophage		
methadone HCl	Dolophine	methysergide maleate	Sansert
methamphetamine HCl	Desoxyn		
		Meticorten	prednisone
methazolamide	Neptazane	metoclopramide HCl	Reglan
methenamine combination	Urised		
		metolazone	Diulo
methenamine hippurate	Hiprex		Zaroxolyn
		Metopirone	metyrapone
Methergine	methylergonovine maleate	metoprolol succinate SR	Toprol XL
methicillin sodium (W)	Staphcillin (W)	metoprolol tartrate	Lopressor
methimazole	Tapazole	MetroGel-Vaginal	metronidazole vaginal gel
methocarbamol	Robaxin		
methohexital sodium	Brevital Sodium	*metronidazole*	Flagyl
		metronidazole SR	Flagyl ER
methotrexate	Mexate	metronidazole vaginal gel	MetroGel-Vaginal
methotrexate, preservative-free inj	Folex PFS		
		metyrapone	Metopirone
		metyrosine	Demser
methotrexate sodium tablets	Rheumatrex	Mevacor	lovastatin
		Mexate	methotrexate
methoxamine HCl	Vasoxyl	mexiletine HCl	Mexitil
		Mexitil	mexiletine HCl
methoxsalen	Oxsoralen	Mezlin	mezlocillin
methscopamine bromide	Pamine	mezlocillin	Mezlin
		Miacalcin	calcitonin-salmon
methyclothiazide	Enduron		
methyldopa	Aldomet	mibefradil dihydrochloride (W)	Posicor (W)
methyldopa; hydrochlorothiazide	Aldoril		
		Micardis	telmisartan
methylergonovine maleate	Methergine	Micro K	potassium chloride SR
methylphenidate HCl	Ritalin	miconazole nitrate	Monistat
methylphenidate SR	Ritalin SR	Micronase	glyburide
		Micronor	norethindrone

Microzide	hydrochloro-thiazide	molindone HCl	Moban
		mometasone furoate topical	Elocon
Midamor	amiloride HCl		
midazolam HCl	Versed	Mometasone furoate monohydrate nasal spray	Nasonex
midodrine HCl	ProAmatine		
Migranol	dihydroergota-mine mesylate nasal spray		
		Monistat	miconazole nitrate
milrinone lactate	Primacor		
Miltown	meprobamate	Monocid	cefonicid sodium
Minipress	prazosin HCl		
Minocin	minocycline HCl	Monopril	fosinopril sodium
minocycline HCl	Minocin		
minoxidil tablets	Loniten	montelukast sodium	Singulair
minoxidil topical	Rogaine		
Mintezol	thiabendazole	Monurol	fosfomycin tromethamine
Miochol E	acetylcholine ophth		
		moricizine	Ethmozine
Mirapex	pramipexole dihydrochloride	morphine sulfate	Roxanol
		morphine sulfate, immediate release concentrated oral soln	Roxanol-T
Mircette	desogestrel; ethinyl estradiol and ethinyl estradiol		
		morphine sulfate inj	Duramorph
		morphine sulfate SR	Kadian MS Contin Oramorph SR Roxanol SR
mirtazapine	Remeron		
misoprostol	Cytotec		
Mithracin	plicamycin		
mitomycin	Mutamycin		
mitotane	Lysodren		
mitoxantrone HCl	Novantrone	Motrin	ibuprofen
		MS Contin	morphine sulfate SR
Mivacron	mivacurium chloride		
		Mucomyst	acetylcysteine
mivacurium chloride	Mivacron	mupirocin nasal ointment	Bactroban
M-M-R II	measles, mumps, rubella vaccines, combined	muromonab-CD3	Orthoclone OKT3
		Muse	alprostadil urethral suppository
Moban	molindone HCl		
modafinil	Provigil		
Moduretic	amiloride HCl; hydrochloro-thiazide	Mustargen	mechlorethamine HCl
		Mutamycin	mitomycin
		M.V.I.-12	vitamin, multiple inj
moexipril HCl	Univasc		
moexipril HCl; hydrochlorothiazide	Uniretic	Myambutol	ethambutol HCl
		Mycelex	clotrimazole

Mycifradin Sulfate	neomycin sulfate oral soln
Myciguent	neomycin sulfate ointment and cream
Mycolog Cream	nystatin; triamcinolone cream
mycophenolate mofetil	CellCept
Mycostatin	nystatin
Mydriacyl	tropicamide
Myleran	busulfan
Mylicon	simethicone
Myochrysine (WA)	gold sodium thiomalate
Myoscint	imciromab pentetate
Mysoline	primidone

N

nabumetone	Relafen
nadolol	Corgard
Nafcil (W)	nafcillin sodium
nafcillin sodium	Nafcil (W)
	Unipen
nalbuphine HCl	Nubain
Nalfon	fenoprofen calcium
nalidixic acid	NegGram
nalmefene HCl	Revex
naloxone HCl	Narcan
naltrexone	ReVia
nandrolone phenpropionate	Durabolin
nandrolone decanoate	Deca-Durabolin
naphazoline ophth soln	Vasocon
Naprelan	naproxen sodium SR

Naprosyn	naproxen
naproxen	Naprosyn
naproxen sodium	Anaprox
naproxen sodium SR	Naprelan
naratriptan HCl	Amerge
Narcan	naloxone HCl
Nardil	phenelzine sulfate
Naropin	ropivacaine HCl
Nasacort	triamcinolone acetonide nasal inhaler
Nasalcrom	cromolyn sodium
Nascobal	cyanocobalamin nasal gel
Nasonex	Mometasone furoate monohydrate nasal spray
Navane	thiothixene
Navelbine	vinorelbine tartrate
Nebcin	tobramycin sulfate
NebuPent	pentamidine isethionate aerosol
nedocromil inhalation	Tilade
nefazodone HCl	Serzone
NegGram	nalidixic acid
nelfinavir mesylate	Viracept
Nembutal	pentobarbital sodium
Neo-Synephrine	phenylephrine HCl
neomycin sulfate ointment and cream	Myciguent
neomycin sulfate oral soln	Mycifradin Sulfate
Neoral	cyclosporine microemulsion capsules and oral soln

Neosar	cyclophospha-mide	nifedipine	Adalat Procardia
Neosporin Cream	polymyxin; neomycin	nifedipine SR	Adalat CC Procardia XL
Neosporin Ointment	polymyxin; neomycin; bacitracin	Nilandron nilutamide Nimbex	nilutamide Nilandron cisatracurium besylate
Neosporin ophth Ointment	polymyxin; neomycin; bacitracin	nimodipine Nimotop	Nimotop nimodipine
Neosporin ophth soln	polymyxin; neomycin	Nipent Nipride	pentostatin inj nitroprusside sodium
neostigmine methylsulfate	Prostigmin	nisoldipine SR	Sular
Neptazane	methazolamide	Nitrek	nitroglycerin transdermal
Nesacaine	chloroprocaine HCl	Nitro-Bid Nitro-Dur	nitroglycerin SR nitroglycerin transdermal
netilmicin sulfate Netromycin	Netromycin netilmicin sulfate	nitrofurantoin macrocrystals	Macrodantin
Neumega	oprelvekin	nitrofurantoin	Macrobid
Neupogen	filgrastim	macrocrystals	
Neurolite	technetium Tc- 99m bicisate kit	and monohydrate	
Neurontin	gabapentin	nitrofurazone	Furacin
Neutrexin	trimetrexate	nitroglycerin	Transderm-Nitro
nevirapine	Viramune	transdermal	
niacin SR	Niaspan Nicobid	nitroglycerin inj *nitroglycerin ointment*	Tridil Nitrol
Niaspan	niacin SR	nitroglycerin	Nitro-Bid
nicardipine HCl	Cardene	SR	
Niclocide	niclosamide	*nitroglycerin sublingual tablets*	Nitrostat
niclosamide	Niclocide		
Nicobid	niacin SR		
Nicorette	nicotine polacrilex	nitroglycerin transdermal	Nitrek Nitro-Dur
nicotine nasal spray	Nicotrol NS	Nitrol	nitroglycerin ointment
nicotine polacrilex	Nicorette	nitroprusside sodium	Nipride
nicotine transdermal	Habitrol Nicotrol Prostep	Nitrostat	nitroglycerin sublingual tablets
Nicotrol	nicotine transdermal		
Nicotrol NS	nicotine nasal spray	Nix nizatidine	permethrin Axid

Nizoral	ketoconazole	Norvasc	amlodipine besylate
nofetumomab	Verluna		
Nolvadex	tamoxifen citrate	Norvir	ritonavir
Norco	hydrocodone bitartrate; acetaminophen	Novantrone	mitoxantrone HCl
		Novocain HCl	procaine HCl
Norcuron	vecuronium bromide	Novolin 70/30	isophane insulin suspension (NPH) 70%, insulin inj 30% (human)
Nordette	levonorgestrel; ethinyl estradiol		
norepinephrine bitartrate	Levophed	Novolin L	insulin zinc suspension (Lente) (human)
norethindrone	Micronor		
norethindrone acetate; ethinyl estradiol	Estrostep Loestrin	Novolin N	isophane insulin suspension (NPH) (human)
norethindrone; ethinyl estradiol (or mestranol)	Genora Ortho-Novum (products)	Novolin R	insulin inj (human)
		Nubain	nalbuphine HCl
norethindrone acetate; estradiol transdermal	CombiPatch	Numorphan	oxymorphone HCl
		Nupercainal	dibucaine
Norflex	orphenadrine citrate	Nuromax	doxacurium chloride
norfloxacin	Noroxin	Nuprin	ibuprofen
Norgesic	orphenadrine citrate; aspirin; caffeine	Nutropin	somatropin for inj
		Nutropin AQ	somatropin inj
norgestimate; ethinyl estradiol	Tri-Cyclen	Nydrazid	isoniazid
		nylidrin HCl (W)	Arlidin (W)
		nystatin	Mycostatin
norgestrel; ethinyl estradiol	Lo/Ovral Ovral	nystatin topical powder	Nystop
Normiflo	ardeparin sodium	nystatin; triamcinolone cream	Mycolog Cream
Normodyne	labetalol HCl		
Noroxin	norfloxacin	Nystop	nystatin topical powder
Norpace	disopyramide phosphate		
Norplant	levonorgestrel implant		
			O
Norpramin	desipramine HCl		
nortriptyline HCl	Aventyl Pamelor	OctreoScan	indium In-111 pentetreotide

octreotide acetate	Sandostatin
ofloxacin	Floxin
ofloxacin otic soln	Floxin Otic
Ogen	estropipate
olanzapine	Zyprexa
olopatadine HCl ophth soln	Patanol
olsalazine sodium	Dipentum
omeprazole	Prilosec
Omnicef	cefdinir
Omnipaque	iohexol
Oncaspar	pegaspargase
OncoScint	satumomab pendetide
Oncovin	vincristine sulfate
ondansetron	Zofran
Ontak	denileukin diftitox
Ophthaine (WA)	proparacaine
Ophthalgan	glycerin ophth soln
Ophthetic	proparacaine HCl
opium; belladonna suppositories	B & O Supprettes
oprelvekin	Neumega
Opticrom	cromolyn sodium
Optimine	azatadine maleate
Optiray	ioversol
Orabase	benzocaine
Orajel	benzocaine
Oramorph SR	morphine sulfate SR
Orap	pimozide
Oretic	hydrochlorothiazide
Oreton Methyl	methyltestosterone
Organidin NR	guaifenesin
Orgaran	danaparoid sodium
Orinase	tolbutamide
orlistat	Xenical
Ornade Spansules	phenylpropanolamine HCl; chlorpheniramine maleate SR
orphenadrine citrate	Norflex
orphenadrine citrate; aspirin; caffeine	Norgesic
Ortho-Cept	desogestrel; ethinyl estradiol
Ortho-Novum (products)	norethindrone; ethinyl estradiol (or mestranol)
Orthoclone OKT3	muromonab-CD3
Orudis	ketoprofen
Oruvail	ketoprofen SR
Os-Cal 500	calcium carbonate
Osmovist	iotrolan
Otrivin	xylometazoline
Ovral	norgestrel; ethinyl estradiol
Oxandrin	oxandrolone
oxandrolone	Oxandrin
oxaprozin	Daypro
oxazepam	Serax
oxiconazole nitrate cream	Oxistat
Oxilan	ioxilan
Oxistat	oxiconazole nitrate cream
Oxsoralen	methoxsalen
oxtriphylline	Choledyl
oxybutynin chloride	Ditropan
oxychlorosene sodium	Clorpactin WCS-90
oxycodone HCl	Percolone Roxicodone
oxycodone HCl SR	OxyContin

oxycodone HCl; acetaminophen	Percocet Endocet Roxicet
oxycodone HCl; aspirin	Percodan
OxyContin	oxycodone HCl SR
oxymetazoline HCl	Afrin nasal spray Dristan Long Lasting
oxymetholone	Anadrol-50
oxymorphone HCl	Numorphan
oxytocin	Pitocin

P

paclitaxel	Taxol
palivizumab	Synagis
Pamelor	nortriptyline HCl
pamidronate disodium	Aredia
Pamine	methscopolamine bromide
Pancrease	pancrelipase EC
pancrelipase	Cotazym
pancrelipase EC	Cotazym-S Pancrease
pancuronium bromide	Pavulon
Pandel	hydrocortisone buteprate cream
papaverine HCl SR	Pavabid
paracetamol	acetaminophen
Paradione	paramethadione
Paraflex	chlorzoxazone 250 mg
Parafon Forte DSC	chlorzoxazone 500 mg
paramethadione	Paradione

Paraplatin	carboplatin
Parathar	teriparatide acetate
paregoric	camphorated tincture of opium
pargyline HCl	Eutonyl
paricalcitol	Zemplar
Parlodel	bromocriptine mesylate
Parnate	tranylcypromine sulfate
paromomycin sulfate	Humatin
paroxetine HCl	Paxil
Parsidol	ethopropazine HCl
Patanol	olopatadine HCl ophth soln
Pavabid	papaverine HCl SR
Pavulon	pancuronium bromide
Paxil	paroxetine HCl
PBZ	tripelennamine HCl
PCE Dispertab	erythromycin base coated particles
Pediazole	erythromycin ethylsuccinate; sulfisoxazole
PedvaxHIB	haemophilus b vaccine
pegaspargase	Oncaspar
pemoline	Cylert
penicillamine	Cuprimine
penciclovir cream	Denavir
penicillin G benzathine	Bicillin L-A (for IM use only) Permapen (for IM use only)
penicillin G benzathine; penicillin G procaine	Bicillin C-R (for IM use only)

penicillin G procaine	Wycillin (for IM use only)	Peri-Colace	docusate sodium; casanthranol
penicillin V potassium	Pen Vee K	Peridex	chlorhexidine gluconate mouth rinse
pentaerythritol tetranitrate	Peritrate		
pentagastrin	Peptavlon	PerioChip	chlorhexidine gluconate
Pentam 300	pentamidine isethionate inj	Peritrate	pentaerythritol tetranitrate
pentamidine isethionate aerosol	NebuPent	Permapen	penicillin G benzathine (for IM use only)
pentamidine isethionate inj	Pentam 300	permethrin	Nix
Pentaspan	pentastarch	Permitil	fluphenazine HCl
pentastarch	Pentaspan	perphenazine	Trilafon
pentazocine HCl	Talwin	perphenazine; amitriptyline HCl	Etrafon Triavil
pentazocine HCl; naloxone HCl	Talwin Nx		
pentobarbital sodium	Nembutal	Persantine	dipyridamole
pentosan polysulfate sodium	Elmiron	petrolatum, white	Vaseline
		Phenaphen with Codeine (#2, 3, and 4)	acetaminophen 300 mg with Codeine Phosphate (15, 30, and 60 mg)
pentostatin inj	Nipent		
Pentothal	thiopental sodium		
pentoxifylline	Trental	phenazopyridine HCl	Pyridium
Pen Vee K	penicillin V potassium	phendimetrazine tartrate	Plegine
Pepcid	famotidine		
Pepcid RPD	famotidine, oral disintegrating tablet	phenelzine sulfate	Nardil
		Phenergan	promethazine HCl
Peptavlon	pentagastrin		
Percocet	oxycodone HCl; acetaminophen	phenobarbital	phenobarbital
		phenobarbital, ergotamine; belladonna	Bellergal-S
Percodan	oxycodone HCl; aspirin		
Percolone	oxycodone HCl	phenoxybenza- mine HCl	Dibenzyline
perflenapent emulsion	EchoGen		
perflubron	Imagent GI	phentermine HCl	Fastin
Pergonal	menotropins		
Periactin	cyproheptadine HCl	phentermine resin	Ionamin

phentolamine mesylate	Regitine	Plasbumin	albumin human
phenylbutyrate sodium	Buphenyl	plasma protein fraction	Plasma-Plex Plasmanate Plasmatein Protenate
phenylephrine HCl	Neo-Synephrine	Plasma-Plex	plasma protein fraction
phenylpropanol-amine HCl; chlorphenir-amine maleate SR	Ornade	Plasmanate	plasma protein fraction
		Plasmatein	plasma protein fraction
phenylpropanol-amine HCl; guaifenesin SR	Entex LA	Platinol AQ	cisplatin
		Plavix	clopidogrel bisulfate
phenytoin	Dilantin	Plegine	phendimetrazine tartrate
Phospholine Iodide	echothiophate iodide	Plendil	felodipine
Photofrin	porfimer sodium	Pletal	cilostazol
physostigmine ophth ointment	Eserine Sulfate	plicamycin	Mithracin
		pneumococcal vaccine	Pneumovax
physostigmine salicylate	Antilirium	Pneumovax	pneumococcal vaccine
phytonadione	AquaMEPHY-TON	podofilox gel	Condylox
pilocarpine HCl ophth	Isopto Carpine	Polaramine Repetabs	dexchlorphenir-amine maleate SR
pilocarpine HCl tablet	Salagen	poliovirus vaccine inactivated	Ipol
pimozide	Orap	polyethylene glycolelectro-lyte soln	CoLyte GoLYTELY
pindolol	Visken		
pipecuronium bromide	Arduan		
piperacillin sodium	Pipracil	polymyxin B sulfate; trimethoprim ophth soln	Polytrim
piperacillin sodium; tazobactam sodium	Zosyn	polymyxin; neomycin	Neosporin Cream Neosporin ophth soln
Pipracil	piperacillin sodium	polymyxin; neomycin; bacitracin	Neosporin Ointment Neosporin ophth Ointment
piroxicam	Feldene		
Pitocin	oxytocin		
Pitressin	vasopressin		
Placidyl	ethchlorvynol	polystyrene sulfonate sodium	Kayexalate
Plaquenil	hydroxychloro-quine sulfate		

polythiazide	Renese
Polytrim	polymyxin B sulfate; trimethoprim ophth soln
Pondimin (W)	fenfluramine HCl (W)
Ponstel	mefenamic acid
Pontocaine	tetracaine HCl
poractant alpha intratracheal susp	Curosurf
porfimer sodium	Photofrin
Posicor (W)	mibefradil dihydro- chloride (W)
potassium bicarbonate; potassium citrate effervescent	K-Lyte
potassium chloride; potassium bicarbonate effervescent	K-Lyte/Cl
potassium chloride SR	Kaon-Cl K-Dur Klor-Con 10 Slow-K Micro K
potassium chloride; potassium gluconate	Kolyum
potassium gluconate	Kaon
povidone iodine	Betadine
pralidoxime chloride	Protopam
pramipexole dihydrochloride	Mirapex
pramoxine HCl	Tronothane HCl
Prandin	repaglinide
Pravachol	pravastatin sodium

pravastatin sodium	Pravachol
prazosin HCl	Minipress
Precose	acarbose
prednisolone syrup	Prelone
prednisone	Deltasone Meticorten
Prelone	prednisolone syrup
Premarin	estrogens, conjugated
Premphase Prempro	estrogens, conjugated; medroxyproges- terone acetate
Prepidil	dinoprostone gel
Preven Emergency Contraceptive Kit	levonorgestrel; ethinyl estradiol
Prevacid	lansoprazole
Preveon	adefovir dipivoxil
Prevpac	lansoprazole; amoxicillin; clarithromycin
Priftin	rifapentine
Prilosec	omeprazole
Primacor	milrinone lactate
Primaxin	imipenemcila- statin sodium
primidone	Mysoline
Principen	ampicillin
Prinivil	lisinopril
Priscoline	tolazoline
ProAmatine	midodrine HCl
Pro-Banthine	propantheline bromide
probenecid	Benemid
probenecid; colchicine	ColBENEMID (W)
procainamide	Pronestyl
procainamide HCl SR	Procan SR Procanbid
procaine HCl	Novocain HCl
Procan SR	procainamide HCl SR

Procanbid	procainamide HCl SR	napsylate; acetaminophen	Propacet-100
procarbazine HCl	Matulane	propranolol HCl	Inderal
Procardia	nifedipine	propranolol HCl; hydrochlorothiazide	Inderide
Procardia XL	nifedipine SR		
prochlorperazine	Compazine	Propulsid	cisapride
Procrit	epoetin alfa	Proscar	finasteride tablets 5 mg
procyclidine HCl	Kemadrin		
progesterone gel	Crinone	ProSom	estazolam
progesterone micronized	Prometrium	ProstaScint	capromab pendetide
Prograf	tacrolimus	Prostep	nicotine transdermal system
ProHance	gadoteridol		
ProHIBiT	haemophilus b vaccine		
		Prostigmin	neostigmine methylsulfate
Prokine (WA)	sargramostim		
Proleukin	aldesleukin	Prostin E$_2$	dinoprostone vaginal suppositories
Prolixin	fluphenazine HCl		
Proloid (W)	thyroglobulin (W)		
		Prostin VR	alprostadil
promazine HCl	Sparine	protamine sulfate	protamine sulfate
promethazine HCl	Phenergan		
		Protenate	plasma protein fraction
Prometrium	progesterone micronized		
		Protopam	pralidoxime chloride
Pronestyl	procainamide		
Propacet-100	propoxyphene napsylate; acetaminophen	protriptyline HCl	Vivactil
		Protropin	somatrem
		Protropin II	somatropin for inj
propafenone HCl	Rythmol		
propantheline bromide	Pro-Banthine	Proventil	albuterol
		Proventil HFA	albuterol sulfate inhalation aerosol
proparacaine HCl	Ophthaine (WA) Ophthetic		
Propecia	finasteride tablets 1 mg	Proventil Repetabs	albuterol SR
Propine	dipivefrin	Provera	medroxyprogesterone acetate
propofol	Diprivan		
propoxyphene HCl	Darvon	Provigil	modafinil
		Prozac	fluoxetine HCl
propoxyphene HCl; acetaminophen	Wygesic	pseudoephedrine HCl	Sudafed
propoxyphene HCl; aspirin; caffeine	Darvon Compound 65	pseudoephedrine HCl; bromphiramine maleate	Drixoral Syrup
propoxyphene	Darvocet-N 100	psyllium	Konsyl-D

Pulmicort Turbuhaler	Metamucil budesonide inhalation powder	rabies immune globulin, human	Hyperab Imogam
Pulmozyme	dornase alfa	rabies vaccine, adsorbed	rabies vaccine, adsorbed
Purinethol	mercaptopurine	rabies vaccine for human use	RabAvert
Pyridium	phenazopyridine HCl	raloxifene HCl	Evista
pyridostigmine bromide	Mestinon	ramipril	Altace
pyrimethamine	Daraprim	ranitidine bismuth citrate	Tritec
		ranitidine HCl	Zantac
		Raxar	grepafloxacin HCl

Q

		Rebetol	ribavirin
		Rebetron	ribavirin; interferon alfa-2b
Quadramet	samarium SM 153 lexidronam	Recombivax HB	hepatitis B vaccine
Quarzan	clidinium bromide	Redux (W)	dexfenfluramine HCl (W)
Questran	cholestyramine	Refludan	lepirudin
quetiapine fumerate	Seroquel	Regitine	phentolamine mesylate
Quinaglute	quinidine gluconate SR	Reglan	metoclopramide HCl
quinapril HCl	Accupril	Regranex	becaplermin gel
quinethazone	Hydromox	Regroton	chlorthalidone; reserpine
Quinidex Extentabs	quinidine sulfate SR	Relafen	nabumetone
quinidine gluconate SR	Quinaglute	Remeron	mirtazapine
quinidine sulfate	quinidine sulfate	Remicade	infliximab
quinidine sulfate SR	Quinidex Extentabs	remifentanil HCl	Ultiva
		Renese	polythiazide
		Renova	tretinoin topical
		Renovue 65	iodamide meglumine
		ReoPro	abciximab
		repaglinide	Prandin
		Repronex	menotropins
		Requip	ropinirole HCl
		Rescriptor	delavirdine mesylate

R

		reserpine	Serpasil
RabAvert	rabies vaccine for human use	RespiGam	respiratory syncytial virus

R
Rx

	immune globulin intravenous (human)	Riopan	magaldrate
		risedronate sodium	Actonel
respiratory syncytial virus immune globulin intravenous (human)	RespiGam	Risperdal	risperidone
		risperidone	Risperdal
		Ritalin	methylphenidate HCl
		Ritalin SR	methylphenidate SR
Restoril	temazepam	ritodrine HCl	Yutopar
Retavase	reteplase	ritonavir	Norvir
reteplase	Retavase	Rituxan	rituximab
Retin-A	tretinoin topical	rituximab	Rituxan
Retin-A Micro	tretinoin gel	rizatriptan benzoate	Maxalt
Retrovir	zidovudine		
Revex	nalmefene HCl	rizatriptan oral disintegrating tablet	Maxalt-MLT
ReVia	naltrexone		
Rezulin	troglitazone		
R-Gene	arginine HCl	Robaxin	methocarbamol
Rheumatrex	methotrexate sodium tablets	Robinul	glycopyrrolate
		Robitussin	guaifenesin
Rhinocort	budesonide nasal inhaler	Robitussin A-C	guaifenesin; codeine phosphate
RH$_O$ (D) immune globulin	RhoGAM		
RH$_O$ (D) immune globulin IV (human)	WinRho SD	Robitussin-DM	guaifenesin; dextromethorphan
		Rocephin	ceftriaxone sodium
RhoGAM	RH$_O$ (D) immune globulin	Roferon-A	interferon alfa-2a
		Rogaine	minoxidil topical
ribavirin	Rebetol Virazole	Romazicon	flumazenil
		ropinirole HCl	Requip
ribavirin; interferon alfa-2b	Rebetron	ropivacaine HCl	Naropin
		Rotashield	rotavirus vaccine, live, oral, tetravalent
Ridaura	auranofin		
Rifadin	rifampin		
Rifamate	isoniazid; rifampin	rotavirus vaccine, live, oral, tetravalent	Rotashield
rifampin	Rifadin Rimactane		
		Rowasa	mesalamine
rifapentine	Priftin	Roxanol	morphine sulfate
Rilutek	riluzole	Roxanol SR	morphine sulfate SR
riluzole	Rilutek		
Rimactane	rifampin	Roxanol-T	morphine sulfate, immediate
rimantadine	Flumadine		
rimexolone	Vexol		

	release concentrated oral soln	Santyl	collagenase
Roxicet	oxycodone HCl; acetaminophen	saquinavir mesylate	Invirase
Roxicodone	oxycodone HCl	saquinavir soft gel capsule	Fortovase
rubella virus vaccine live attenuated	Meruvax II	sargramostim	Leukine Prokine (WA) OncoScint
Rubex	doxorubicin HCl	satumomab pendetide	
Rythmol	propafenone HCl	Sclerosol	talc, sterile aerosol
		scopolamine hydrobromide ophth	Isopto Hyoscine
		scopolamine transdermal	Transderm Scop

S

		Sectral	acebutolol HCl
		Seldane (W)	terfenadine (W)
		Seldane D (W)	terfenadine; pseudoephedrine HCl (W)
sacrosidase	Sucraid	selegiline HCl	Carbex Eldepryl
Saizen	somatropin		
Salagen	pilocarpine HCl tablet	selenium sulfide	Selsun Blue
		Selsun Blue	selenium sulfide
salbutamol sulfate	albuterol sulfate	senna	Ex Lax Senokot
salmeterol xinafoate	Serevent	senna concentrates	Senokot
salmeterol xinafoate inhalation powder	Serevent Diskus	Senokot	senna concentrates
		Septra	sulfamethoxazoletrimethoprim
salsalate	Disalcid		
Sal-Tropine	atropine sulfate tablets	Ser-Ap-Es	hydralazine; hydrochlorothiazide; reserpine
Saluron	hydroflumethiazide		
samarium SM 153 lexidronam	Quadramet	Serax	oxazepam
		Serentil	mesoridazine
		Serevent	salmeterol xinafoate
Sandimmune	cyclosporine		
Sandoglobulin	immune globulin intravenous	Serevent Diskus	salmeterol xinafoate inhalation powder
Sandostatin	octreotide acetate		
Sanorex	mazindol	sermorelin acetate	Geref
Sansert	methysergide maleate		
		Seromycin	cycloserine

Serpasil	*reserpine*	sulfacetamide	
Serlect	sertindole	lotion	
Seroquel	quetiapine fumerate	sodium tetradecyl	Sotradecol
sertindole	Serlect	sulfate	
sertraline HCl	Zoloft	Solganal	aurothioglucose
Serzone	nefazodone HCl	Solu-Cortef	hydrocortisone sodium
sevoflurane	Ultane		succinate
short chain fatty acids enema	Colomed	Solu-Medrol	methylpredniso-lone sodium
sibutramine HCl monohydrate	Meridia		succinate
sildenafil citrate	Viagra	Soma	carisoprodol
Silvadene	silver	somatostatin	Zecnil
	sulfadiazine	somatrem	Protropin
silver	Silvadene	somatropin for inj	Genotropin Humatrope
sulfadiazine			Nutropin
simethicone	Mylicon		Protropin II
Simulect	basiliximab		Saizen
simvastatin	Zocor	somatropin inj	Nutropin AQ
Sinemet	levodopa; carbidopa	Soriatane	acitretin
		sotalol	Betapace
Sinemet CR	levodopa; carbidopa SR	Sotradecol	sodium tetradecyl
Sinequan	doxepin HCl		sulfate
Singulair	montelukast sodium	sparfloxacin	Zagam
Skelid	tiludronate disodium	Sparine	promazine HCl
Slo-bid	theophylline SR	stavudine	Zerit
		spectinomycin HCl	Trobicin
Slo-Phyllin	theophylline	spironolactone	Aldactone
Slow Fe	ferrous sulfate SR	spironolactone; hydrochlorothi-	Aldactazide
Slow-K	potassium	azide	
	chloride SR	Sporanox	itraconazole
Slow-Mag	magnesium	Stadol	butorphanol
	chloride SR		tartrate
sodium citrate; citric acid	Bicitra		inj
sodium fluoride	Luride	Stadol NS	butorphanol tartrate nasal
sodium	Amvisc		spray
hyaluronate	Healon	stanozolol	Winstrol
	Hyalgan	Staphcillin	methicillin
sodium	Buphenyl		sodium
phenylbutyrate		Stelazine	trifluoperazine
sodium	Klaron		HCl

Stilphostrol	diethylstilbestrol diphosphate	Synthroid	levothyroxine sodium
Streptase	streptokinase	Synvisc	hylan G-F 20
streptokinase	Streptase		
streptomycin sulfate	streptomycin sulfate		
streptozocin	Zanosar		
Stromectol	ivermectin		
Sublimaze	fentanyl citrate		
succinylcholine chloride	Anectine		

Sucraid	sacrosidase	TACE (W)	chlorotrianisene (W)
sucralfate	Carafate	tacrine HCl	Cognex
Sudafed	pseudoephedrine HCl	tacrolimus	Prograf
		Tagamet	cimetidine HCl
Sufenta	sufentanil citrate	talc, sterile aerosol	Sclerosol
sufentanil citrate	Sufenta		
Sulamyd sodium	sulfacetamide sodium ophth	Talwin	pentazocine HCl
		Talwin Nx	pentazocine HCl; naloxone HCl
Sular	Nisoldipine SR		
sulfacetamide sodium ophth	Sulamyd sodium	Tambocor	flecainide acetate
		tamoxifen citrate	Nolvadex
sulfamethoxazole	Gantanol	tamsulosin HCl	Flomax
sulfamethoxazole-trimethoprim	Bactrim Cotrim co-trimoxazole Septra	Tapazole	methimazole
		Taractan (W)	chlorprothixene
		Tarka	trandolapril; verapamil SR
sulfasalazine	Azulfidine		
sulfinpyrazone	Anturane	tarzarotene gel	Tazorac
sulindac	Clinoril	Tasmar	tolcapone
Sultrin	triple sulfa vaginal cream	tasosartan	Verdia
		Tavist	clemastine fumarate
sumatriptan	Imitrex		
Surmontil	trimipramine maleate	Taxol	paclitaxel
		Taxotere	docetaxel
Sumycin	tetracycline HCl	Tazicef	ceftazidime
Suprane	desflurane	Tazidime	ceftazidime
Suprax	cefixime	Tazorac	tarzarotene gel
Surfak	docusate calcium	technetium Tc-99m bicisate kit	Neurolite
Survanta	beractant		
Sustiva	Efavirenz	technetium Tc-99m red blood cell kit	Ultratag
Symmetrel	amantadine HCl		
Synagis	palivizumab	technetium Tc-99m teboroxime kit	Cardiotec
Synalar	fluocinolone acetonide		
Synkayvite	menadiol sodium diphosphate	Teczem	enalapril

	maleate; diltiazem malate	tetracaine HCl *tetracycline HCl*	Pontocaine Achromycin (WA)
Tegretol	carbamazepine		Sumycin
Teldrin	chlorpheniramine maleate SR	tetrahydrozoline HCl ophth	Collyrium Visine Extra
Telepaque	iopanoic acid	Tetramune	diphtheria and
telmisartan	Micardis		tetanus
temazepam	Restoril		toxoids;
Tenex	guanfacine HCl		pertussis
teniposide	Vumon		vaccine,
Tenoretic	atenolol; chlorthalidone		adsorbed and haemophilus b
Tenormin	atenolol		conjugate
Tensilon	edrophonium chloride	Teveten	vaccine eprosartan
Tenuate	diethylpropion HCl	thalidomide	mesylate Thalomid
Terazol	terconazole	Thalomid	thalidomide
terazosin HCl	Hytrin	Tham	tromethamine
terbinafine HCl	Lamisil	Theo-Dur	theophylline SR
terbutaline sulfate aerosol	Brethaire	theophylline	Elixophyllin Slo-Phyllin
terbutaline sulfate tablets and inj	Brethine Bricanyl	theophylline SR	Slo-bid Theo-Dur
terconazole	Terazol	TheraCys	BCG intravesical
terfenadine (W)	Seldane (W)	Theragran-M	vitamins;
terfenadine; pseudoephe- drine HCl (W)	Seldane D (W)	thiabendazole thiethylperazine maleate	minerals Mintezol Torecan
teriparatide acetate	Parathar	thioguanine thiopental	thioguanine Pentothal
Teslac	testolactone	sodium	
Teslascan	mangofodipir trisodium	Thioplex thioridazine HCl	thiotepa Mellaril
Testoderm	testosterone transdermal	thiotepa thiothixene	Thioplex Navane
Testoderm TTS	testosterone transdermal	Thorazine thyroglobulin (W)	chlorpromazine Proloid (W)
testolactone	Teslac	thyroid	thyroid
testosterone cypionate SR	DEPO- Testosterone	Thyrogen Thyrolar	thyrotropin alpha liotrix
testosterone transdermal	Androderm Testoderm	thyrotropin thyrotropin	Thytropar Thyrogen
	Testoderm TTS	alpha	
tetanus immune globulin (human)	Hyper-Tet	Thytropar tiagabine HCl	thyrotropin Gabitril

Tiamate	diltiazem maleate SR	TobraDex	tobramycin; dexamethasone oint and susp
Tiazac	diltiazem HCl SR	tobramycin sulfate	Nebcin
Ticar	ticarcillin disodium	tobramycin sulfate ophth	Tobrex
ticarcillin disodium	Ticar	tobramycin; dexamethasone oint and susp	TobraDex
ticarcillin; clavulanic acid	Timentin	tobramycin soln for inhalation	TOBI
TICE BCG	BCG intravesical		
Ticlid	ticlopidine	Tobrex	tobramycin sulfate ophth
ticlopidine	Ticlid		
Tigan	trimethobenz-amide HCl	tocainide HCl	Tonocard
		Tofranil	imipramine HCl
Tilade	nedocromil inhalation	tolazamide	Tolinase
tiludronate disodium	Skelid	tolazoline	Priscoline
		tolbutamide	Orinase
Timentin	ticarcillin; clavulanic acid	tolcapone	Tasmar
		Tolectin	tolmetin sodium
timolol maleate ophth soln	Timoptic		
timolol maleate ophth soln, gel forming	Timoptic-XE	Tolinase	tolazamide
		tolmetin sodium	Tolectin
		tolnaftate	Tinactin
timolol maleate	Blocadren	tolterodine tartrate	Detrol
timolol maleate; dorzolamide HCl	Cosopt		
		Tonocard	tocainide HCl
Timoptic-XE	timolol maleate ophth soln, gel forming	Topamax	topiramate
		Topicort	desoximetasone
		topiramate	Topamax
Timoptic	timolol maleate ophth soln	topotecan HCl	Hycamtin
		Toprol XL	metoprolol succinate SR
Tinactin	tolnaftate		
Tine Test Tuberculin Old	tuberculin, old	Toradol	ketorolac tromethamine
Tine Test PPD	tuberculin, purified protein derivative	Torecan	thiethylperazine maleate
		toremifene citrate	Fareston
tioconazole	Vagistat-1	Tornalate	bitolterol mesylate
tirofiban HCl	Aggrastat		
tizanidine HCl	Zanaflex	torsemide	Demadex
TOBI	tobramycin soln for inhalation	Totacillin-N	ampicillin sodium

Tracrium	atracurium besylate	triazolam	Halcion
tramadol HCl	Ultram	Tricor	fenofibrate
Trandate	labetalol HCl	Tri-Cyclen	norgestimate; ethinyl estradiol
trandolapril	Mavik		
trandolapril; verapamil SR	Tarka	Tridesilon	desonide
Transderm Scop	scopolamine transdermal	Tridil	nitroglycerin inj
Transderm-Nitro	nitroglycerin transdermal	Tridione	trimethadione
Tranxene	clorazepate dipotassium	trifluoperazine HCl	Stelazine
tranylcypromine sulfate	Parnate	trifluridine	Viroptic
trastuzamab	Herceptin	trihexyphenidyl HCl	Artane
Trasylol	aprotinin	Tri-Immunol	diphtheria and tetanus toxoids and pertussis vaccine, adsorbed
Travasol	amino acid inj		
trazodone HCl	Desyrel		
Trecator-SC	ethionamide	Trilafon	perphenazine
Trental	pentoxifylline	Tri-Levlen	levonorgestrel; ethinyl estradiol
tretinoin cream 0.025%	Avita		
tretinoin gel	Retin-A Micro	Trilisate	choline magnesium trisalicylate
tretinion topical	Renova Retin-A		
tretinoin capsules	Vesanoid	trimethadione	Tridione
triamcinolone acetonide	Aristocort Kenalog	trimethaphan camsylate	Arfonad
triamcinolone acetonide aerosol	Azmacort	trimethobenza- mide HCl	Tigan
		trimetrexate	Neutrexin
triamcinolone acetonide nasal inhaler	Nasacort	trimipramine maleate	Surmontil
		Trimox	amoxicillin
triamterene	Dyrenium	Triostat	liothyronine sodium inj
triamterene 37.5 mg; hydro- chlorothiazide 25 mg	Maxzide -25MG Dyazide	Tripedia	diphtheria & tetanus toxoids & acellular pertussis vaccine
triamterene 75 mg; hydro- chlorothiazide 50 mg	Maxzide		
		tripelennamine HCl	PBZ
Triavil	perphenazine; amitriptyline HCl	Triphasil	levonorgestrel; ethinyl estradiol

triple sulfa vaginal cream	Sultrin	Tylenol with Codeine (#2, 3, and 4)	acetaminophen 300 mg with Codeine Phosphate (15, 30, and 60 mg)
triprolidine HCl; pseudoephedrine HCl	Actifed		
Tritec	ranitidine bismuth citrate	Typhim Vi	typhoid vaccine
		typhoid vaccine	Typhim Vi
Tri-Vi-Flor	vitamins A, D, & C; fluoride	tyropanoate sodium	Bilopaque

U

Trobicin	spectinomycin HCl
troglitazone	Rezulin
tromethamine	Tham
Tronothane HCl	pramoxine HCl
TrophAmine	amino acid inj
Tropicacyl	tropicamide
tropicamide	Mydriacyl Tropicacyl
trovafloxacin	Trovan tablets
Trovan tablet	trovafloxacin mesylate
Trovan inj	alatrovafloxacin mesylate IV
Trusopt	dorzolamide HCl
tuberculin, old	Tine Test, Tuberculin Old
tuberculin, purified protein derivative	Tine Test PPD
tuberculin skin test	Aplisol
tubocurarine	tubocurarine
Tucks	witch hazel pads
Tums	calcium carbonate
Tussi-Organidin NR	guaifenesin; codeine phosphate
Tussionex	hydrocodone polistirex; chlorpheniramine
Tylenol	acetaminophen

Ultane	sevoflurane
Ultiva	remifentanil HCl
Ultralente U	insulin zinc suspension, extended (beef)
Ultram	tramadol HCl
Ultratag	technetium Tc-99m red blood cell kit
Ultravist	iopromide
Unasyn	ampicillin sodium; sulbactam sodium
Unipen (WA)	nafcillin sodium
Uniretic	moexipril HCl; hydrochlorothiazide
Univasc	moexipril HCl
Urecholine	bethanechol chloride
Urised	methenamine combination
Urispas	flavoxate HCl
urofollitropin for inj	Fertinex
urokinase	Abbokinase
URSO	ursodiol

ursodiol	Actigall
	URSO

V

Vagistat-1	tioconazole
valacyclovir	Valtrex
Valium	diazepam
valproate sodium inj	Depacon
valproic acid	Depakene
valsartan	Diovan
Valtrex	valacyclovir
Vancenase	beclomethasone dipropionate
Vancenase AQ Nasal	beclomethasone dipropionate
Vanceril	beclomethasone dipropionate
Vancocin	vancomycin HCl
vancomycin HCl	Vancocin
Vantin	cefpodoxime proxetil
Vaponefrin	epinephrine racemic
Vaqta	hepatitis A vaccine, inactivated
varicella virus vaccine	Varivax
Varivax	varicella virus vaccine
Vascor	bepridil
Vaseline	petrolatum, white
Vaseretic	enalapril maleate; hydrochloro-thiazide
Vasocon	naphazoline ophth soln
Vasodilan	isoxsuprine HCl
vasopressin	Pitressin
Vasotec	enalapril maleate
Vasoxyl	methoxamine HCl
vecuronium bromide	Norcuron
Velban	vinblastine sulfate
Velosef	cephradine
Velosulin Human	insulin inj (human)
venlafaxine HCl	Effexor
venlafaxine HCl SR	Effexor XR
Ventolin	albuterol
VePesid	etoposide
verapamil HCl	Isoptin
verapamil HCl SR	Calan SR
	Verelan
verapamil HCl SR bedtime formulation	Covera HS
Verdia	tasosartan
Verelan	verapamil HCl SR
Verluna	nofetumomab
Vermox	mebendazole
Versed	midazolam HCl
Vesanoid	tretinoin capsules
Vexol	rimexolone
Viagra	sildenafil citrate
Vibramycin	doxycycline hyclate
Vicodin	hydrocodone bitartrate; acetaminophen
Vicoprofen	hydrocodone bitartrate 7.5 mg; ibuprofen 200 mg
vidarabine monohydrate	Vira-A
Videx	didanosine
vinblastine sulfate	Velban
vincristine sulfate	Oncovin

vindesine sulfate	Eldisine
vinorelbine tartrate	Navelbine
Vioform	clioquinol
Vira-A	vidarabine monohydrate
Viracept	nelfinavir mesylate
Viramune	nevirapine
Virazole	ribavirin
Viroptic	trifluridine
Visine Extra	tetrahydrozoline HCl ophth
Visipaque	iodixanol
Visken	pindolol
Vistaril	hydroxyzine pamoate
Vistide monohydrate	
Viracept	nelfinavir mesylate
Viramune	nevirapine
Virazole	ribavirin
Viroptic	trifluridine
Visine Extra	tetrahydrozoline HCl ophth
Visipaque	iodixanol
Visken	pindolol
Vistaril	hydroxyzine pamoate
Vistide	protriptyline HCl
Vitravene	fomivirsen sodium inj
Vivelle	estradiol transdermal system
Volmax	albuterol SR
Voltaren	diclofenac sodium
Voltaren-XR	diclofenac sodium SR
Vumon	teniposide

W

warfarin sodium	Coumadin

Wellbutrin	bupropion HCl
Wellbutrin SR	bupropion HCl SR
Wellcovorin	*leucovorin calcium*
WinRho SD	RH_O (D) immune globulin IV (human)
Winstrol	stanozolol
witch hazel pads	Tucks
Wyamine	mephentermine sulfate
Wycillin (for IM use only)	penicillin G procaine (for IM use only)
Wydase	hyaluronidase
Wygesic	propoxyphene HCl; acetaminophen
Wymox	amoxicillin
Wytensin	guanabenz acetate

XYZ

Xalatan	latanoprost
Xanax	alprazolam
Xeloda	capecitabine
Xenical	orlistat
Xylocaine HCl	lidocaine HCl
xylometazoline	Otrivin
Xyrem	gamma hydroxybutyrate
Yutopar	ritodrine HCl
zafirlukast	Accolate
Zagam	sparfloxacin
zalcitabine	Hivid
Zanaflex	tizanidine HCl
Zanosar	streptozocin
Zantac	ranitidine HCl
Zarontin	ethosuximide

Zaroxolyn	metolazone	zolmitriptan	Zomig
Zecnil	somatostatin	Zoloft	sertraline HCl
Zemplar	paricalcitol	zolpidem tartrate	Ambien
Zenapax	daclizumab	Zomig	zolmitriptan
Zerit	stavudine	Zonegran	zonisamide
Zestoretic	lisinopril; hydrochloro-thiazide	zonisamide	Zonegran
		Zosyn	piperacillin so-dium; tazobac-tam sodium
Zestril	lisinopril		
Zetar	coal tar product	Zovirax	acyclovir
Ziac	bisoprolol fumarate; hydrochloro-thiazide	Zyban	bupropion HCl SR
		Zyflo	zileuton
zidovudine	Retrovir	Zyloprim	allopurinol
zidovudine; lamivudine	Combivir	Zyprexa	olanzapine
		Zyrtec	cetirizine HCl
zileuton	Zyflo		
Zinacef	cefuroxime sodium		
zinc acetate	Galzin		
Zinecard	dexrazoxane		
Zithromax	azithromycin		
Zocor	simvastatin		
Zofran	ondansetron		
Zoladex	goserelin acetate implant		

References

1. Facts and comparisons. St. Louis: Facts and Comparisons, Inc. (published monthly)
2. Billup NF, Billup SM. American drug index. St. Louis: Facts and Comparisons, Inc. (published yearly)
3. Physicians GenRx. St. Louis: Mosby. (published yearly)
4. Reynolds JEF, ed. Martindale: The extra pharmacopeia. London: 31st edition. The Pharmaceutical Press. 1996

Chapter 6

Normal Laboratory Values*

In the following tables, normal reference values for commonly requested laboratory tests are listed in traditional units and in SI units. The tables are a guideline only. Values are method dependent and "normal values" may vary between laboratories.

Blood, Plasma or Serum		
	Reference Value	
Determination	**Conventional Units**	**SI Units**
Ammonia (NH₃)	10–80 μg/dl	5–50 μmol/L
Amylase	≤130 units/L	≤130 units/L
Antinuclear antibodies	negative at 1 : 10 dilution of serum	negative a 1 : 10 dilution of serum
Antithrombin III (AT III)	18–30 mg/dl	18–30 mg/dl
Bilirubin: conjugated	≤0.2 mg/dl	≤4 μmol/L
total	0.1–1 mg/dl	2–18 μmol/L
Calcitonin:	<100 ng/L	<100 ng/L
Calcium: female <50 years old	8.8–10 mg/dl	2.2–2.5 mmol/L
female >50 years old	8.8–10.2 mg/dl	2.2–2.56 mmol/L
male	8.8–10.3 mg/dl	2.2–2.58 mmol/L
Carbon dioxide content	22–28 mEq/L	22–28 mmol/L
Carcinoembryonic antigen	<3 ng/ml	<3 μg/L
Chloride	95–105 mEq/L	95–105 mmol/L
Coagulation screen:		
Bleeding time	2.9 min	60–540 sec
Prothrombin time	10–12 sec	10–12 sec
Partial thromboplastine time (activated)	33–45 sec	35–45 sec
Protein C	0.4 mg/dl	4 g/L
Protein S	2.3 mg/dl	2.3 g/L
Copper, total	70–140 μg/dl	11–22 μmol/L
Corticotropin (ACTH)	20–100 pg/mL	4–22 pmol/L
Cortisol: 0800 hr	4–19 μg/dl	110–520 nmol/L
1800 hr	2–15 μg/dl	40–410 nmol/L
2400 hr	<5 μg/dl	<140 nmol/L
Creatine phosphokinase, total (CK, CPK)	≤150 units/L	≤150 units/L
Creatine phosphokinase isoenzymes, MB fraction	>5% in MI	>0.05 fraction of 1
Creatinine	0.6–1.2 mg/dl	50–110 mcmol/L
Fibrinogen (coagulation factor I)	150–350 mg/dl	1.5–3.5 g/L
Follicle stimulating hormone (FSH):		
female	2–15 mIU/mL	2–15 IU/L
peak production	20–50 mIU/mL	20–50 IU/L
male	1–10 mIU/mL	1–10 IU/L

*1998 by Facts and Comparisons. Used with permission from *Drug Facts and Comparisons, 1998 ed.* St. Louis: Facts and Comparisons, Inc.

Normal Laboratory Values (Cont.) Blood

Blood, Plasma or Serum (Cont.)		
	Reference Value	
Determination	**Conventional Units**	**SI Units**
Glucose fasting	70–110 mg/dl	3.9–6.1 mmol/L
Haptoglobin	50–220 mg/dl	0.5–2.2 g/L
Hematologic tests:		
Hematocrit (Hct), female	33%–43%	0.33–0.43 fraction of 1
male	39%–49%	0.39–0.49 fraction of 1
Hemoglobin (Hb), female	11.5–15.5 g/dl	115–155 g/L
male	14–18 g/dl	140–180 g/L
Leukocyte count (WBC)	3200–9800/mm^3	3.2–9.8 × 10^9/L
Erythrocyte count (RBC), female	3.5–5 10^6/mm^3	3.5–5 × 10^{12}/L
male	4.3–5.9 10^6/mm^3	4.3–5.9 × 10^{12}/L
Mean corpuscular volume (MCV)	76–100 μm^3/cell	76–100 fl/cell
Mean corpuscular hemoglobin (MCH)	27–33 pg/RBC	27–33 pg/RBC
Mean corpuscular hemoglobin concentration (MCHC)	33–37 g/dl	330–370 g/L
Erythrocyte sedimentation rate (sedrate, ESR): female	≤30 mm/hr	≤30 mm/hr
male	≤20 mm/hr	≤20 mm/hr
Ferritin	18–300 ng/mL	18–300 μg/L
Folic acid: normal	>3.8 ng/mL	>8.4 nmol/L
Platelet count	130–400 × 10^3/mm^3	130–400 × 10^9/L
Vitamin B$_{12}$:	200–1000 pg/mL	150–750 pmol/L
Iron		
female	60–160 μg/dl	11–29 mcmol/L
male	80–180 μg/dl	14–32 mcmol/L
Iron binding capacity	250–460 μg/dl	45–82 μmol/L
Lactic acid (lactate)	0.5–2 mEq/L	0.5–2.2 mmol/L
Lactic dehydrogenase	50–150 units/L	50–150 units/L
Lead (toxic levels)	≤60 μg/dl	≤2.9 μmol/L
Lipids:		
Triglycerides		
Desirable	<250 mg/dL	<2.82 mmol/L
Borderline	250–500 mg/dL	2.82–5.65 mmol/L
High	>500 mg/dL	>5.65 mmol/L
LDL Cholesterol		
Desirable	<130 mg/dL	<3.36 mmol/L
Borderline	130–159 mg/dL	3.36–4.11 mmol/L
High	>159 mg/dL	>4.11 mmol/L
HDL Cholesterol		
High	<35 mg/dL	<0.91 mmol/L
Total Cholesterol		
Desirable	<200 mg/dL	5.17 mmol/L
Borderline	200–239 mg/dL	5.17–6.18 mmol/L
High	>239 mg/dL	>6.18 mmol/L
Triglycerides	<460 mg/dL	<5.3 mmol/L
Magnesium	1.6–2.4 mEq/L	0.8–1.2 mmol/L
Osmolality	280–300 mOsm/kg	280–300 mmol/kg
Oxygen saturation (arterial)	96%–100%	0.96–1 fraction of 1

Normal Laboratory Values (Cont.) Blood

	Blood, Plasma or Serum (Cont.)	
	Reference Value	
Determination	**Conventional Units**	**SI Units**
PCO₂, Arterial	35–45 mm Hg	4.7–6 kPa
pH, Arterial	7.35–7.45	7.35–7.45
PO₂, Arterial: breathing room air	75–100 mm Hg	10–13.3 kPa
Phosphatase (acid)	2–11 IU/L	3–183 mckat/L ≤16.1 units/L
Phosphatase alkaline (ALP)	25–100 IU/L	4–1.7 mckat/L
Phosphorus, inorganic (phosphate)	2.5–5 mg/dl	0.8–1.6 mmol/L
Potassium	3.5–5 mEq/L	3.5–5 mmol/L
Progesterone: Follicular phase Luteal phase	 <2 ng/mL 2–20 ng/mL	 <6 nmol/L 6–64 nmol/L
Prolactin	<20 ng/mL	<20 μg/L
Protein: Total Albumin Globulin	5.5–9 g/dl 3.5–5 g/dl 2–3 g/dl	55–90 g/L 35–50 g/L 20–30 g/L
Rheumatoid factor	<80 IU/ml	<80 kIU/L
Sodium	135–147 mEq/L	135–147 mmol/L
Testosterone: female male	<0.6 ng/mL 4–8 ng/mL	<2 nmol/L 14–28 nmol/L
Thyroid Hormone Function Tests: Thyroid-stimulating hormone (TSH) Thyroxine-binding globulin capacity Total triiodothyronine (T₃) Total thyroxine by RIA (T₄) T₃ resin uptake	 2–11 μ units/mL 15–28 μg T₄/dl 75–220 ng/dl 4–11 μg/dl 25%–35%	 2–11 mU/L 150–360 nmol/L 1.2–3.4 nmol/L 52–142 nmol/L 0.25–0.35 fraction of 1
Transaminase, AST (Aspartate aminotransferase, SGOT)	≤35 units/L	≤35 units/L
Transaminase, ALT (Alanine aminotransferase, SGPT)	≤35 units/L	≤35 units/L
Urea nitrogen (BUN)	8–18 mg/dl	3–6.5 mmol/L
Uric acid	2–7 mg/dl	120–420 μmol/L
Vitamin A (retinol)	10–50 μg/dl	0.35–1.75 μmol/L
Zinc	75–120 μg/dl	11.5–18.5 μmol/L

Normal Laboratory Values-Drug Levels

		Drug Levels†	
		Reference Value	
Drug Determination		**Conventional Units**	**SI Units**
Aminoglycosides (peak levels)	Amikacin	16–32 µg/mL	nd
	Gentamicin	4–8 µg/mL	nd
	Kanamycin	15–40 µg/mL	nd
	Netilmicin	6–10 µg/mL	nd
	Streptomycin	20–30 µg/mL	nd
	Tobramycin	4–8 µg/mL	nd
Anti-arrhythmics	Amiodarone	0.5–2.5 µg/mL	nd
	Bretylium	0.5–1.5 µg/mL	nd
	Digitoxin	9–25 µg/L	11.8–32.8 nmol/L
	Digoxin	0.5–2.2 ng/mL	0.6–2.8 nmol/L
	Disopyramide	2–8 µg/mL	6–18 µmol/L
	Flecainide	0.2–1 µg/mL	nd
	Lidocaine	1.5–6 µg/mL	4.5–21.5 µmol/L
	Mexiletine	0.5–2 µg/mL	nd
	Procainamide	4–8 µg/mL	17–34 µmol/L
	Propranolol	50–200 ng/mL	190–770 nmol/L
	Quinidine	2–6 µg/mL	4.6–9.2 µmol/L
	Tocainide	4–10 µg/mL	nd
	Verapamil	0.08–0.3 µg/mL	nd
Anti-convulsants	Carbamazepine	4–12 µg/mL	17–51 µmol/L
	Phenobarbital	15–40 µg/mL	65–172 µmol/L
	Phenytoin	10–20 µg/mL	40–80 µmol/L
	Primidone	5–12 µg/mL	25–46 µmol/L
	Valproic acid	50–100 µg/mL	350–700 µmol/L
Anti-depressants	Amitriptyline	110–250 ng/mL	nd
	Amoxapine	200–500 ng/mL	nd
	Bupropion	25–100 ng/mL	nd
	Clomipramine	80–100 ng/mL	nd
	Desipramine	125–300 ng/mL	nd
	Doxepin	100–200 ng/mL	nd
	Imipramine	200–350 ng/mL	nd
	Maprotiline	200–300 ng/mL	nd
	Nortriptyline	50–150 ng/mL	nd
	Protriptyline	100–200 ng/mL	nd
	Trazodone	800–1600 ng/mL	nd
Antipsychotics	Chlorpromazine	30–500 ng/mL	nd
	Fluphenazine	0.13–2.8 ng/mL	nd
	Haloperidol	5–20 ng/mL	nd
	Perphenazine	0.8–1.2 ng/mL	nd
	Thiothixene	2–57 ng/mL	nd
Miscellaneous	Amantadine	300 ng/mL	nd
	Amrinone	3.7 µg/mL	nd
	Chloramphenicol	10–20 µg/mL	31–62 µmol/L
	Cyclosporine[1]	250–800 ng/mL (whole blood, RIA)	nd
		50–300 ng/mL (plasma, RIA)	nd
	Ethanol[2]	0 mg/dl	0 mmol/L
	Hydralazine	100 ng/dl	nd
	Lithium	0.5–1.5 mEq/L	0.5–1.5 mmol/L
	Salicylate	100–200 mg/L	724–1448 µmol/L
	Sulfonamide	5–15 mg/dl	nd
	Terbutaline	0.5–4.1 ng/mL	nd
	Theophylline	10–20 µg/mL	55–110 µmol/L
	Vancomycin (peak)	30–40 mg/mL	nd

†The values given are generally accepted as desirable for achieving therapeutic effect without toxicity for most patients. However, exceptions are not uncommon.
[1]24 hour trough values. [2]Toxic: 50–100 mg/dl (10.9–21.7 mmol/L).
nd—No data available.

Normal Laboratory Values-Urine

URINE				
	Reference Value			
Determination	**Conventional Units**		**SI Units**	
Catecholamines: Epinephrine Norepinephrine	<10 μg/day <100 μg/day		<55 nmol/day <590 nmol/day	
Creatinine: female male	14–22 mg/kg/24 h 20–26 mg/kg/24 h		0.12–0.19 mmol/kg/day 0.18–0.23 mmol/kg/day	
Potassium (diet dependent)	25–100 mEq/day		25–100 mmol/day	
Protein, quantitative	<150 mg/day		<0.15 g/day	

Steroids:	Age (yrs)	(mg/day)		(μmol/day)	
		male	female	male	female
17-Ketosteroids	10	1–4	1–4	3–14	3–14
	20	6–21	4–16	21–73	14–56
	30	8–26	4–14	28–90	14–49
	50	5–18	3–9	17–62	10–31
	70	2–10	1–7	7–35	3–24
17-Hydroxycorticosteroids (as cortisol): female male		2–8 mg/day 3–10 mg/day		5–25 μmol/day 10–30 μmol/day	

Please forward additional meanings for these abbreviations, additional abbreviations and their meanings, or corrections to the author so that the list can be updated. Thank you.

Dr. Neil M Davis
1143 Wright Drive
Huntingdon Valley, PA 19006-2721
FAX (215) 938 1937
E-mail med@neilmdavis.com

Additions

_____

_____

_____

_____

_____

_____

_____

_____

_____

_____

_____

_____

_____

_____

_____

_____

_____

_____